# Praise for Hormones and Human P...

*"This book is an absolute must read for anyone with an interest in the fascinating links between our hormones and overall health. It is grounded in easy to understand science and offers practical and empowering advice that everyone can apply. Nicky is a fountain of knowledge and I love the fact that she has poured all of that into this incredible book."*

Chrissie Wellington OBE
FOUR TIMES IRONMAN TRIATHLON WORLD CHAMPION

*"Hormones are integral to our health and performance. Nicky is one of the most authoritative voices in this specialist area of hormones and how to harness their potential. This is a must read for us all, healthcare professionals and non-professionals alike."*

Renee McGregor
CLINICAL DIRECTOR AND SPORTS DIETICIAN, UK

*"In an era bubbling with misinformation on hormones and how to 'balance' them, this straight-talking, evidence-based book by Dr Nicky Keay could not have arrived at a better time."*

Dr Hazel Wallace
DOCTOR AND REGISTERED ASSOCIATE NUTRITIONIST,
FOUNDER OF THE FOOD MEDIC, UK

*"The influence hormones have on the performance of a dancer is crucial, both in regard to injury mitigation and performance optimisation. Nicky's knowledge of endocrinology coupled with her insight and enthusiasm for dance make her a leading voice in this field."*

Martin Lanfear
HEAD OF PERFORMANCE MEDICINE SCOTTISH BALLET

*"Our hormones are tremendously powerful and all too often they're an overlooked piece in the puzzle of health and performance. Nicky Keay's work has been instrumental in disseminating essential information in a way that's easy to understand, but also easy to act upon, and expertly tailored to individual circumstances."*

Michelle Arthurs-Brennan
DIGITAL EDITOR, CYCLING WEEKLY, UK

*"Dr Keay's book is an excellent resource for those hoping to enhance both their health and sporting performance. In this case, knowledge is power so understanding the role of hormones in sport and everyday life enables us to harness their potential to the fullest effect.*

*Relative Energy Deficiency in Sport (RED-S) is a huge barrier to performance at both elite and recreational level. It is often under-recognised however Dr Keay's work in this area continues to revolutionise both the understanding and management of this condition to the benefit of athletes worldwide."*

Dr Eddie Craghill
WOMEN'S TEAM SUPPORT DOCTOR
MANCHESTER UNITED FC

*"Athletic peak performance requires health and a good balance between training load and recovery. Hormones are an essential part of maintaining this balance and they are part of body mass regulation, aging, and so much more. This book provides key information for these processes, so I highly recommend reading it to anyone trying to achieve results in recreational or top level sport."*

Dr Iva Jurov.
KLINIČNI INŠTITUT ZA MEDICINO DELA, PROMETA IN ŠPORTA
LJUBLJANA, SLOVENIA.

*"Nicky has been one of the primary pioneers in advocating, researching and educating, especially to the broader community on the importance of hormones for optimal performance and health. Her knowledge and expertise in this area, especially in female athletes, is second to none. This book will be an exceptional recourse for women to improve their health and be empowered to understand their bodies better."*

Dr Isobelle Smith
MEDICAL DOCTOR, AUSTRALIA

*"Hormones are such an important topic for women and men, and yet there is still a dearth of top-class, accurate information in the area. I am so grateful for the work that Dr Nicky Keay does in this area, shining a very well-informed light on the subject, and this book is extremely welcome and highly recommended. Thanks Nicky, so many people will benefit from your expertise."*

Simon Mundie
THE TODAY PROGRAMME, BBC RADIO 4,
TODAY AT WIMBLEDON, BBC TV SPORT

*"As a professional cyclist, without a medical background, Nicky's help and guidance over the years has thoroughly helped my understanding of how training load, fuelling and recovery influence my performance and my body's wellbeing as a whole."*

Harry Tanfield
PROFESSIONAL WORLD TOUR RIDER WITH QHUBEKA-ASSOS

*"Hormones, Health and Human Potential is a fantastic tool for anyone wanting to understand their body better and use it to their advantage. As an athlete who has hugely benefitted from Dr Keay's extensive research and practical expertise in order to overcome RED-S and reach the highest levels in sport, I can confidently say there is no one better to write this book. By sharing her insight with others, Dr Keay can help us all feel more educated and empowered with every chapter."*

Pippa Woolven
FORMER GB ATHLETE

*"Nicky's extensive expertise helps athletes understand that the endocrine system is critical to successful training, overall well-being and the ability to participate long term. Her work is an invaluable guide for every coach, as well as athletes of all sexes and all ages."*

Jill Colangelo
PSYCHOLOGY RESEARCHER, ITALY

*"Nicky is one of those professionals that you always want to have near. She is easy to reach and with so great an expertise, that she can really help you to understand 'the hormone world'. She has collaborated with us in a study with the Female FC Barcelona football team. Female sport and especially female football is in continuous growth, that not only is in need of great players, but of*

*good healthcare professionals too. Understanding what takes place in the woman body, its physiology and the response when playing football is essential to continue developing knowledge. Nicky has been a perfect partner in this challenge, and I look forward to working together in future studies."*

*Dr Eva Ferrer*
Medicina de l'esport. Sports medicine doctor
Departament Medic. Barça. Barcelona Football Club, Spain

"A brilliant book that will be invaluable for athletes and dancers looking to optimise their health and performance."

*Anita Bean*
Registered Nutritionist, UK

# Hormones, Health and Human Potential

Every possible effort has been made to ensure that the information contained in this book is accurate at the time of going to press. The publishers and author(s) cannot accept responsibility for any errors and omissions, however caused. No responsibility for loss or damage occasioned to any person acting, or refraining from action, as a result of the material contained in this publication can be accepted by the editor, the publisher or the author.

First published in 2022 by Sequoia Books

Apart from fair dealing for the purposes of research or private study, or criticism or review, as permitted under the Copyright, Designs and Patents act 1988, this publication may only be reproduced, stored or transmitted, in any form or by any means, with the prior permission in writing of the publisher, or in the case of reprographic reproduction in accordance with the terms and licenses issued by the CLA. Enquiries concerning reproduction outside these terms should be sent to the publisher using the details on the website www.sequoia-books.com

©Nicola Keay

The right of Dr Nicola Keay to be identified as editor of this work has been asserted in accordance with the Copyright, Designs and Patents act 1988.

ISBN
Print: 9781914110207
EPUB: 9781914110214

A CIP record for this book is available from the British Library

Library of Congress Cataloguing-In-Publication Data

Name: Dr Nicola Keay
Title: Hormones, Health and Human Potential/ Dr Nicola Keay
Description: 1st Edition, Sequoia Books UK 2022
Subjects: R5920 Medicine (general)
Print: 9781914110207
EPUB: 9781914110214

Library of Congress Control Number: 2022917530

Print and Electronic production managed by Deanta Global

Cover designed by Kelly Miller, logo by Lucy Milligan

# Hormones, Health and Human Potential

A Guide to Understanding Your Hormones to Optimise Your Health and Performance

**Dr Nicky Keay**

# Author Background

Nicky is an Honorary Clinical Lecturer in the Division of Medicine, University College London. She lectures and researches in areas of exercise endocrinology, with publications in this field. Nicky's clinical endocrine work is mainly with exercisers, dancers and athletes, with a focus on relative energy deficiency in sport (RED-S) and female exercisers, including women experiencing perimenopause and menopause. Nicky is the medical advisor to Scottish Ballet.

Nicky studied medicine at Cambridge University. Following international clinical attachments and gaining membership of the Royal College of Physicians, London, UK, Nicky was a Research Fellow at St Thomas' Hospital, London, where she was part of the international medical team that developed an anti-doping test for growth hormone. While CMO of Forth, Nicky contributed her medical expertise towards developing a potential clinical tool to deliver personalised female hormone health by employing artificial intelligence techniques to model female hormones over the menstrual cycle.

Nicky is the lead author of the *British Association of Sport and Exercise Medicine* (BASEM) educational website Health4Performance.co.uk on RED-S. She frequently writes articles for the *British Journal of Sport Medicine* (BJSM). Nicky is a member of the British Menopause Society.

Nicky practises ballet and enjoys cycling, swimming and windsurfing.

*Dr Nicola Keay, BA, MA, MB, BChir (Cantab), MRCP*

# Thanks

My thanks to my husband Gavin. Ever since we first met at St John's College, Cambridge, Gavin has been my steadfast support. This includes all the time and patience he has put in to help me with the analysis and writing of research papers and now this book. Gavin has a clarity of expression that has been invaluable in shaping my ideas into something that I hope is both informative and engaging.

# Acknowledgments

Thanks to Lucy Milligan who provided the artwork of "the jump" on the cover and throughout the book to represent the vitality that our hormones can bring us.

Figures marked with an asterisk (*) are were created by Dr Nicky Keay and are reproduced with the kind permission of the BJSM.

# Contents

**Prelude**     1

*"If we could give every individual the right amount of nourishment and exercise, not too little and not too much, we would have found the safest way to health."*
*Hippocrates*

**Act 1**     5

Scene 1: What is Health?     7
*"Health is a state of complete physical, mental and social well-being and not merely the absence of disease or infirmity."*
*World Health Organisation, 1948*

Scene 2: Hormones for Health     13
*"Setting in motion"*
ὁρμῶν *(hormon)*

Scene 3: Harnessing Hormones     34
*"Walking is man's best medicine."*
*Hippocrates*

Scene 4: It's all in the Timing     52
*"Not just a question of what, rather when we eat, sleep and exercise"*
*Dr N Keay BJSM blog*

Scene 5 XY: Of Mice and Men     70
*Testosterone rex?*

Scene 5 XX: Of Mice and Men . . . and Women!     82
Ὁρμή *(Horme)*
*Goddess of effort, energy and action*

Scene 6: Hormone Supermodels — 102
*"The practice of medicine is an art."*
*Sir William Osler*

Scene 7: Bare Bones — 115
*"Make no bones about it."*

Scene 8: Mind the Gut — 134
*"Let food be thy medicine and medicine be thy food."*
*Hippocrates*

Scene 9: A Balancing Act — 148
*"All parts of the body which have a function, if used in moderation and exercised in labours in which each is accustomed, become thereby healthy, well developed and age more slowly, but if unused they become liable to disease, defective in growth and age quickly."*
*Hippocrates*

Scene 10: In the Red — 161
*"Before you heal someone, ask him if he's willing to give up the things that make him sick."*
*Hippocrates*

# Entr'acte — 187

*"All the world's a stage,*
*And all the men and women merely players;*
*They have their exits and their entrances;*
*And one man in his time plays many parts,*
*His acts being seven ages."*
*Shakespeare, As You Like It*

# Act 2    189

Scene 1: Infancy    191
*"At first the infant,*
*Mewling and puking in the nurse's arms."*
*Shakespeare*

Scene 2: Childhood    202
*"And then the whining school-boy with his satchel*
*And shining morning face, creeping like a snail,*
*Unwillingly to school."*
*Shakespeare*

Scene 3: Teenager    212
*"And then the lover,*
*Sighing like furnace, with a woeful ballad,*
*Made to his mistress' eyebrow"*
*Shakespeare*

Scene 4: Young Man (and Young Woman!)    226
*"Then a soldier,*
*Full of strange oaths, and bearded like the pard,*
*Jealous in honour, sudden and quick in quarrel,*
*Seeking the bubble reputation*
*Even in the cannon's mouth"*
*Shakespeare*

Scene 5: Middle Age    249
*"And then the justice,*
*In a fair round belly, with good capon lin'd,*
*With eyes severe, and beard of formal cut,*
*Full of wise saws, and modern instances."*
*Shakespeare*

Scene 6: Old Age     270

*"The lean and slipper'd pantaloon,*
*With spectacles on nose and pouch on side,*
*His youthful hose, well sav'd, a world too wide*
*For his shrunk shank, and his big manly voice,*
*Turning again toward childish treble, pipes*
*And whistles in his sound."*
*Shakespeare*

Scene 7: Dotage     284

*"Second childishness and mere oblivion,*
*Sans teeth, sans eyes, sans taste, sans everything."*
*Shakespeare*

## Coda     294

*"If we could give every individual the right amount of nourishment and exercise, not too little and not too much, we would have found the safest way to health."*
*Hippocrates*

*References*     295

*Glossary*     325

# Prelude

*"If we could give every individual the right amount of nourishment and exercise, not too little and not too much, we would have found the safest way to health."*

*Hippocrates*

**Subtitle:** The rationale for this book is to redefine the concept of personalised optimal human health and performance. Our understanding of the human body has vastly increased since the times of ancient Greece. Furthermore, our modern lifestyle is very different. Recognising and harnessing hormones, as the link between our lifestyle behaviours and our health, can lead the way to personalised optimal health and attainment of our full potential.

Was Hippocrates right? Hippocrates was born in the fifth century BC, living through the golden age of Athens. He was a contemporary of Sophocles, Herodotus, Plato and Socrates, who produced some of the most influential and enduring aspects of Western culture. On the face of it, the advice of Hippocrates appears to be as appropriate to us today as it was to the people of ancient Greece.

Although we live in a very different modern environment, we share a lot in common with the ancient Greeks. Our human physiology is much the same as it was 2,500 years ago. The plays and historical texts of his contemporaries resonate with human thoughts and desires that are familiar to us. The Olympians of today still want to be citius, altius, fortius (faster, higher, stronger). We all pursue goals and ambitions both inside and outside the sports arena.

A marked contrast in the modern lifestyle is the extension of life expectancy. In ancient times, living into old age was an achievement, largely down to avoiding plague, pestilence and war. Today much of the burden of healthcare is devoted to the elderly, who face diseases and disabilities of old age that would have been largely unknown in classical times.

The most significant change has been in our understanding of health. Hippocrates knew what to do, but he did not know why. We had to wait two millennia until, just over a hundred years ago, the first hormone was described. In homage to Hippocrates, the word "hormone" is derived from ancient Greek, meaning "setting in motion". Modern medicine benefits from a detailed knowledge of how our lifestyle behaviours affect hormones and set in motion our path to health.

The purpose of this book is to explore the clandestine work of hormones. It uncovers the roles of hormones in maintaining an optimal internal environment and in controlling how our behaviours, including our "nourishment and exercise", determine our health and human performance.

Hormones are dynamic players whose roles form an interwoven plot, worthy of any of the Greek playwrights. Act 1 describes the vital role of hormones in bringing our DNA to life. It explores the intricate mechanisms by which our hormones strive to maintain our bodies in a healthy state. The hormone control centre is the hypothalamus, located in the brain. The hypothalamus acts as the neuroendocrine gatekeeper: monitoring external and internal physical factors and our psychological interpretation of events. In other words, the hypothalamus brings together body and mind and directs the conductor of the endocrine orchestra: the pituitary gland. The endocrine orchestra includes the hormone-producing glands, the hormones and their complex control systems. The performers include a vast array of hormones, all working in concert. These include insulin, growth hormone and its family members, thyroid hormones, steroid hormones like testosterone and oestrogen and many more. Each hormone axis keeps time, using its own biological clock, working in synchrony with other hormone networks to support the smooth running of our body systems, whose processes define life. These life processes include the generation of energy from nutrition, as well as movement, growth, development and reproduction. The symphony of life is conducted by hormones performing at the right time and at the right rate for the individual.

Hormones act as the link between our interactions with the external environment, characterised by our lifestyle behaviours, and our internal physical and mental health. Through our behaviours, we can harness our hormones positively to optimise health. On the other hand, imbalances in our lifestyle choices and mistiming between our actions and internal hormone biological clocks can derail the intricate interactions and timing of hormone networks.

To refine advice about nutrition, exercise and sleep for the individual, we can now monitor our own hormone networks. Artificial intelligence techniques are being increasingly used in medicine to personalise healthcare. This opens exciting possibilities for optimising hormone health.

Act 2 relates to the changing roles of hormones over our lifespan. "Hormones stories" illustrate the subtleties of hormone function on personalised health and human performance at different stages of life. Each scene explores practical ways to avoid hormone disruption and maintain a healthy hormone network throughout life.

The Coda assesses why Hippocrates was right and what we can apply to our lives today to optimise our hormone health and attain our personal full potential.

A glossary explains terms used in the book.

## Note

Throughout this book, the terms female or woman/women refer to the biological sex of a person with the XX karyotype, and the terms male or man/men refer to the biological sex of a person with the XY karyotype.

British spelling is used throughout this book. For example, the hormones oestradiol and oestrogen have American equivalents estradiol and estrogen.

The information in this book explains how hormones affect health. This should not be used for medical diagnostic purposes and is not a substitute for seeking medical advice. The characters in all the hormone stories are fictitious.

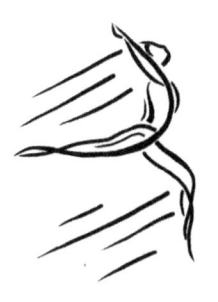

# Act 1

# Scene 1
## What is Health?

> *"Health is a state of complete physical, mental and social well-being and not merely the absence of disease or infirmity."*
> *World Health Organisation, 1948*

**Subtitle:** Health is a dynamic, positive state of optimal personal physical, mental and social well-being. Hormones are the link between external lifestyle behaviours and intrinsic genetic factors that determine health. Personalisation of health and disease prevention is possible by focusing on hormones, which determine gene expression and set DNA in motion.

Britain's Nation Health Service was founded in 1948 to provide free healthcare to all. In the same year, the World Health Organisation (WHO) published the statement that opens this chapter. In addition to conveying a sense of positivity after the suffering of the Second World War, it reflected the multi-faceted nature of well-being.

Attitudes to health have changed over the years. The WHO added a social aspect to the healthy mind in a healthy body, expressed in the writings of Decimus Junius Juvenalis during the first century AD: "mens sana in corpore sano". But the world has changed in many ways since the mid-twentieth century. Global demographics have recorded a huge increase in population, a reduction in infant mortality and a dramatic increase in expected lifespan. Advances in pharmaceutical and medical techniques are now available to treat many life-threatening conditions. Computer technology has led to the decoding of the human genome, the study of the microbiome and the increased application of artificial intelligence to the field of medicine. These factors have enabled a shift away from generalised methods towards a more personalised approach.

Critics of the WHO's description of health suggest that it creates an unrealistic ideal that is unattainable for the increasingly large proportion of older people or those suffering from a chronic illness or disability. In fact, no one can expect to avoid illness or injury throughout an entire lifetime. When combined with medical advances, the ideal of "perfect health" can create a sense of entitlement allied with an abrogation of personal responsibility for one's health. An update of our portrayal of health is long overdue.

## A dynamic interaction with our environment

A first step is to accept that overall well-being is dynamic, perpetually changing over the course of our life, rather than being a fixed, static state[1]. Our health is dynamic because we interact with the ever-shifting environment around us. We must adapt in order to stay alive. Our health reflects our ability to manage ourselves and address challenges to well-being. These challenges might include physical injury, environmental stress, infection, malnutrition, social or mental stress.

Our bodies are equipped with finely tuned biological self-regulatory systems that keep us healthy by maintaining optimal function of vital physiological processes. Many of these processes rely on factors, such as body temperature, blood pressure or blood glucose levels, remaining within narrow ranges. Homeostasis is a negative feedback system that preserves these variables within range. Allostasis is the process by which the body maintains physiological processes in the face of external challenges. When the allostatic load becomes too great, our bodies are unable to adapt to the stress we are undergoing. Ill health and disease ensue as a consequence[2].

Ultimately, our health relies on the effectiveness of our body's internal self-regulatory systems, which are predominantly managed by hormone networks. Hormones are chemical messengers. Hormones are the crucial link between our external environment and internal processes.

The tricky aspect is that these systems do not work in isolation; they form part of an intricate network of all the other processes going on in the body, including the brain. Our health is affected by the ways in which we interpret our internal body function and how we think about ourselves. For example, the state of mind of a young person who is uncertain, reflected in anxiety about their body weight and shape, can in turn impact their physiology and health. Harnessing this important connection between brain and body in a positive way is why cognitive behavioural therapy (CBT) can be helpful in many health conditions, including those where the health issue lies in the miscuing and mistiming within hormone networks. It is no coincidence that the controller of the hormone networks, the hypothalamus, is located in the brain where our thought processes occur. The hypothalamus is described as the neuroendocrine gatekeeper, keeping a watching brief on our external and internal milieu and our psychological assessment of these: the crossroads where body, brain and emotion meet.

Our personal internal health management systems make every one of us unique. This explains why some people seem to have a more robust constitution and higher levels of mental and physical resilience than others. This calls for a more personalised approach.

## Nature or nurture

The revolutionary progress of mapping the human genome is truly amazing. It is now possible to associate genes or clusters of genes with a wide range of medical conditions. In a few instances, the existence of a faulty gene, or lack of a gene, leads inevitably to a specific outcome. This is why newborn babies have a heel prick blood test to exclude so-called "inborn errors of metabolism", where the inherited version of a faulty gene causes the malfunction of a particular enzyme (biological catalyst) and a log jam in the production of a specific protein.

However, harmful single-gene faults are rare. In the vast majority of cases, genetic analysis provides only a partial explanation of the variation of a particular condition. For example, a study seeking a genetic link to the age of menopause found a group of genes that explained 10% of the variation in the timing of the cessation of ovarian responsiveness. This was widely reported in the press as a revolutionary breakthrough, in spite of the fact that the researchers themselves recognised that this left 90% of the variation unexplained: "missing heritability". The authors of the study advised against using this type of genetic testing as a clinical tool[3].

Among twins with identical genes, it is quite possible for one to suffer from a condition or disease, while the other does not. The reason is epigenetics. Epigenetics describes the way that the environment can modify the behaviour of genes in the short term, in response to life events. This works through a mechanism called methylation of DNA. A methyl group attaches itself to a segment of DNA, a gene, to alter the production of the protein encoded by that gene[4]. This adds another layer of complexity to the body's web of genetic interactions. However, in isolation, DNA is inert; it only has an effect when its genes are expressed and specific proteins are produced.

## Personalisation of health

> *"It is more important to know what sort of person has a disease, than to know what sort of disease a person has."*
>
> *Hippocrates*

Although your DNA provides a blueprint, it does not determine your fate. Most disease states result from a combination of various genetic elements and environmental factors. The extensive use of genetic testing generally reveals only partial associations and correlations with health outcomes, leaving a great deal of uncertainty unexplained. Figure 1.1 shows that the normal range of every population is made up of subgroups. If a test is able to categorise you as a member of a subgroup, what practical use is this when it comes to disease prevention[5]?

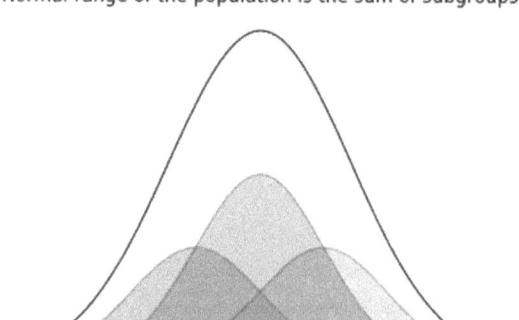

Normal range of the population is the sum of subgroups

**Figure 1.1:** A population of subgroups.*

For example, although there is a genetic element to developing type 2 diabetes mellitus, the more powerful driver comes from adverse lifestyle choices. So general recommendations about "healthy" lifestyle choices around nutrition and exercise are actually more effective than targeted recommendations based on genetics[6].

We have a significant level of control over the influence of environmental factors on our health, through our choice of behaviours and lifestyle. In other words, we have the ability, and arguably a personal responsibility, to manage ourselves and to address challenges to well-being. However, each of us is different in our personal biological responses to the behavioural and lifestyle choices we make. Rather than a doctor prescribing a medication, the healthcare provider must act as an advisor to empower the individual to make informed choices that are beneficial to health.

## Hormones as the directors of health

This book is about the crucial link in our understanding of health that has been overlooked. How do our lifestyle choices determine the expression of our DNA, whether for illness or health? Identifying the nature of the linkage between our behaviours and our gene expression would certainly help us in our quest to personalise health and disease prevention. Identifying and harnessing the mobiliser of selective gene expression would allow us to optimise health and performance, empowering individuals to make positive, informed choices. Figure 1.2 shows the central role of hormones in determining our health. We need to understand and manage our hormones.

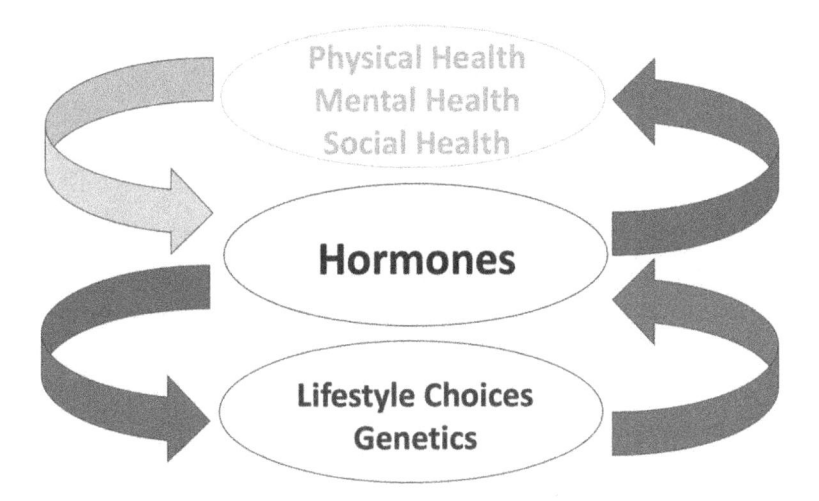

**Figure 1.2:** Hormone feedback loops

Hormones are responsible for the self-regulatory processes of homeostasis and allostasis that keep us alive and determine our ability to adapt to environmental stress. Hormones control the expression of our genes, setting in motion the messages encoded in our DNA. Hormones are directly affected by our behaviour and lifestyle choices, providing the link between nature and nurture.

Understanding our hormones and how to harness them positively is a sure way to optimise personal health. In striving for a fulfilling life, optimal health is a prerequisite for each of us in attaining our full potential.

# Scene 2
# Hormones for Health

*"Setting in motion"*

ὁρμῶν (hormon)

**Subtitle:** Hormones set in motion and govern the physiological processes determining health, by bringing to life our genetic code. We explore the intricate biological control systems that ensure hormones are produced at the right time and in the required amount to support health.

Although the word hormone is derived from ancient Greek, it was not until 1905 that the term was coined by the British physiologist Ernest Henry Starling. He and his brother-in-law, William Bayliss, had been studying a substance produced by glands in the intestine, called secretin, which regulates water concentration throughout the body. Starling drew upon a classical education to name the body's internal chemical messengers, recognising the fact that they do more than simply deliver instructions. Rather than choosing the noun ὁρμή (*horme*) which means "that which sets in motion", he chose the verb which conveys action ὁρμᾶν (*horman*) which means "to set into motion". Furthermore, he chose the form of the verb that invokes the sense of continuous, ongoing action, namely the present participle ὁρμῶν (*hormon*) which means *"setting into motion"*.

The reason to emphasise this point is not to delve into ancient Greek grammar but rather to demonstrate that hormones are more than mere messengers. They actually put the instructions into action and perform follow-up checks to ensure the message has been implemented. In other words, hormones dynamically adjust and regulate all aspects of physiological processes. They do this throughout our lives: from conception to death.

## Setting in motion

Deoxyribonucleic acid (DNA) contains the blueprint of life. It encodes the instructions for making all the proteins required to build and maintain a functioning body. In isolation, DNA is inert. It only comes to life when it is in the nucleus of a cell, surrounded by the biological machinery that can convert the genetic code into a range of essential proteins. The cells in different organs, such as the heart, liver or skin, have specialised functions requiring particular proteins. Gene regulatory networks play an important role in the creation and function of body structures, by ensuring that the right proteins are produced in the correct cells at the appropriate time.

Many of the proteins produced in a cell act as enzymes. These biological catalysts speed up certain metabolic pathways, enabling the physiological processes of life: growth, reproduction, cellular respiration (conversion of food to energy), excretion, movement, reaction to stimuli and assimilation of food (digestion). But these processes cannot simply operate on autopilot, because every individual must interact with their environment, in order to survive and reproduce.

Hormones are key players in the gene regulatory networks that allow the body to adapt to its environment. They do this by sending instructions to specific cells, triggering the expression of genes encoded in the DNA, to produce particular proteins. Often these proteins are enzymes that promote further reactions to ensure that physiological processes continue to operate optimally. An example is the production of insulin after a meal, to maintain glucose levels in the optimal range. We shall meet many similar instances in this book.

## Quo vadis?

Hormones are molecules that are produced by ductless glands. This means they are free to wash over adjacent cells and enter the bloodstream, allowing them to reach more distant other organs or tissues. Depending on how far a hormone travels, its action can be described as autocrine, paracrine or endocrine. Autocrine is when a hormone has an effect on the cell that produced it; paracrine describes a hormone exerting influence on neighbouring cells; and endocrine is when the chemical message enters the bloodstream, in order to reach more distant target cells.

Hormones bind to specific receptor proteins on the outside of their target cells. But then they need to pass their messages on to the nucleus of a cell to direct gene expression, a process known as signal transduction. How the hormone gains access to the DNA code depends on its type.

Hormones are generally either water soluble (hydrophilic) or lipid soluble (lipophilic). Peptide and protein hormones, such as insulin, are water soluble, so they are unable to cross the cell membrane. However, the action of binding to the outside of the cell triggers a cascade of secondary messengers inside the cell wall, which enter the nucleus, resulting in gene expression. Steroid hormones, such as testosterone, being lipid soluble, are able to shimmy through the membrane and go to the nucleus, where they directly unlock the DNA code.

## Time dimension

The chemical messages employed by the hormone system are slower and more persistent than the electrical messages used by the nervous system. Hormones are typically produced in response to chemical information delivered to an endocrine (hormone-producing) gland. Each hormone needs to be made and released. Even if a hormone has been prepared in advance, its release is still much slower than the instantaneous generation of an electrical nerve signal. There is also a time difference in the delivery speed of these biological messages. Electrical nerve conduction easily beats the speed of hormone delivery via the bloodstream, even if over a short distance.

Once messages have been delivered, the response time is also different. A nerve impulse arriving at a muscle causes rapid contraction and movement. A hormone needs to get into the cell nucleus and switch on gene transcription to make the desired protein. Although doting grandparents marvel that their grandchildren have "shot up overnight", in reality, the hormones determining growth rate act over much longer time scales.

The "let down reflex", in breastfeeding, is an example of a hybrid neuroendocrine response, where a neural electrical impulse triggers the rapid release of a prepared hormone. A suckling baby stimulates nerve cells in the nipple, causing the brain to release oxytocin, which in turn facilitates the "let down" of breast milk.

## Hormone message subtleties

In contrast to the digital nature of a nerve signal, which is either on or off, hormones use an analogue system. This gives hormones a repertoire of messages to fine-tune the cell response and overall physiological function. In the first instance, a particular hormone could vary in concentration in the bloodstream. This determines the response elicited in the target cells and tissues. High levels of insulin facilitate the entry of glucose from the bloodstream into the cell. Conversely low levels of insulin allow glucose to remain circulating in the bloodstream. This is the principle of a "sliding scale" (variable-rate intravenous insulin infusion) of an insulin pump infusion used in hospital, when diabetic patients present with excessive levels of blood glucose. The aim is to mimic the physiological variation of insulin production according to blood glucose levels and so maintain blood glucose in an optimal range.

Another subtlety of hormone communication is that the tempo of hormone release can be varied. Some hormones, such as cortisol, exhibit diurnal variation over a 24-hour period. The female hormones that control menstrual cycles rise and fall in close coordination over a time period of roughly one month.

Follicle-stimulating hormone (FSH) released from the pituitary gland in the brain is part of the hormone network that regulates the timing of women's menstrual cycles. FSH release varies in timing and concentration. Rather than a continuous monotone, the hormone message has the texture of tempo and volume, with many levels of complexity compared to the on/off message of a nerve impulse.

## Location-specific response to hormones

Hormones can bind to more than one type of target cell, eliciting different responses. This explains why a single hormone can have multiple physiological effects. For example, the sex steroid oestradiol (the most active form of oestrogen) binds to alpha receptors in the tissues of the female reproductive tract, thickening the lining of the uterus. Oestradiol also binds to beta receptors in bones, the brain and the heart, resulting in a number of other effects.

## Endocrine system

The term endocrine system describes the ductless glands producing the hormones, the target cells and tissues, their response and monitoring of the effects on physiological processes, which, in turn, determine the next round of hormone messages. The smooth running of the endocrine system is based on sophisticated, biological feedback mechanisms. When a physiological process is pushed out of equilibrium, it is the ability of the endocrine system to adjust via a negative feedback loop that brings it back into balance.

## Hormone network control systems

Biological systems run smoothly in a "Goldilocks" environment that is maintained within certain limits. The body should be not too hot, not too cold. Biochemical molecules should be not too concentrated, not too dilute. Metabolic rate should be not too high, not too low. This is challenging because our interactions with the world are dynamic.

Self-driving cars can also operate quite well in Goldilocks environments. But the driving performance and passenger experience can become much more problematic when there are external challenges to deal with, like changes in traffic conditions, diversions, unusual weather, other drivers making errors and many more. In Figure 2.1 the onboard computer control system must account for these environmental factors, while monitoring its own internal status, in order to adapt the vehicle's speed and direction, within appropriate safety margins. When this is done effectively, the car performs well and the passengers are happy.

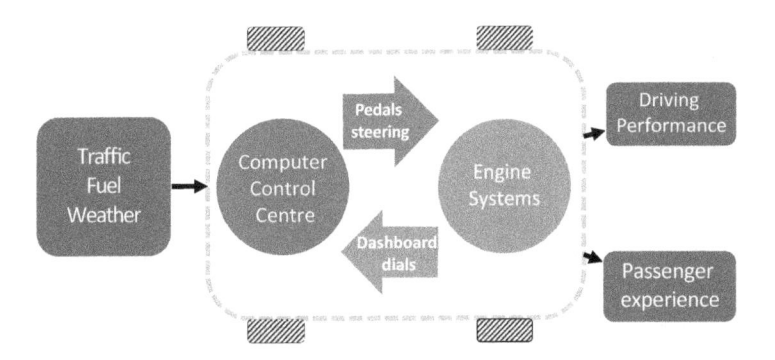

**Figure 2.1:** Self-driving car

In Figure 2.2 the endocrine system operates as the physiological control centre of the human body. It has to deal with environmental stresses, such as variations in exercise, nutrition or sleep, while monitoring the body's own internal feedback signals. Hormones are produced in order to maintain blood glucose concentrations, metabolic rate, blood pressure, production of red blood cells and many other biological variables within safety margins. When your hormones are working well, you feel physically and mentally fit, with a positive sense of well-being.

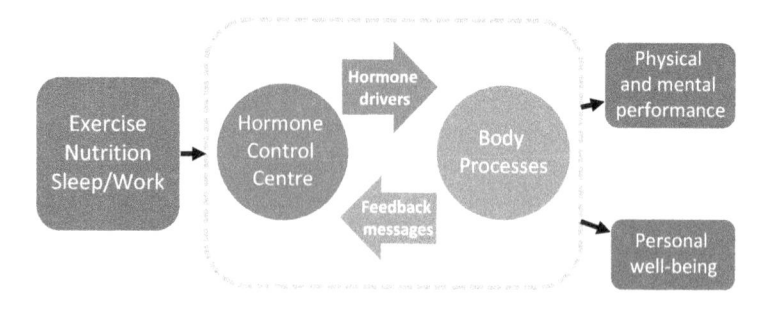

**Figure 2.2:** Self-driving human body

In addition to maintaining an optimal internal steady state of homeostasis, hormones control the longer-term allostatic adaptations to external events. Hormones networks are the key players in these control systems, often operating through negative feedback loops. Hormones drive changes in physiology by controlling gene expression. The resulting production of proteins and resultant molecules feeds back messages to regulate further hormone production.

There are many examples of negative hormone feedback loops that maintain optimal function across a wide range of physiological processes.

## *Blood glucose regulation*

The concentration of glucose in the blood needs to be maintained within certain limits for optimal physiological function. Elevated blood glucose levels are detected by the beta cells of the Islets of Langerhans, located in the pancreas. These cells release insulin, which promotes the absorption of glucose from the blood into the cells, thereby reducing blood sugar levels. When blood glucose falls back into range, the stimulus for insulin release stops, preventing continued fall in blood glucose.

In the inverse situation, when blood glucose is too low, glucagon is released by the alpha cells of the Islets of Langerhans. Glucagon is an antagonistic hormone to insulin; in other words, it has the opposite effect to insulin. It causes the breakdown of glycogen, the storage form of glucose, which goes into the blood, resulting in an increase of blood glucose concentrations. Production of glucagon ceases when blood glucose levels are restored. Figure 2.3 shows how the interplay of these two hormones in negative feedback loops maintains homeostasis of blood glucose.

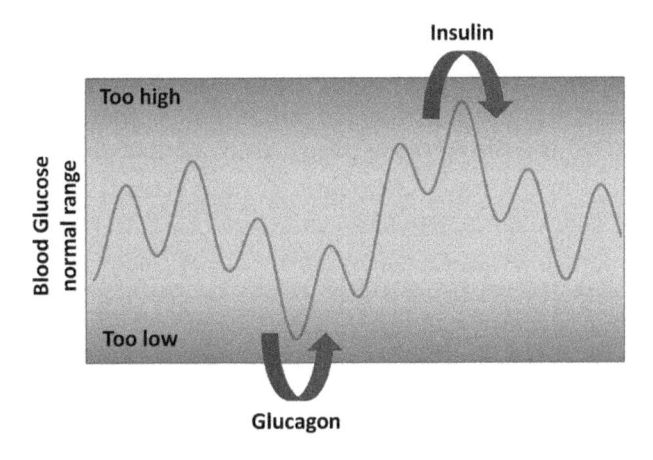

**Figure 2.3:** Hormones and blood glucose homeostasis

## EPO for oxygen

Red blood cells produced in the bone marrow contain the oxygen-carrying molecule, haemoglobin. Since internal energy production (cellular respiration) requires oxygen, it is essential to maintain a consistent level of red blood cells circulating at all times. This is the job of the hormone erythropoietin (EPO) produced in the kidney.

At first, it may seem strange that a hormone produced in the kidney is involved in red cell production in the bone marrow. After oxygenated blood leaves the left ventricle of the heart in the aorta, one of the first calling points in the body is the kidneys. High blood flow to the kidney is required to fulfil its main function of "filtering" the blood. The other advantage of being high in the pecking order of freshly oxygenated blood delivery is that the kidney has a first look at these oxygenation levels.

Low blood oxygen levels trigger the release of additional EPO, which travels to bone marrow, in order to stimulate red blood cell production. The restoration of optimal blood oxygen levels causes EPO production to return to normal. This negative feedback loop maintains red blood cell homeostasis.

It is sometimes necessary to supplement this hormone regulation system. For example, in chronic kidney disease, both the filtering system and EPO production are impaired, so patients on renal dialysis may also receive EPO injections.

EPO has also been a favoured choice of "doping" for endurance athletes, with the aim of increasing the oxygen-carrying capacity of blood flowing to exercising skeletal muscles. This carries the significant health risk that supraphysiological levels of red blood cells make the blood very viscous: like adding a thickener. Many endurance athletes have a slow heart rate, reflecting efficiency of the heart muscle pumping action. Doping with EPO puts these individuals at risk of thick, slow-moving blood, which tends to clot, resulting in serious consequences, including stroke and pulmonary embolism. This shows that the replacement of a hormone to physiological levels is beneficial for health, whereas excessive hormone levels disrupt the normal control feedback loops and may have grave health outcomes.

### Stones, bones, groans and psychic moans

The title of this section is the medical student mnemonic for the four symptoms caused by high levels of parathyroid hormone (PTH), produced as a result of overactive parathyroid glands. Hyperparathyroidism is the third most common endocrine condition after diabetes mellitus and thyroid disease, most often seen in menopausal women. The four symptoms are caused by high levels of calcium.

PTH is responsible for calcium homeostasis. This hormone is released by the parathyroid glands sitting next to the thyroid gland in the neck. The target cells for PTH are bone (calcium store), the kidneys (calcium excretion) and the gut (calcium absorption). In this way PTH can regulate both supply and demand, to ensure steady blood calcium levels.

If the feedback mechanism breaks down, PTH can be produced in an uncontrolled manner. This causes bones to be eaten away and high levels of circulating calcium to be deposited as kidney stones. Elevated levels of calcium are also associated with psychological issues.

## The endocrine orchestra

All the hormone negative feedback loops described above involve direct communication between the hormone and the concentration of something in the bloodstream that needs to be maintained in an optimal range for physiological function. These are a bit like individual components of a self-driving car that do something like turning the steering wheel to the left or right if the vehicle is off course.

The hypothalamic-pituitary axis (HP axis) represents a whole new level of sophistication. This involves multiple hormones operating on several levels, in conjunction with internal feedback and adaptation to external environmental changes. This is an important control unit in the endocrine system.

## *Neuroendocrine gatekeeper*

The hypothalamus is the neuroendocrine gatekeeper of the endocrine system. The hypothalamus is located in the brain, ideally situated to monitor inputs originating from outside the body, including external "stressors" such as lack of sleep, high demands from work, exercise, family or social interactions. This endocrine gland is also continually surveying internal feedback from within the body, particularly hormone levels.

The hypothalamus integrates all these inputs and is in close communication with the pituitary gland via an exclusive blood supply. This communication is written in the language of hormones called hypothalamic releasing factors that target the pituitary gland. Like a never-ending musical score, it defines the frequency and amplitude of the subsequent production of hormones. The score continuously adapts, illuminating the fine detail of the intended flow of chemical messages.

## *Conductor of the endocrine orchestra*

The pituitary gland is the conductor of the endocrine orchestra, marshalling the various hormone players, according to the score delivered by the hypothalamus. The pituitary releases trophic hormones that specifically target other endocrine glands, employing the variables of frequency and amplitude to add further nuance to its messages. The third level of control in this chain of command is the target endocrine gland, which releases its hormone to cause a physiological functional effect.

A multi-tiered feedback monitoring system adds to the complexity of this hierarchical hormone control system as shown in Figure 2.4. The effector hormone released by the target endocrine gland has a negative feedback effect on both the hypothalamus and the pituitary gland. In some cases, there are also short-range negative hormone feedback loops between the pituitary and hypothalamus. The net effect of this intricate HP axis chain of command and control is that the physiological processes of our body self-regulate to maintain homeostasis and allostasis for optimal health.

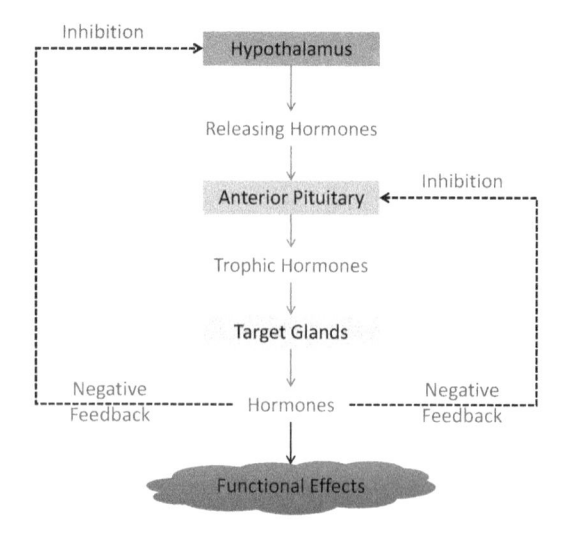

**Figure 2.4:** Hormone feedback loop of the hypothalamic-pituitary axis

## The protagonists of the hypothalamic-pituitary axis

There are several physiological processes under the regulation of the HP axis. Each is dependent on messages being passed down a hierarchy and feedback coming back up, somewhat reminiscent of A. A. Milne's poem "The King's Breakfast".

### *Reproductive axis*

The reproductive axis in men and women starts with the pulsatile, episodic release of gonadotrophin-releasing hormone (GnRH) from the hypothalamus, which instructs the pituitary to release luteinising hormone (LH) and/or follicle-stimulating hormone (FSH) at the rate and level encoded in the GnRH message. LH and FSH act on the gonads (ovaries in women and testes in men) to produce the sex steroid hormones oestradiol (most active form in the oestrogen family) and testosterone. Being steroid hormones, oestradiol and testosterone pass through cell membranes to the nucleus to cause physiological effects throughout the body.

The expected negative feedback loops are in place to regulate hormone levels. However, in the female HP axis, there is also an unusual positive feedback loop that causes ovulation. This is discussed in more detail in "Scene 5XX: Of Mice,

Men . . . and Women". The female reproductive axis is the most finely tuned of all the endocrine axes, with its own complex intrinsic timing and subtle nuances between individual women. With deep understanding of these temporal aspects, it is possible to mathematically model these hormones. As discussed in "Scene 6: Hormone Supermodels", this can help women navigate their female hormone fluctuations from cycle to cycle and over their lifetime.

The reproductive hormone network in men, and especially women, is particularly sensitive to both external behaviours and internal stressors. This offers the possibility to optimise these hormones and health. On the downside, imbalances in external behaviours can lead to functional disruption of the HP axis, which is discussed in "Scene 10: In the Red".

## Stress response axis

Another process under the control of the HP axis involves the production of the stress response hormone, cortisol. This follows a diurnal rhythm of secretion. Cortisol is higher in the morning, prompting a wakening response that helps get us ready for the day ahead.

The hypothalamus is continuously on the alert for external and internal sources of stress. Upon detection, corticotrophin-releasing hormone (CRH) is released, which acts on the pituitary to cause the production of adrenocorticotrophic hormone (ACTH). ACTH travels in the bloodstream to the adrenal cortex (the outer layer of the adrenal glands situated on top of the kidneys) resulting in cortisol production.

Cortisol puts the body on alert to be able to respond to sources of stress. This is an expected physiological response. However, when stress levels from internal and/or external sources are maintained, cortisol tends to lose its expected diurnal variation and can downregulate other hormone axes. This situation is discussed in "Scene 9: A Balancing Act" and "Scene 10: In the Red".

Rarely the intrinsic control system goes wrong, resulting in either an underproduction of cortisol (Addison's disease) or an overproduction (Cushing's disease). In Addison's disease, the adrenal cortex cannot produce adequate cortisol in response to "stress". On the other hand, continuous high levels of cortisol are not a good thing either. Some medical historians believe that Henry VIII suffered from Cushing's disease. If you conjure up an image of this monarch in his later life, you get a good idea of what someone with this endocrine condition might look like.

## Thyroid axis: regulator of metabolic rate

The hypothalamic-pituitary-thyroid axis works to control resting metabolic rate. This is the rate at which energy is utilised to maintain all the physiological processes working at an optimal rate, while at rest. Its regulation is achieved in the modus operandi of the HP axis: the hypothalamus releases thyrotrophin-releasing hormone (TRH), to request the pituitary to produce thyroid-stimulating hormone (TSH) that travels to the thyroid gland which obliges by producing thyroxine (T4) and the more active hormone sibling triiodothyronine (T3). Negative feedback loops ensure that T4 is kept in optimal range for ensuring a steady resting metabolic rate.

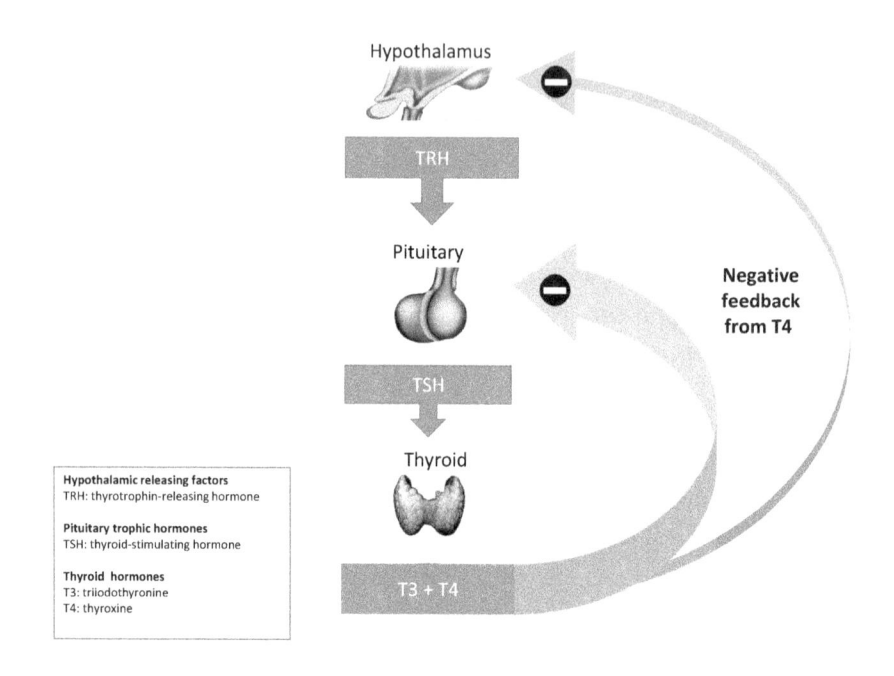

**Figure 2.5:** Hypothalamic-pituitary-thyroid axis.*

## An unusual family member: prolactin

In the family of anterior pituitary hormones, there is an unusual member: prolactin. Prolactin is kept at a steady level by the negative control of dopamine, a neurotransmitter, which is a short-range messenger molecule between neurons. The stability of prolactin can be disturbed by external stress. In fact, in a stressful situation, such as high exercise training, both cortisol and prolactin can often be seen at the upper end of the range. The negative inhibition by dopamine on prolactin release can be overcome by the influence of hormones such as TRH or oestradiol. Oestradiol is high during pregnancy and after giving birth, so prolactin is able to rise, facilitating lactation.

### Oxytocin sets love in motion

The posterior pituitary is the source of two hormones with diverse actions. One is oxytocin, which as mentioned earlier is responsible for the release of breast milk when the baby suckles and for bonding. This occurs via the neuroendocrine reflex where the suckling action of the baby causes nerve impulses to travel to the posterior pituitary and release oxytocin. In addition to "letting down" of breast milk, oxytocin also stimulates the contraction of the uterus. This is why a woman breastfeeding her baby in the first few days/weeks after birth may actually feel her uterus contracting.

### Holding onto water

The other hormone released by the posterior pituitary gland is anti-diuretic hormone (ADH) also known as vasopressin. The role of this hormone is osmolarity homeostasis: the maintenance of the concentration of dissolved substances in the bloodstream at a steady level. When you are dehydrated your kidneys "hold on" to water and you may notice your urine looks very dark. On the other hand, if you drink a lot of water your kidneys let some of this pass out in the urine, and you may notice that your urine looks paler.

The mechanism behind this regulation involves ADH. In the hypothalamus, specialised osmoreceptors monitor the concentration of dissolved substances in the blood. If the blood is very concentrated, these receptors stimulate the release of ADH, which acts on the collecting ducts in the kidneys to allow more water to be reclaimed from in the urine. This decreases the osmolarity of the blood, and the good news is reported back to the osmoreceptors. Satisfied that the status quo has been restored, no more ADH is released, completing the negative feedback loop.

## Interactions of hormone networks

None of the intricate hormonal negative feedback loops works in isolation. There are interactions. For example, cortisol suppresses other hormone axes. The evolutionary explanation is that when the body is presented with a stressful situation, priorities need to be set to focus on overcoming the challenge. This could be an internal or external challenge. For example, if you have not eaten enough to cover energy demand, the resulting internal metabolic stress signals increase cortisol levels, which can downregulate the thyroid axis or the reproductive axis to "save energy".

This hormone interaction is harnessed in clinical situations: a patient presenting in "thyrotoxic storm" (a massively overactive thyroid) is given medication to slow the heart rate and steroids, which have an action similar to cortisol in preventing the conversion of T4 to T3. This prevents the "over-revving" effect of excess T4 production.

## Spotlight on some hormone axes

Although the intricate network of hormone feedback loops generally functions very reliably, there are nevertheless some medical conditions where control systems go awry.

### *"Sweet" diabetes*

Insulin is a peptide hormone whose role is to promote the absorption of glucose from the blood into the cells. When insulin is not doing its job effectively, blood glucose control is compromised, leading to diabetes mellitus (DM). Mellitus means sweet, specifically referring to the sweet taste of urine (don't ask!). The reason why urine becomes sweet is that, in the absence of the normal action of insulin, blood levels of glucose rise and overflow into the urine.

Fortunately, we have more sophisticated testing methods today than taste. It is straightforward to measure blood glucose levels with finger-prick blood samples or to perform continuous monitoring via skin sensors.

There are two types of DM depending on the level of insulin malfunction. In type 1 DM, there is insufficient production of insulin from the pancreas. Typically, the onset of this type of DM is early in life. It is thought to be an autoimmune disease, in other words, the body produces antibodies to its own beta cells in the Islets of Langerhans.

DM has been described as starvation in the face of plenty. During one of my early jobs working in the Brighton Hospital casualty unit, I remember a young boy coming in really short of breath. Initially it sounded like asthma and that is what the boy and his parents thought. However, listening to his breathing there was no sign of wheeze or anything else amiss. The boy mentioned that he had lost some weight and was feeling really thirsty.

## Scene 2: Hormones for Health

This type of human puzzle is why I chose to focus on hormones for my medical career. The explanation hinges on small clues from the patient's story and on testing for hormones that I suspected may be the culprit for symptoms. As hormones never work in isolation and have multiple effects, it is important to put all the pieces of evidence together to solve the mystery.

Why had the young boy been losing weight without reducing what he ate? How could he be short of breath, yet have perfectly healthy lungs? Without insulin, blood glucose climbs, but it is unable to enter the cells. The cells are literally starving in the face of plenty, so the person often loses weight. Cells have to resort to an inefficient way of making energy. This results in the production of ketones and hydrogen ions, which are very acidic and whose concentration determines pH. So, the body has several problems to deal with. The cells are starving yet due to the lack of insulin, the blood and urine are overflowing with glucose and the person needs to urinate a lot (osmotic diuresis) and feels really thirsty. The production of acid reduces blood pH, threatening the function of enzymes, which can only withstand a small degree of disruption of pH homeostasis. The body needs a way to offload this acidic load. The lungs play an important role in trying to restore acid-base balance. The person starts breathing rapidly (Kussmaul breathing) to dispose of the acid load in the form of carbon dioxide (an acidic gas).

The boy's symptoms were due to type 1 DM. I treated him acutely by providing fluid and insulin in a drip to rehydrate and get glucose into his starving cells. In the long term, he would need insulin injections to substitute for the lack of his own insulin production.

Type 2 DM, although also presenting with high blood glucose readings, has a totally different aetiology. In this type of DM, there is enough insulin, but the cells become resistant to its action, so glucose remains in the bloodstream. Typically, this type of DM is a result of lifestyle factors, so initial management is always directed at increasing activity levels and limiting food intake. Medication may also be required and in some cases insulin injections as with those with type 1 DM.

Why is running a high glucose level a problem? Aside from the short-term effects of feeling unwell, there are long-term medical complications. Having consistently high blood glucose levels damages the blood vessels, specifically, the arteries delivering oxygenated blood from the left side of the heart around the body. Damage of the larger-sized arteries results in macrovascular complications. Organs such as the kidneys, brain and heart cannot get their fair share of oxygen, resulting in an increased risk of kidney malfunction, stroke and heart attack. Damage to the smaller-diameter arteries is also problematic, with microvascular complications impacting the blood vessels supplying the retina of the eye and peripheries of the hands and feet. This can lead to visual and circulatory problems[1]. On a positive note, improved ways of monitoring and keeping blood glucose levels in a healthy range reduce the risk of circulatory complications.

Exercise is an important lifestyle choice for those with type 2 diabetes. The most effective exercise is something that the person finds enjoyable. During my time working in diabetic clinics, I found that rather than giving a "prescription" to do a certain type and amount of exercise, it was far better to start the conversation with what type of exercise the person enjoyed. If the answer was "none", then we would explore what might at least be a starting point, perhaps a walk around the block, and build from there. For some, exercising in a group might be more appealing.

For those with sporting aspirations, DM can present challenges to reach their full athletic potential. When a first-year university rower presented with newly diagnosed type 1 diabetes, we worked together to personalise practical strategies to manage his diabetes to enable him to continue to train and compete[2]. Doing exercise requires energy and tends to lower blood glucose. Being prepared and planning ahead become even more important for a diabetic athlete. For example, for a rower out training in the middle of a river, having readily available sources of glucose is a priority. The same applies to road cyclists, where the long duration of exercise needs a fuelling strategy. These factors need particular attention to detail for each individual athlete with DM. This is possible and there is a professional cycling team where all the riders have type 1 diabetes.

The challenges of DM where blood glucose regulation is not working effectively highlight what an amazing self-regulating control system the body has in place. Endocrine feedback loops are in constant action to maintain blood glucose homeostasis. Nevertheless, increasing our understanding of these hormone regulation mechanisms means that it is possible to provide the best clinical advice and support for individuals with DM.

### *To treat or not to treat? Thyroid axis*

Figure 2.5 shows the feedback loops involved in the thyroid gland's role in regulating the body's metabolic rate. When the thyroid gland is working as expected, the control feedback loops maintain TSH from the pituitary and thyroxine T4 in central zone of the graph shown in Figure 2.6. However, if the thyroid gland starts to become sluggish at producing thyroxine, TSH levels start to rise in an attempt to get the thyroid gland back on track. Initially this might result in compensation, shown in the subclinical zone on the right side of the central healthy zone. Subclinical means the person feels fine, but the blood test shows the TSH a bit high in normal range and T4 a bit low in the normal range, like dance partners getting out of step. If the thyroid gland continues to misbehave, it can become a primary underactive thyroid. This is defined according to National Institute of Clinical Excellence (NICE) guidelines where TSH levels rise above 10 mIU/L, warranting thyroxine replacement. Response to treatment can be monitored by TSH dropping back into the normal range[3].

Conversely, if the thyroid gland becomes too frisky, producing high levels of T4 above the normal range, then TSH falls. An overactive thyroid may require treatment to bring TSH and T4 back in range.

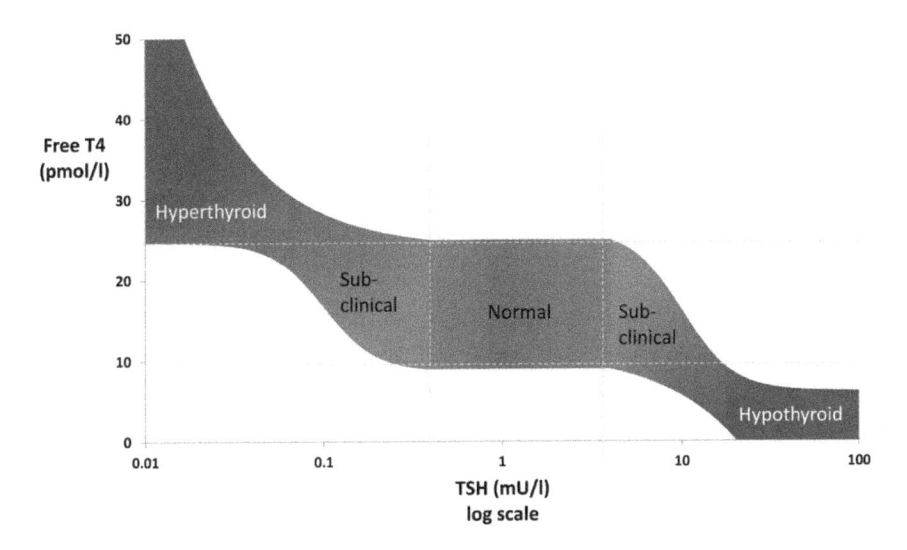

**Figure 2.6:** Thyroid function. After "What should be done when thyroid function tests do not make sense?" Mark Gurnell, David J. Halsall, V. Krishna Chatterjee, Clinical Endocrinology, Volume 74, Issue 6, June 2011, Pages 673–678

So, you might think that thyroid function is relatively straightforward to assess. In essence, look at TSH and T4 to see if they are in step. Things become complicated if you fail to look at both hormones in the feedback loop and do not take into account clinical context[4]. Recently an aspiring 25-year-old amateur cyclist came to see me. He explained that he had been training hard and reducing his food intake in order to reach "race weight". He was feeling tired and had been told he had an "underactive thyroid" as his T4 was at the lower end of the range and that he should take thyroxine medication. In fact, what he really needed to do is to reassess his balance of exercise and nutrition. Although T4 was indeed at the lower end of range, TSH was not raised as one would expect of primary underactive thyroid. What was going on?

There was in fact nothing wrong with the thyroid gland per se. Rather the hypothalamus had detected external and internal stress caused by an imbalance of exercise (energy expenditure) and nutrition (energy intake) causing an energy deficit. Therefore, quite sensibly the hypothalamus had instructed the pituitary to reduce the TSH signal sent to the thyroid. Clearly, TSH was not at the level set by NICE to qualify as an underactive thyroid, requiring thyroxine replacement. Although thyroxine is not on the World Anti-Doping Authority (WADA) list of banned substances, nevertheless prescribing unwarranted medication of any sort can present a risk to health. Over-riding the physiological health-preservation mechanism of functional downregulation of the thyroid axis can potentially have adverse effects on long-term health. The same applies to taking thyroxine in order to lose/control weight where there is no clinical indication of an underactive thyroid based on TSH levels.

When I was working in an NHS endocrine clinic in London, a 30-year-old woman came presenting with fatigue. She told me that wishing to lose weight she had taken thyroxine and cortisol (steroid tablets). As she had neither an underactive thyroid nor Addison's disease, taking these medications had shut down her own internal production of these hormones. The usual feedback loops had been overridden. So, in an attempt to feel better, the dose had been increased resulting in a further internal shut down of hormone production, leaving her dependent on these external hormones. We had to gradually wean her off external hormones. Stopping abruptly would be too much of a challenge for her own hormone networks to reboot. This is why if you ever need a course of steroids to dampen inflammation, you must gradually reduce the dose and never stop suddenly.

The bottom line is that if there is a definitive clinical indication for hormone replacement this should, of course, be swiftly prescribed, and the dose titrated for the individual. However, if the hormone levels do not meet the clinical criteria for diagnosis, then external hormones should not be given, as they disrupt internal control mechanisms, in some cases, permanently.

## Growth hormone is not just about "growth"

Growth hormone (GH) is a key player in the endocrine repertoire. GH is not just important for growth in childhood; it plays a key role in maintaining health throughout life. It helps ensure favourable body composition, supporting lean body mass, such as skeletal muscle rather than adipose tissue. GH helps to regulate metabolic health issues associated particularly with visceral fat: the type of fat that is found around organs. The control of GH release is via the HP axis shown in Figure 2.7. Once released from the pituitary, GH is converted to the more active IGF-1 (insulin-like growth factor 1) which acts on a broad range of tissues with receptors for this hormone.

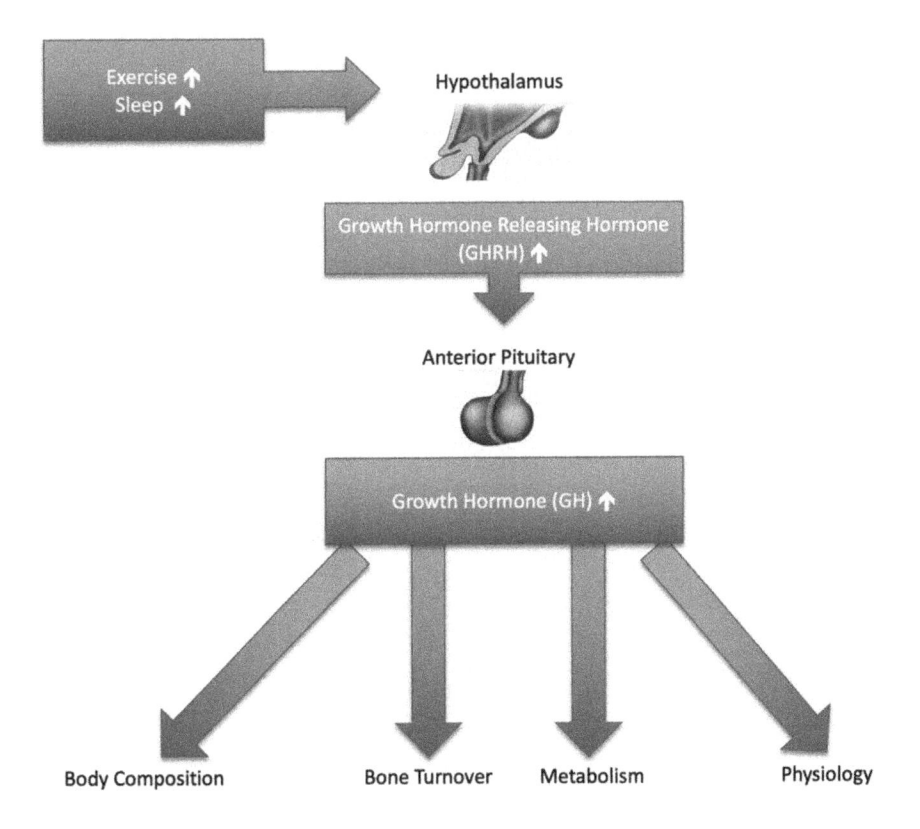

**Figure 2.7:** Growth hormone.*

An unfortunate consequence of GH producing several positive biological effects and potential improvements in human athletic performance is that GH has been used by some athletes as an illicit way to enhance performance. Although GH might appear to offer the promise of an elusive gold medal, there are potential serious health consequences of taking external (exogenous) GH, which are demonstrated by the clinical condition of acromegaly. In acromegaly, the pituitary goes haywire and secretes high levels of GH. In children this results in excessive vertical growth, in adults this causes growth of parts of skeleton that can still increase in size. Rather quaintly as medical students we were advised to ask about any increase in glove and hat size, in reference to times when these items of clothing were worn every day, not just for playing sport. The jaw also has the potential to grow in presence of excess GH in adults and can give people a distinctive facial appearance. Other potential consequences of excessive GH levels (whether from endogenous or endogenous sources) are increased risk of high blood glucose levels, which can lead to the development of type 2 DM and increased risk of cancer.

## Anti-doping

Despite these potential health risks, sometimes some athletes are so desperate for success that they resort to "doping". To safeguard athlete health, the World Anti-Doping Authority (WADA) maintains a list of banned substances, which is updated every year. As hormones play such a crucial role in health and performance, these have the unsolicited notoriety of accounting for 75% of adverse analytical findings reported by WADA in 2014.

Developing an anti-doping test for a peptide hormone like GH is not straightforward, as I found out as part of the international medical team at St Thomas' Hospital, London, commissioned with this task by the International Olympic Committee. The first challenge was to establish the normal range for athletes, given that the two main stimuli for GH release are exercise and sleep. We suspected athlete ranges may differ from the broader population. This heralded journeys to various sporting venues, often armed with a portable centrifuge to take blood samples from a cross-section of athletes in various sports. We also needed to understand the timescales over which GH release was stimulated as a result of taking exercise. To quantify this, we spent many evenings testing people running on a treadmill and taking blood samples.

The next challenge was to decide what to measure. You might think that would be simple: just measure GH? Unfortunately, that is not a practical solution as GH has a very short half-life. In other words, GH has perfected a physiological disappearing act. GH is very rapidly converted to the "business" molecule IGF-1 which immediately gets bound to various protein transport vehicles and sped off to mobilise action in muscle, bone and other tissues. In other words, GH is the hormone equivalent of Macavity: the mystery cat.

However, GH does leave its calling card in terms of ongoing effects on tissues, in particular bone. Although bone might seem like a rather boring, static tissue, actually it is continuously being recycled. Bone is broken down and reformed in a process known as bone turnover. There are specific blood markers to indicate the rate of this turnover. Crucially this rate is over a far longer time scale than the disappearing act of GH. Furthermore, the effect on bone lasts far longer than the initial nudge given by GH.

So, could these bone turnover markers be surrogate candidates for indicating GH doping? To answer this question, we turned to the "gold standard" double-blind randomised controlled trial study. We recruited some reasonably fit men and women and injected each participant with "dummy" (placebo) or GH. We then measured blood markers, body composition and their exercise performance. The double-blind aspect meant that neither the participants nor I, as the doctor conducting the UK part of the study, knew who was receiving the placebo or GH, in case this might bias the results. Only when all the results were in was the "safe unlocked", and we could break the code to see who had received what. Strikingly those who had received the real deal GH had significant increases in their bone turnover markers. This was an exciting discovery and using bone turnover markers became a method to detect athletes doping with GH[5].

The good news is that there are legal and safe ways of promoting and harnessing your hormones, without having to resort to doping. We discuss how to do this through lifestyle choices shortly.

## Time to shine

Hormones play a key role in health by bringing to life the instructions encoded in DNA. The complex control systems of endocrine networks orchestrate this process. There is a score determining how the hormone symphony plays out over an individual's lifetime, which is discussed in Act 2. This begins in utero, when the developing baby is exposed to the mother's hormones through the placenta, where only one cell thickness separates maternal and foetal blood. Following birth, during infancy and childhood the child's endocrine system goes solo. This eventually culminates in the growth spurt and puberty. Adulthood sees the endocrine system continue to react to external lifestyle behaviours and support reproduction. Moving into middle age and beyond, the endocrine system starts to wind down.

We can influence how this hormone symphony plays out to a large extent through our choice of behaviours, which is the topic of the next scene: "Harnessing Hormones".

# Scene 3
# Harnessing Hormones

*"Walking is man's best medicine."*

*Hippocrates*

**Subtitle:** Hormones are the instigators and regulators of our internal physiology. They manage the biological processes that maintain life. Given their crucial role in optimising all aspects of health, what regulates the hormones? Internally, hormones can regulate themselves through feedback mechanisms. But hormones are also influenced by external factors, including our lifestyle choices. What is the best combination of lifestyle behaviours to harness our hormones for optimal health?

## Hormones, homeostasis and health

The action of hormones is to maintain homeostasis. The resulting stable internal state is optimal for all the biological processes that allow our bodies to function. Why is homeostasis so important for our health?

The day-to-day business of the body is based on chemical reactions. Proteins, called enzymes, are essential to make these reactions occur fast enough to have a physiological effect. The blueprint of each of these biological catalysts is encoded in our DNA. Hormones manage our physiology by regulating the expression of DNA to make enzymes.

Homeostasis is important because proteins are fussy operators. Just as a fair-weather cyclist like me only ventures out on warm, sunny days, proteins only operate in conditions that are just right: not too hot, not too cold, not too acidic and not too alkaline. We can see what happens to proteins every time we boil an egg: they change in structure and lose their function in a process known as denaturing. Since enzymes are proteins, any denaturing compromises their ability to catalyse biological processes. This becomes a major problem for our physiology and health.

Hormones maintain homeostasis at multiple levels. For example, the hormone insulin maintains blood glucose homeostasis. This is important for the optimal functioning of other hormone-enzyme partnerships. A lack of insulin activity allows a sustained rise in blood glucose which forces cells to generate energy via a different pathway. This causes internal cellular acidity to increase, disrupting pH homeostasis, which in turn disrupts the function of interdependent enzymes. This includes disturbance of enzyme function in the mitochondria, the "powerhouses" of cells, involved in generating energy for use in the body. Hormone dysfunction can produce knock-on effects that further destabilise homeostasis.

## Hormone networks: mediators of health via internal feedback loops

Hormones maintain homeostasis through feedback loops that ultimately determine our health. The top half of Figure 3.1 shows internal feedback loops where hormones affect health and health affects hormones.

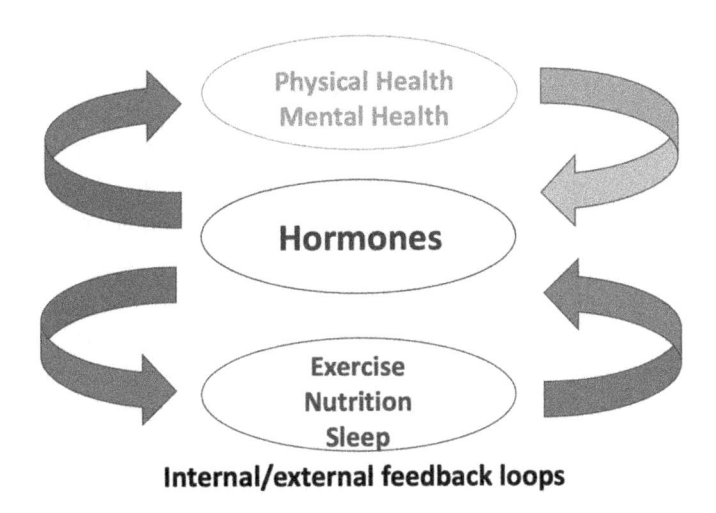

**Figure 3.1:** Hormone networks – mediators of health

## Challenging the status quo

We do not live in hermetically sealed boxes. Our bodies are continually challenged by external perturbations, simply as a result of going about our daily lives. The weather, a dog barking in the night and other day-to-day inconveniences are largely outside our control. However, we are all able to make personal decisions on the key lifestyle factors of exercise, nutrition and sleep. Hormones are the mediators between our lifestyle choices and our health.

## Hormone networks: mediators of health via external feedback loops

Well-functioning hormone networks are essential in order to gain the beneficial health effects of good lifestyle choices. These positive gains feed back to support the effectiveness of hormone networks. The positive interaction between external behaviours and internal hormone networks is shown in the lower half of Figure 3.1. On the other hand, poor lifestyle choices can create negative feedback effects. Too little, or indeed too much exercise, nutrition or sleep can have adverse impacts on hormone function, with detrimental health consequences. Figure 3.1 shows how hormones connect our interactions with the external environment and our internal physical and mental health.

## How hormones connect exercise and internal physiology

There is irrefutable evidence that regular exercise supports health and plays an important role in disease prevention[1]. On the other hand, insufficient exercise, and sometimes excessive exercise, can have adverse effects on health. We are told that exercise is good for us, but we are not told why. How exactly does exercise bring about changes in the body?

When we exercise, the metabolically active tissues of the muscle, bone and gut release a cocktail of molecules, including peptides, nucleic acids and metabolites, known as exerkines[2]. These exerkines drive the recognised beneficial adaptive changes of exercise, across a range of body systems. Although exerkines are not produced by the glands of the endocrine system, they act as hormones, serving as chemical messengers over different dimensions of time and space. The initial effects are local: on the cell itself (autocrine) or crosstalk with neighbouring cells (paracrine)[3]. In this hierarchy of control, the broader and longer-term

*Scene 3: Harnessing Hormones*

effects of hormones from endocrine glands drive beneficial adaptive changes in physiology for both health and exercise performance.

Crucially, these positive hormone-driven changes occur *after* exercise, during recovery and especially during sleep. With appropriate refuelling, you actually become healthier and fitter when you are asleep, rather than while you are exercising. By repeating a cycle of exercise, nutrition and recovery, over time you reap the rewards in a stepwise fashion. This positive adaptative response is shown by the feedback arrow on the left in Figure 3.2.

On the other hand, insufficient or excessive exercise results in a lack of response or an overload of the endocrine system, leading to maladaptation. This negative adaptive response is shown by the feedback arrow on the right in Figure 3.2, representing at best no beneficial effect or at worst a negative impact on health from an inappropriate amount of exercise.

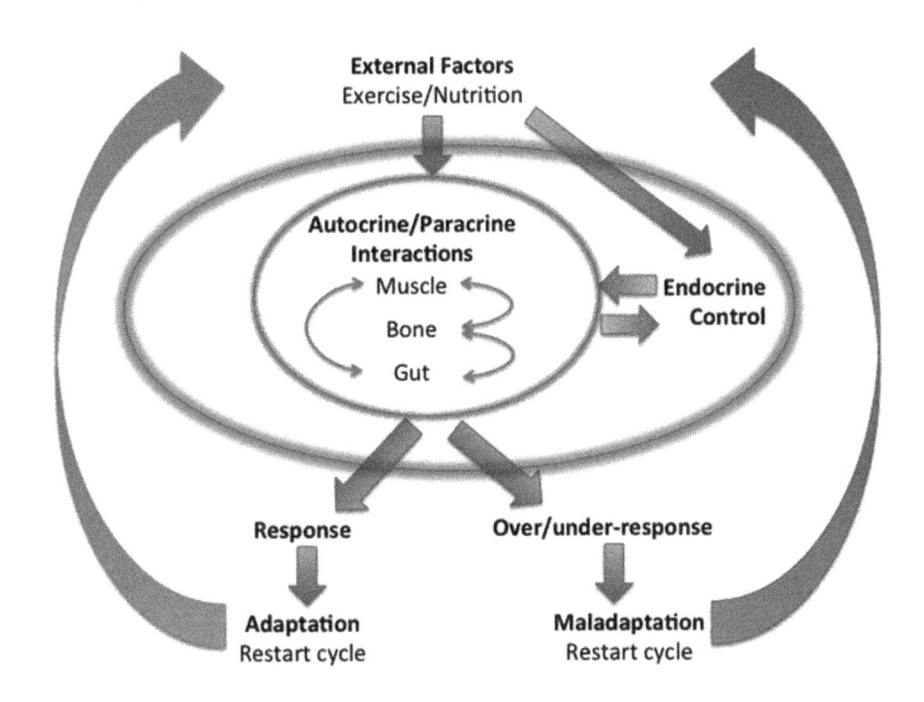

**Figure 3.2:** Interaction of external and internal factors

*Effects of exercise and hormones: body composition*

Being overweight has adverse effects on health. Global obesity has tripled over the last 40 years according to the World Health Organisation. Exercise has been advocated as a way to control body weight and to reduce the body mass of the overweight. However, in a study, 150 minutes or more of brisk walking per week increased life expectancy by 3.4–4.5 years, independent of body weight[4]. In other words, exercise is beneficial for health and disease prevention, even when it does not reduce body weight. This finding also indicates that focusing just on change in body weight as a positive outcome of exercise can overlook the beneficial effects of exercise on body composition, hormone health and psychological well-being[5].

Body mass index (BMI) has the advantage of taking body height into account, but this still does not account for body composition or hormone health. BMI is generally considered to be in the "healthy" range if this falls between 18.5 and 24. However, this metric does not tell the full story about internal health. Lean mass (especially metabolically active muscle) is both better for metabolic health and denser than fat. This means that a very muscular 25-year-old rugby player may record a high "obese range" BMI. On the other hand, a 25-year-old female athlete might record a "healthy" BMI of 20, even if she is not having menstrual periods, a clear indication that her hormone networks are not healthy.

Delving further into the details of body composition, different types of fat also have different health implications. Subcutaneous tissue fat is the type of fat most of us are familiar with, lying just beneath the skin. This can be measured using skinfold callipers. On the other hand, visceral fat found deep within the body around organs can only be measured using the imaging technique of dual X-ray absorptiometry (DXA). High levels of visceral fat are more informative in terms of potential adverse effects on metabolic and psychological health[6].

The big fat story does not end there. "White" fat, whether subcutaneous or visceral, is metabolically inert, whereas "brown" fat is the complete opposite, being highly metabolically active. Irisin is a relatively newly identified exerkine hormone that has been implicated in "fat browning"[7]. It is thought to be responsible for the hormone-driven alchemy of turning metabolically inactive white fat into its metabolically active sibling, brown fat. In older age groups, exercise has been found to mitigate the cognitive decline, mediated by irisin[8]. So, we have another link between exercise, hormones and health.

The more established hormone mechanism for exercise-induced improvements in body composition is through the anabolic action of hormones secreted from endocrine glands, which are released, particularly in response to resistance exercise. The term "anabolic" refers to increasing the amount of active metabolic tissue like muscle and bone. Natural, exercise-induced increases in growth hormone (GH) and androgenic sex steroids (such as testosterone) have anabolic effects, especially if supported by a good protein intake.

Improvements in body composition can slightly raise weight, due to an increased proportion of metabolically active, lean mass versus fat. However, because muscle is more compact and denser than fat, a change in body shape may give a slimmer waistline. Waist circumference is a surrogate measure of visceral fat. Remember that the figure displayed on the weighing scales is just a measure of gravity, not hormone health[9].

To understand how exercise improves health, we need to look beyond anthropometric measures of weight and height, to account for the effects of hormone networks.

*Effects of exercise and hormones: metabolic health*

Exercise acts through internal hormone networks to improve the ability to maintain energy homeostasis in the face of stressors. This involves modifications of the neuroendocrine response of hormones relating to energy storage and production. For example, the protagonists in regulating the homeostasis of blood glucose levels include adrenaline, the duet of insulin and glucagon, insulin-like growth factor 1 (IGF-1) and cortisol. Furthermore, exercise increases the sensitivity of tissues to these key hormones. Exercise training is recognised to increase insulin sensitivity. Given that insulin resistance is the underlying cause of type 2 diabetes mellitus, exercise is an important therapeutic tool in the prevention and management of this increasingly common metabolic disease[10].

Exercise can also harness hormones to improve metabolic health by increasing metabolic flexibility. Metabolic flexibility is the ability to switch between carbohydrate and fats as a fuel source, depending on availability. Inability to do so, metabolic inflexibility, is a feature in chronic disease conditions such as obesity and type 2 diabetes. A sedentary lifestyle can impair metabolic flexibility, even if some exercise is being performed, causing the body to use carbohydrate, rather than fat, as the default energy source. Avoiding long periods of sitting is the most important factor[11]. For those with a sedentary job/lifestyle trying to intersperse exercise "bouts" during the day helps with facets of metabolic flexibility, such as improvement of daily blood glucose control, prevention of sustained high levels of glucose after meals and higher rates of fat oxidation overnight. Being active and taking exercise are important for metabolic health and reducing the risk of heart disease.

*Effects of exercise and hormones: mental health*

Exercise promotes the release of "feel-good" neurotransmitters in the brain. These include endorphins, which are short-range protein hormones released by the pituitary gland. Exercise is also a good "stress" reliever. The reason inevitably comes down to hormones. The acute response to exercise is an increase in the "stress hormone", cortisol, released from the adrenal cortex. However, in the long term, regular exercise helps to modulate this hormone response to stressors[10]. Exposure to chronic environmental stress can dampen the normal 24-hour diurnal variation of the "stress" hormone cortisol. The receptors to cortisol become desensitised to unvarying levels of cortisol. The mechanism is very similar to the way cells become resistant to continuous high levels of insulin, in type 2 diabetes mellitus. A lack of cell responsiveness to continually high levels of cortisol leaves inflammation unchecked. Furthermore, a worldwide study showed that regular and increasing levels of moderate-to-vigorous physical activity decreased depressive symptoms in adults of all ages[12].

## What exercise?

*"Walking is man's best medicine."*

*Hippocrates*

There is strong evidence that Hippocrates was correct about exercise being the best medicine. Now we know why. Exercise supports physical and mental health for all ages, due to the far-reaching effects of hormones.

An ideal form of exercise would be one that supports the beneficial hormone effects on all aspects of health. Dance, as a form of "creative heath", can be valuable in restoring and maintaining health, as outlined in the All-Party Parliamentary Group on Arts for Health and Wellbeing[13]. Dance can stimulate physical, mental and social health. Although ballet happens to be my personal preference, many different sports and activities are available to match personal tastes and objectives. In fact, personal choice is emerging as being just as important as the lifestyle factor itself.

In a fascinating Australian study, allowing participants to select exercise levels was shown to be beneficial in terms of their choice of food[14]. A sample of

58 people was divided in half. One group was given a choice of exercise, while the other group was "prescribed" a specific exercise workout. After the exercise, all the participants were provided with a choice of food at a buffet. What the participants didn't realise was that this was an important part of the study. Those in the group with a free choice of exercise made "healthier" food choices, with relatively lower calorie content. They also reported higher enjoyment and perceived benefit than those who had no exercise choice. This shows how the autonomous choice of exercise not only provides positive reinforcement of exercising but subsequent food choice is improved.

When it comes to exercise for older populations, it can be difficult to distinguish between the effects of ageing and loss of fitness[15]. However, this does not mean that a supportive and inclusive approach should be abandoned when it comes to exercise for health, throughout life. Rather, encouraging people to participate in decision-making, which they feel leads to options that are realistic and beneficial, is the approach most likely to work, especially in the long term.

When exploring different types of exercise, including a variety that supports all the various aspects of fitness, is a good starting point. The exact type of exercise and balance of different forms depend not only on personal preference but also on an individual's age and starting point of fitness. This approach can help integrate external exercise behaviours with internal hormone networks to support health and performance[16].

## What are the key elements of fitness that can be supported through exercise-driven hormone adaptations?

*Cardiovascular fitness* is the ability to extract oxygen from air and transport it to exercising muscles for energy production (cellular respiration). As described above, exercise is important for cardiovascular health. Cardiovascular exercise supports hormones that optimise metabolic health and reduce hormones associated with "stress". Beneficial types of exercise include brisk walking, swimming, cycling, running and dancing. These are forms of aerobic exercise, which means that the intensity can be maintained for more than about 20 minutes, with oxygen supply sufficient to meet demand. Cardiovascular fitness can be evaluated in the laboratory by assessing $\dot{V}O_2$ maximum, which measures the utilisation of oxygen in millilitres per minute per kg of body weight. While $\dot{V}O_2$ max is partially genetically determined, this element of fitness certainly can be improved.

*Muscular strength.* Although defined as peak power production (1 repetition maximum for moving/lifting an external weight), in terms of everyday life, muscular strength is important for activities such as carrying shopping, children or suitcases. The best way to ensure muscular strength is through resistance training. Depending on age and ability, this does not necessarily mean free weights in a gym setting. Resistance bands or using everyday objects can be just as valuable.

The anabolic ("body building") hormones that drive the beneficial adaptions to strength exercise include IGF-1 and testosterone, the latter being a powerful anabolic steroid. These anabolic hormones support a favourable body composition: muscle over fat. Strength exercise also has a positive effect on metabolic health. The mechanism is that this type of exercise recruits many muscle units, which being very metabolically active increases metabolic rate, even after stopping exercise. This supports the regulation of blood glucose control and metabolic health[10]. The type of muscle we are talking about is skeletal muscle, which is voluntary muscle attached to bone used in movement. When performing strength exercise, this skeletal muscle exerts a force on bone which strengthens the bone tissue.

*Muscular endurance.* This is the ability to sustain continuous muscular contraction without fatiguing. The hormone mechanism that improves this element of fitness is that, in response to exercise, hormones induce the production of enzymes that make aerobic cellular respiration more efficient and effective. Cellular respiration occurs in cells in the specialist energy conversion organelles, or units, called mitochondria. Glucose and fat molecules from the diet are broken down to generate energy-rich molecules of adenosine triphosphate (ATP), which is the internal energy currency. The by-product of carbon dioxide is easily exhaled.

The ability to generate a plentiful supply of ATP molecules allows you to keep exercising at low to moderate intensity. However, when muscles "run out of steam", or more precisely run out of oxygen, the required enzymes for ATP generation must switch from aerobic respiration to less efficient anaerobic (without oxygen) respiration. Fewer ATP molecules are produced per glucose molecule during anaerobic respiration. Furthermore, the lactic acid by-product is a much trickier customer to deal with. Lactic acid splits into lactate and hydrogen ions. It is these hydrogen ions, rather than lactate acid molecules, that are problematic, because they cause acidity.

A drop in pH due to increased hydrogen ion concentration is very bad news for enzymes. These biological catalysts are all proteins, which become denatured when internal conditions stray outside of a narrow range of pH and/or temperature. Denaturing of proteins is when structural changes render the protein unable to carry out its function. In terms of exercise this means you literally grind to a halt. Regular aerobic exercise helps improve mitochondrial activity[17] and improves the body's ability to deal with potentially harmful waste products. Reactive oxygen species (ROS) are free radicles of oxygen which are produced as a result of physiological stress. Although a certain degree of oxidative stress in response to exercise is helpful in driving beneficial adaptive processes, excessive levels of ROS have been implicated in many disease states. Exercise helps modulate oxidative stress[18].

*Neuromuscular skills.* This type of fitness encompasses the connections between the nervous system and skeletal muscles for movement. Neuromuscular fitness supports the skills of co-ordination, reaction time, agility (ability to change direction of movement quickly and effectively) and proprioception. Proprioception is awareness of where your body is in space, an important component of co-ordinated movement. As we explore in Act 2, this component of fitness becomes especially important during times of hormonal change: during adolescent years, when growth and sex steroid hormones change rapidly, and later in life, when hormones are declining.

*Flexibility.* This type of fitness ensures the maintenance of the range of movement around joints. This does not mean that we should all be aiming for the hyper-mobility of a rhythmic gymnast. However, poor flexibility prevents the joints and soft tissues of muscles, ligaments and tendons from attaining the range of movement required for optimal, effective, efficient movement patterns. Flexibility increases during pregnancy and in the early post-natal period as a result of the aptly named hormone relaxin. Relaxin increases the laxity of collagen structures including the ligaments of the usually fixed joint of the symphysis pubis at the front of the pelvis, which facilitates childbirth.

Flexibility can be maintained and, in some cases, improved through stretching, which is best performed when warmed up. Static stretching consists of holding the muscle group in a stretched position for a minimum of 30 seconds (which can seem like a very long time!). There is another way of stretching called proprioceptive neural facilitation (PNF), which requires a professional, trained in physical therapy, to provide resistance against which the person contracts the muscle group. On releasing the contraction, the trainer gently moves the limb to stretch the muscle. Although PNF is an effective method, there is a risk of injury if it is not performed with a specialist trained in this technique.

*In summary.* We can support health, throughout life, by pursuing a balance of exercise covering each type of fitness. In Act 2 of this book, we explore how the importance of specific types of fitness depends on the changes in the endocrine system as we age. It is helpful to follow the principle of performing bouts of exercise during the day, interspersed with rest/recovery, because the body reacts to change. Perturbations in lifestyle behaviours provoke action by endocrine networks. For athletes this is known as periodised, polarised training. Mixing up higher and lower intensity exercise in a pattern over a longer time frame ensures maximal benefits from exercise.

## How hormones connect nutrition and internal physiology

*"Let food be thy medicine and medicine be thy food."*

*Hippocrates*

Just as medication needs to be adjusted according to the individual, so does food intake. Each of us is different in terms of body size, body composition (where muscle is more metabolically active than adipose tissue) and activity levels. Furthermore, for an individual, requirements change according to personal internal physiology linked with age, changes in hormones and according to external factors of lifestyle behaviours, especially activity levels, over their lifespan.

Nevertheless, there are some guiding principles that can help support healthy hormone networks. Aim to include all food groups in the diet[19], with rough percentages of total dietary intake shown in brackets to indicate the segment portion size of these food groups on a plate[20]:

Complex carbohydrates found in bread, potatoes, cereals, rice and other similar foods (30%)
Fruit and vegetables (30%)
Protein found in meat, fish, eggs and some plants (15%)
Dairy products, or alternatives (15%)
Fats and sugars: simple carbohydrates (7%)

Total energy intake needs to match the demands of physical activity on top of the energy demand of basic metabolism that keeps hormone networks functioning optimally. The body has evolved to maintain homeostasis, so slight deviations and short-term mismatches are well managed. However, sustained surplus or insufficient energy intake have a negative impact on hormone networks and health in the long term. Chronic excess intake relative to requirement (overeating) can lead to hormone network disruption and metabolic syndrome. Metabolic syndrome is a constellation of symptoms that greatly increases the risk of cardiovascular disease, including poor blood glucose control, adverse cholesterol profile, high blood pressure and high abdominal visceral fat[21]. Conversely, chronic insufficient energy intake relative to requirement (undereating) results in prolonged low energy availability with consequent adverse health consequences, seen in both men and women[22]. Female hormone networks are particularly sensitive to energy deficits[23]. This topic is discussed in detail in "Scene 9: A Balancing Act" and "Scene 10: In the Red".

Eating in a consistent manner, with some degree of flexibility according to age and personal lifestyle behaviours, helps to avoid imbalances in energy intake and demand. This has the benefit of helping maintain optimally functioning hormone networks. While it is important to keep a balance, some food groups deserve particular attention. Including optimal, personalised levels of complex carbohydrates supports sex steroid hormone networks. Adequate protein intake provides the "building blocks" to support favourable body composition in terms of lean tissue[24]. The optimal timing of eating and exercise is also an important consideration. For example, to reap the beneficial effects of exercise, post-exercise fuelling with carbohydrate and protein supports hormone actions to replenish glycogen stores and aid muscle repair[25]. The timing of external lifestyle behaviours to synchronise with internal hormone timing is explored in more detail in the next "Scene 4: It's all in the Timing".

## How hormones connect sleep and internal physiology

*"Sleep is the chief nourisher in life's great feast"*

Shakespeare, Macbeth

Sleep[26] is essential in supporting the lifestyle choices of exercise and nutrition. It is when you are asleep that your hormone networks work their magic of supporting health and performance. Sleep is one of the key stimuli for the release of hormones such as growth hormone (GH). LH pulsatility increases overnight to support the production of the sex steroids oestradiol and testosterone. These hormones are particularly important for muscle and bone repair, as well as metabolism. You get fitter while you are asleep (provided of course you have done some exercise and balanced your energy intake during the day). This positive, hormone-directed process is supported by taking on some protein before bedtime: milk, for example, is ideal. Milk contains casein, a protein for providing the building blocks of the hormone-driven process of muscle repair. Milk also contains tryptophan which is a precursor molecule for making the sleep hormone melatonin.

Exercise during the day can help achieve a good night's sleep. "Sleep pressure" builds up during the day from the build-up of adenosine which is a brain neuronal waste product. Exercise can add to this accumulation of chemical "sleep pressure", provided you don't exercise too close to bedtime, in which case exercise could be more of a stimulating influence to keep us awake.

Good sleep patterns allow hormone networks to stimulate health benefits. These include both the direct benefits, on body composition and metabolism, and indirect effects, such as improved functional immunity and cognitive function. How much sleep do we need? Although there is some individual variation, adults generally need around 8 hours (minimum 7 hours) on a regular basis[27]. There is a gradated scale for younger age groups: up to 1 year minimum 12 hours sleep; 1–2 years minimum 11 hours; 3–5 years minimum 10 hours; 6–12 years minimum 9 hours; 13–18 years minimum 8 hours sleep. Youngsters clocking up at least this minimal sleep time ensure healthy hormone networks and benefit from improved cognitive function: learning and memory, mood, mental and physical health and overall good quality of life[28].

However, it is not just a question of how much, there is also the important factor of timing. Ideally, sleep and other lifestyle behaviours should be synchronised with our internal biological clocks. The hormone networks of the endocrine system are particularly sensitive, as discussed in more detail in "Scene 4: It's All in the Timing". Disrupted sleep patterns have negative consequences on hormone networks and consequently on health. For children, insufficient sleep can store up health problems for adult life. Among adults, shift workers, whose sleeping patterns fall out of sync with their hormonal biochronometers, have an increased risk of health problems, such as metabolic syndrome.

In the short term, a lack of sleep impairs your quality of life. When I worked as a (very) junior doctor in medicine many years ago in various hospitals, I can attest to that! I personally experienced a lull in hormones around 2 am, snatching a few minutes rest lying down fully dressed, only to be started to attention by a bleep. I found myself devouring a bowl of cereal around 5 in the morning. However, it was the next day that was the worst. This was in the dark ages, before doctors' hours were regulated. So as a 24-year-old, being "on call" for medicine meant that you would work during the day on the ward, in clinics and in A&E holding the "crash bleep" in addition to your designated bleep. Then overnight you would work covering medical emergency admissions, usually without any sleep. Your reward would then be to work the following day, which is when the wheels would start to come off, especially if you knew that you had to also cover that night and the next day.

To avoid the adverse effects of suboptimal sleep patterns on hormones and health, there are some practical strategies. Sleep hygiene describes actions you can take to help ensure good sleep patterns in terms of timing, duration and quality of sleep. These include exploring ways to "wind down" for sleep and avoiding late evening computer work (of which I am guilty). This allows your nocturnal hormone networks to make the most of whatever exercise and nutrition you enjoyed during the day.

## Harnessing hormones for health through balanced lifestyle behaviours

Although I have described the key lifestyle behaviours of exercise, nutrition and recovery separately, in practice we need to consider the combined effects of these external factors on our internal hormone networks. To gain the maximal beneficial health effects, it is important to balance the triumvirate[29]. The zone in the centre of Figure 3.3 represents the ideal balance between lifestyle factors. Slipping into the peripheral zones, represents an imbalance: either too much or too little of any of the three elements.

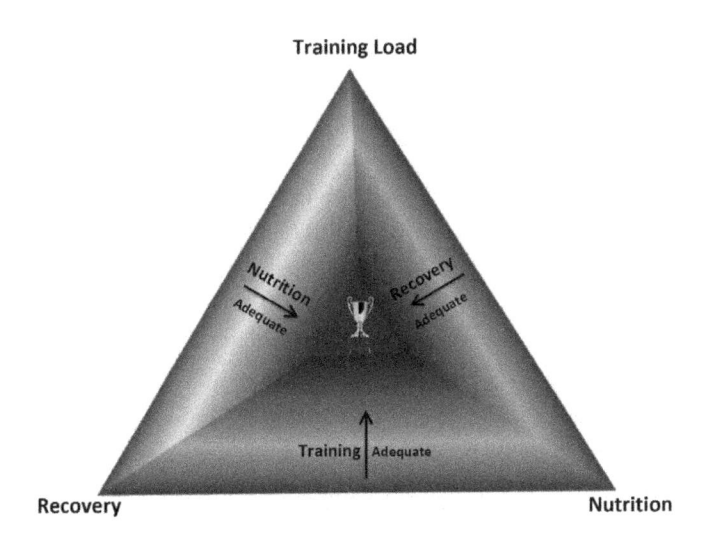

**Figure 3.3:** Triumvirate of lifestyle behaviours.*

Balancing lifestyle behaviours is the most effective way to harness hormones for many aspects of health. To illustrate this approach, let's consider cardiovascular health, metabolic health and body composition.

## *Harnessing hormones for cardiovascular health through combined lifestyle behaviours*

Although diet is certainly an important consideration in improving cardiac health and reducing the risk of heart disease, the combination of diet with exercise has an additive effect. The cause of heart disease is blockage of the coronary arteries supplying oxygen to the hard-working cardiac muscle. In the process of atherosclerosis, the artery wall becomes roughened, accumulating deposits of cholesterol that cause turbulent blood flow. This can result in the formation of a clot, atherothrombosis, which causes critical restriction of blood flow to the heart muscle.

A healthy diet of fresh, non-refined produce is beneficial in mitigating the risk of heart disease. However, there are other factors at play. Specifically, the inflammatory process, which helps fight infections, can be an aggravating factor in processes such as heart disease[30,31]. This is where combining diet with exercise can have a synergistic positive effect. An optimal combination is more effective than either lifestyle factor in isolation, in keeping inflammation at bay. The combination of a varied diet and regular exercise can improve quality of life, life expectancy, optimise all aspects of health and reduce the risk of heart disease[30].

## *Harnessing hormones for metabolic health through balancing lifestyle behaviours*

Obesity, and specifically adverse body composition with a large amount of abdominal, visceral fat, is an increasing health concern. Increasing fat metabolism (utilisation/oxidation) helps reduce fat as a component of body composition. To achieve this, let's revisit the effects of the lifestyle factors of nutrition and exercise.

Considering dietary options: calorie-restricted diets result in weight loss; however, this reduction includes loss in both skeletal muscle and fat. What are the solutions to target fat metabolism and fat loss over muscle?

The effects of diets low in carbohydrate with high fat have been studied. Although this may seem counter-intuitive, eating more fat in place of carbohydrate did increase fat metabolism in two studies. Effectively the body was given no choice but to use fat as an energy source. However, exercise performance, especially at high intensity, decreased[32,33]. This could be because fat needs more oxygen compared with carbohydrate to be metabolised and converted to internal energy. Another proposed reason is that the body gets used to using fat as an energy source. The enzymes required for utilising carbohydrate as the main energy source during high exercise intensity take a break. This might not be a problem, or indeed may be helpful for ultra-endurance athletes. "Ketogenic" diets (very high in fat intake) may be useful in some medical conditions like early Alzheimer's disease to prevent cognitive decline[34]. On the other hand, if you are aiming to improve your high-intensity exercise performance, this might be a poor dietary choice.

Rather than artificially forcing the body to use a particular energy source, having a degree of metabolic flexibility is a valuable physiological asset. This is the ability to make effective use of a variety of energy sources, to match the energy demand from exercise. Metabolic flexibility is the ability to metabolise fat for low intensity, long-duration exercise, then to switch to carbohydrates for higher intensity, shorter-duration exercise. This illustrates why nutrition needs to be considered in conjunction with exercise and personalised depending on the individual and their objectives.

Returning to exercise strategies for weight and body composition control: "fat-burning" aerobic exercise is accepted as a good approach. This contrasts with higher intensity exercise, where carbohydrate is the preferred energy source. A key hormone driving this exercise effect on the reduction of visceral fat is growth hormone (GH). GH release is stimulated by exercise and promotes fat breakdown[35]. Revisiting the post-exercise hormone effects on metabolic health and body composition provides some interesting insights.

In a study of overweight individuals, as anticipated, lifestyle interventions, including exercise, produced weight loss through increased fat oxidation. However, after stopping the study, although all participants maintained an increased rate of fat oxidation, some sustained a lower body weight, while others regained weight. This outcome appeared to be due to differences in the rate of fat deposition, dictated by differences in hormone network's responses occurring after exercise[36]. In other words, both sides of the fat metabolism equation need to be considered: the balance between fat utilisation and fat deposition. The long-term effects of exercise on this fat balance are hormone-driven but subject to individual hormone responses to exercise.

This observation would explain why intense exercise, although not a "fat-burning" type of exercise, can reduce fat. The acute activity increases post-exercise metabolic rate. Specifically, the skeletal muscle, recovering from exercise competes for the available energy with the energy required to lay down fat. Muscle wins. In other words, energy from food intake is preferentially diverted to muscles for growth and repair, rather than towards fat deposition. The importance of the nature and timing of post-exercise refuelling is discussed further in the next scene. The exercised muscles also "demand" energy from fat stores through anabolic hormone-mediated signals. This mechanism also explains why strength training, engaging many muscle groups, has a positive post-exercise effect on metabolic activity and inhibits fat deposition[37].

Ultimately, there is an interactive effect of exercise and diet on health. There are no shortcuts with "One road to Rome" for optimal hormone function and health.[38] A recently published paper reported that to personalise advice on balanced lifestyle behaviours, it is important to identify "the optimal hormonal profile associated with fat loss and the most appropriate exercise and diet program required to achieve such a hormonal profile"[39]. Quod erat demonstrandum.

## Conclusions for harnessing hormones for health

Hormones can be effectively harnessed through the choice of a balanced combination of exercise, nutrition and sleep. However, a prescriptive approach to lifestyle factors could be counter-productive. Discussing options and encouraging individuals to make their own informed and personal choices are far more likely to enable them to take responsibility for their health and adhere to changes in lifestyle that are beneficial for their health.

## Strategies for harnessing your hormones

### *Exercise*

- Aim to include exercise that encompasses activities to support all areas of fitness
- Choose exercise options that you enjoy where possible

### *Nutrition*

- Aim to include a range of food types that cover your personal requirements according to your age and activity levels
- Be aware that your intake varies depending on your lifespan and according to changes in activity levels
- A food-first approach, choosing options that you like is important

## *Sleep*

- Timing, quality and quantity of sleep are crucial to support healthy hormone networks
- Explore the areas of "sleep hygiene" behaviours for good sleep patterns
  - Aim for eight hours of sleep per night. Go to bed and get up at consistent times – set an alarm for bedtime, well before midnight!
  - Establish a bedtime routine to ensure good sleep hygiene
  - Explore what helps you wind down: reading, listening to music, taking a bath
  - A milk drink at bedtime contains tryptophan to make the sleep hormone melatonin and the protein casein to aid muscle repair and formation
  - Avoid electronic devices close to bedtime, as the frequency of light disrupts the production of melatonin
  - Avoid alcohol or stimulants such as caffeine, nicotine or late exercise
  - Sleep in a well-ventilated room

# Scene 4
# It's all in the Timing

*"Not just a question of what, rather when we eat, sleep and exercise"*
*Dr N Keay BJSM blog*

**Subtitle:** Biochronometers are internal biological clocks. Each hormone system runs according to its own timekeeper. Fast-acting processes take seconds, while others proceed over timescales measured in years. The calibration of these biochronometers can change over one's lifespan; some may slow down or stop completely. Integrating the timing of our external behaviours with our internal endocrine biochronometers allows us to gain maximal health and performance benefits.

## Biochronometers: biological clocks

In 2017, the Nobel Prize in Physiology or Medicine was awarded to scientists who revealed the mechanisms behind the internal biological clocks that enable all living organisms to anticipate and synchronise with the day/night cycle due to the Earth's rotation[1].

Innate biological timekeeping determines the timetable of internal physiological processes. This ensures that body systems are prepared to meet the varying demands at different chronological times, throughout the lifespan of an organism. These internal biological clocks, known as biochronometers, run across a range of different time scales: from seconds, to days, to years. Biological clocks possess a degree of adaptability that allows the body to deal with changes in environment and behaviours. Hormone networks are key players in ensuring that all biological processes operate on a time schedule that maintains homeostasis and enables adaptation[2].

Figure 4.1 shows a range of biological timescales, from a short daily circadian rhythm to the seasons of the year, which may correspond to an annual exercise programme, out to the longest biological time scale of all: the lifespan of an individual.

*Scene 4: It's all in the Timing*

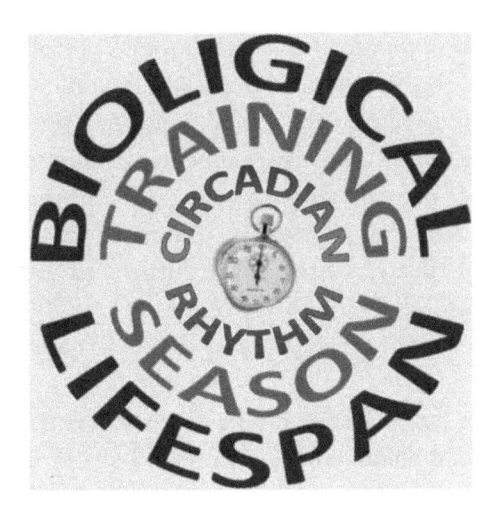

**Figure 4.1:** Biological timescales.*

## Hormone biochronometers

Accurate biological timekeeping aligns our internal physiology with the rotation of the earth and its circulation around the sun. In stable conditions, the timing and pattern of hormone release are determined by innate biochronometers. Changes in external environmental factors or behaviours impact the operation of hormone networks, causing them to release hormones that can trigger gene expression impacting the calibration of biological clocks. This continual fine-tuning forms part of a negative feedback loop. The endocrine system plays a crucial and unique role in biological time keeping, both as servant and master of biochronometers[3].

## Hormone timing control

Many of the time-sensitive hormone release patterns are governed by the hypothalamic-pituitary axis. The central circadian (daily) pacemaker, called the supra chiasmic nucleus (SCN), is located in the hypothalamus. The SCN issues instructions to the hypothalamus, which in turn controls the timed release of hormones. The hypothalamus delivers hormone-releasing factors to the neighbouring pituitary gland, which conducts hormone release patterns from the endocrine glands across the body. The SCN is located just above the crossover point of the optic nerves coming from each eye, allowing it to pick up external light levels. The SCN transmits this information to the hypothalamus via short-range hormones (paracrine action) and neural signals.

The hypothalamus acts as the neuroendocrine gatekeeper, the link between external factors and internal hormone networks. This gatekeeping capacity allows the hypothalamus to conduct the timing of the endocrine orchestra. Like all great conductors, the hypothalamus listens to the feedback, making it an integrated control and monitoring centre. It keeps biological time while gathering information from outside the body to modify intrinsic, internal pacemakers.

The action of the hypothalamic-pituitary axis allows the endocrine system to fulfil the dual role of maintaining homeostasis and responding to changes in the timing of environmental factors or behaviours relating to exercise, food and sleep.

## Daily hormone variations

Circadian derives from Latin "circa", meaning around, and "diem" day. Circadian rhythm is a biochronometer with roughly a 24-hour periodicity, regulating the sleep-wake cycle. Circadian timing is generated intrinsically and occurs independently of external cues, known as Zeitgebers (time-givers), such as light, temperature or food. For example, the circadian rhythm of sleep and wake patterns tends to be maintained, even in the absence of daylight. However, circadian patterns can be influenced and entrained by the environment. When travelling over time zones, although we often experience jet lag, ultimately our circadian clock and sleep/wake cycles reset.

Diurnal variation describes the changes in a physiological measurement over the 24-hour light-dark cycle, with the zenith and nadir being about 12 hours apart. In contrast to circadian rhythms, diurnal timing is dependent on external environmental "time givers". An example of the diurnal variation is the secretion of the steroid hormone cortisol.

The timings of peak release of hormones over a 24-hour period are shown in Figure 4.2.

*Scene 4: It's all in the Timing*

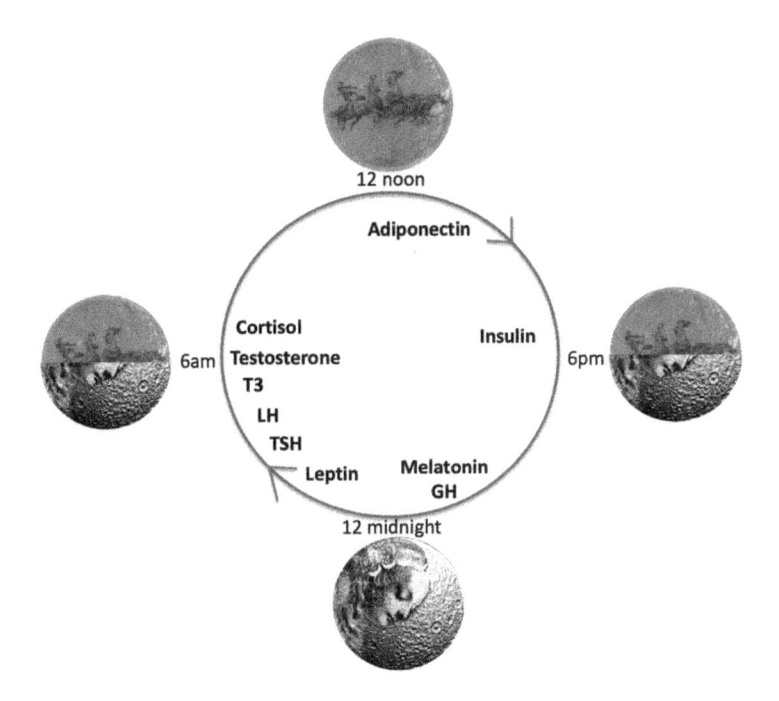

**Figure 4.2:** Circadian release of hormones.*

## Hormone timing overnight

Dropping light levels at dusk are detected by the SCN. This prompts the pineal gland located deep in the brain to release the hormone, melatonin. Melatonin prepares us for sleep by lowering body temperature and blood pressure. The timing of melatonin release helps integrate external changes in the length of daylight according to the season, with internal endocrine time keeping. Looking at the screens of electronic devices late in the evening disrupts the release of melatonin and subsequent sleep onset. The frequency of light emitted by these devices miscues the SCN into delaying the signal for melatonin release.

After melatonin has kicked in, the production of growth hormone (GH) ramps up. GH is secreted by the anterior pituitary gland, in response to growth hormone-releasing hormone (GHRH) from the hypothalamus. GH is not just important for growth in children. GH is converted peripherally to insulin-like growth factor-1 (IGF-1), which as the name suggests has an action similar to insulin, in being an anabolic hormone (building tissue and energy stores) to support favourable body composition (muscle relative to fat) and muscle repair. IGF-1 also contributes to bone health. The nocturnal peak production of GH is the main reason why, if you want to benefit from exercise, you should make sure to have good sleep patterns. Remember, you get fitter while you are asleep!

The thyroid function hormones, thyroid-stimulating hormone (TSH), thyroxine (T4) and T3 (triiodothyronine), control metabolic rate: the rate at which food energy is converted to internal "biological" energy. These metabolic control hormones display circadian variation, under the control of the SCN, the circadian pacemaker-in-chief. The conditions known as hyperthyroidism (overactive thyroid) and hypothyroidism (under active thyroid) disrupt the pattern of thyroid function hormones. The cells in thyroid cancers have been found to express faulty versions of intrinsic thyroid cell "clock genes" (cellular clocks are discussed in more detail shortly). This provides further evidence that hormone networks play a dual role in circadian alignment as pacemakers and responders to biological timing[4].

Another hormone, related to metabolism and closely linked to reproduction hormone production, also shows a temporal pattern of secretion. Leptin is a hormone produced by adipose tissue. It plays several roles. Leptin is the satiety part of the appetite hormone duo, along with ghrelin the "hungry hormone". An increase in leptin during sleep prevents you from waking up hungry and, importantly, supports the night-time action of the reproductive hormone axis. Leptin regulates the reproductive axis in a permissive way.

During sleep, luteinising hormone (LH) emphasises its pulsatile, episodic release. By varying the frequency and amplitude of its signal, LH prompts the gonads to ramp up sex steroid production: testosterone in the testes of men and oestradiol and progesterone in the ovaries of women. This can become rather obviously apparent to men when they wake up. This is why the number of early morning erections per week can be used as surrogate indicator of healthy daily physiological variation of testosterone in men[5]. As sleep is the time when the reproductive hormone axis is most active, unsurprisingly, lack of sleep has been linked to fertility issues in both men and women[6].

Acting on a different timescale, an uptick in the overnight activity of LH heralds the start of puberty and continues into adulthood.

## Hormone timing over the day

Cortisol levels show a diurnal variation and start to rise towards the end of sleep, peaking first thing in the morning shortly after waking. This is the cortisol awakening response. This catabolic hormone (breaking down internal energy stores to release energy) prepares us for the day ahead. Cortisol is released from the adrenal glands, under the control of the hypothalamic-pituitary-adrenal axis. The pituitary releases adrenocorticotrophic hormone (ACTH) to trigger the adrenals to increase cortisol production. After the morning peak, cortisol gradually declines throughout the day.

Adiponectin is a late riser, reaching its zenith between noon and 2 pm. Adiponectin is part of the adipokine family of hormones produced by adipose tissue. Adiponectin is thought to help sensitise the body to the peak of insulin production occurring around 5 pm. Insulin is an anabolic hormone, promoting energy storage in the form of fat and glycogen in preparation for the overnight fast when asleep. In contrast, insulin is at its lowest around 4 am, to allow the mobilisation of stored nutrients, while we are effectively in an overnight fast, during sleep.

## Infradian rhythms

Infradian rhythms have time scales longer than a day, for example, a lunar month seen in the menstrual cycle. The intrinsic hormone timing of the menstrual cycle is discussed in detail in "Scene 5XX: Of Mice, Men... and Women".

## Lifespan time scales

Premature and small-for-date babies can experience intrauterine reprogramming of the hypothalamic-pituitary axis which increases the risk of long-term endocrine and metabolic dysfunction[7]. This is discussed in further detail in Act 2 "Scene 1: Infancy". At the other end of the biological time scale, faltering biological timekeeping occurs with increasing age, as discussed in Act 2 "Scene 7: Dotage".

## Integration of internal and external periodisation

The reason for describing, in some detail, the role of hormones, in the timing of your body's internal biological processes, is that you have the ability either to optimise or disrupt these processes according to the way you choose to schedule your behaviours and lifestyle.

Being aware of internal hormone clocks is very important. It can help you plan activities in ways that maximise the health benefits and allow you to reach your personal best and attain your full potential. Figure 4.3 shows that, below the surface, inside the body, hormone biological processes are driven by hormones over the full range of timescales relevant to an individual. Meanwhile, above the surface, various activities and lifestyle behaviours take place in the form of exercise, nutrition and recovery patterns, over their own corresponding range of timescales. The examples in the figure refer to the activities of an athlete, but the concept of marrying up internal and external timekeeper applies, whatever your objectives, sporting or otherwise. The crucial point is that there is an intimate connection between the timing of what is happening inside and outside your body.

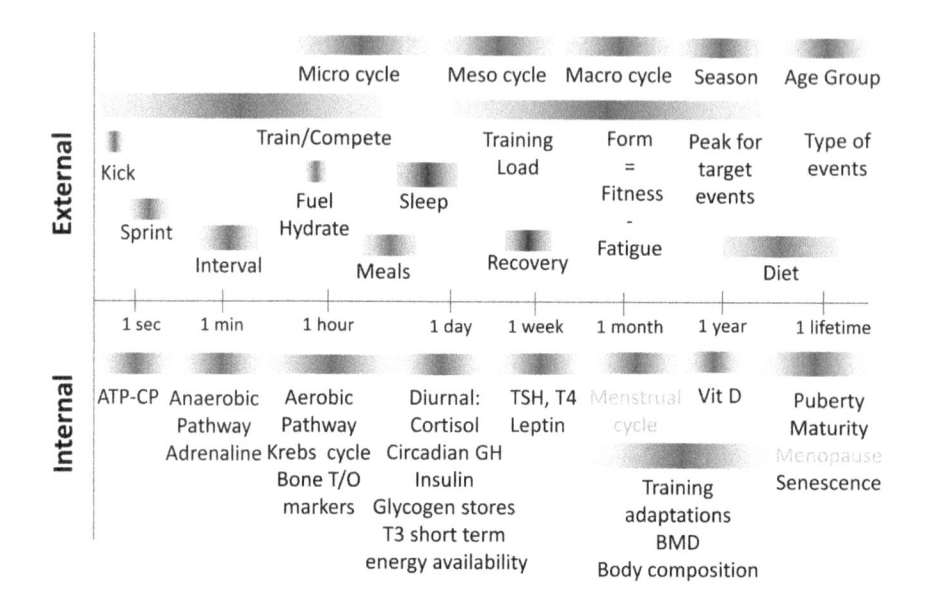

|  | | Micro cycle | | Meso cycle | Macro cycle | Season | Age Group |
|---|---|---|---|---|---|---|---|
| **External** | Kick | Train/Compete | | Training Load | Form = Fitness - Fatigue | Peak for target events | Type of events |
| | Sprint | Fuel Hydrate | Sleep | | | | |
| | | Interval | Meals | Recovery | | | Diet |
| | 1 sec | 1 min | 1 hour | 1 day | 1 week | 1 month | 1 year | 1 lifetime |
| **Internal** | ATP-CP | Anaerobic Pathway Adrenaline | Aerobic Pathway Krebs cycle Bone T/O markers | Diurnal: Cortisol Circadian GH Insulin Glycogen stores T3 short term energy availability | TSH, T4 Leptin | Menstrual cycle Training adaptations BMD Body composition | Vit D | Puberty Maturity Menopause Senescence |

**Figure 4.3:** External and internal periodisation of an athlete

## Short timescales (seconds)

Energy is required to stay alive and to go about daily activities. Hormone networks ensure that the right amount of energy is available, at the right time. The main food groups, carbohydrates, fat and protein, are the source of the fuel substrates used within the cells. Cellular respiration describes the continual process of converting fuel substrates into the biological energy required to sustain life. Cells can convert a range of different types of substrates into energy.

At the shortest time scale, your muscles store enough freely available energy to perform a brief strenuous movement, such as kicking a ball. Creatine phosphate stored in the muscle can be broken down rapidly to produce the cell's energy currency: adenosine triphosphate (ATP). Since rapid availability takes precedence over quantity, supply is limited, lasting only a few seconds.

## Longer timescales (hours)

To perform activities of daily living, including longer and more continuous activity, the body makes use of two types of cellular respiration: aerobic (with oxygen) and anaerobic (without oxygen). The balance between these two forms of energy production depends on exercise intensity and the fitness of the individual. The fitness of the individual, itself dependent on hormone "fitness", determines the efficiency of oxygen delivery to the cells, substrate availability and abundance of enzymes required for cellular respiration.

The neuroendocrine system controls the mixture of fuel substrates used to power the aerobic system and the point at which cells shift towards using predominately anaerobic energy production. The hormones glucagon (released from the endocrine part of the pancreas), the catecholamines (adrenaline and noradrenaline from the adrenal medulla), GH (from the pituitary) and cortisol (from the adrenal cortex) are all involved[8].

The aerobic system can produce large amounts of ATP, by breaking down fuel substrate molecules completely into carbon dioxide and water, in a series of reactions that rely on an ample supply of oxygen being delivered to the cell. This process is powered by glucose, derived from carbohydrates, as well as glycerol and fatty acids, drawn from adipose tissue. In extreme situations, protein can also be used.

Glucose is stored in the form of glycogen in the liver and in the skeletal muscles. It enters the cells through the bloodstream, under the control of insulin. Once inside the cell, enzymes break down the molecule in a process called glycolysis, which produces pyruvate and some ATP energy. The pyruvate passes into the mitochondria, the powerhouses of the cell, where it is converted into acetyl CoA. In the presence of sufficient oxygen, the acetyl CoA enters the Krebs cycle. The Krebs cycle, named after Hans Krebs, consists of a series of reactions to release the stored chemical energy in acetyl CoA. The electron transport system produces prodigious amounts of ATP, with water and exhaled carbon dioxide as by-products.

The aerobic system can also burn fat, which is a dense store of energy with a high energy return per molecule. Glycerol and fatty acids also reach cells through the bloodstream, entering through special channels. Glycerol is broken down into pyruvate. On the other hand, fatty acids are transported into the mitochondria where they undergo β-oxidation to produce acetyl CoA, leading to the production of ATP via the Krebs cycle as before.

In extreme situations when glucose and fat supplies are severely depleted, proteins can be converted to acetyl CoA. Muscle fibres are literally broken down as the fuel of last resort.

The aerobic system makes use of a mix of glucose and fat substrates, but at rest it is predominantly fat. For low to moderate exercise, the heart rate increases and breathing becomes faster and deeper, in order to supply sufficient oxygen to the cells to maintain aerobic respiration. At the same time, the fuel substrate mix shifts in favour of aerobic glycolysis. One possible explanation is that the catecholamines, adrenaline and noradrenaline, divert blood flow to the muscles and away from adipose tissue, thereby reducing the supply of fatty acids.

As exercise intensity increases, the cardiovascular system eventually reaches its maximum rate of oxygen transfer to the cells: $\dot{V}O_2$ max. This is the maximum rate at which oxygen can be supplied to the muscles and converted into mechanical energy[9].

## Intermediate timescales (minutes)

Very intense exercise can be maintained for periods from ten seconds up to a few minutes using the anaerobic system. The duration depends on the level of intensity because, in the absence of available oxygen, anaerobic respiration produces lactic acid as a by-product. Lactic acid dissociates into lactate ions that can be measured in the blood and acidic hydrogen ions that reduce blood pH. These take time to clear, so sustained activity leads to an accumulation of hydrogen ions that disrupt the protein enzymes that drive many systems throughout the body. This acidity is responsible for the burning sensation in the muscles that eventually forces you to slow down.

Anaerobic respiration takes place inside the cell, but outside the mitochondria. It is less efficient than the Krebs cycle, producing fewer units of ATP per glucose molecule. The lactate by-product can be converted back to glycogen or glucose in the liver or muscle.

## Exercise training adaptation timescales

Hormones continue to play a role in the adaptation processes that take place in the recovery period after exercise. Interactions of anabolic hormones, such as GH and the sex steroid hormones, together with catabolic hormones such as cortisol help drive the expression of genes that increase the size and number of mitochondria, build muscle tissue, raise the amounts of available fat and glycogen stored in the muscles, develop the heart muscles and boost the production of red blood cells to transport oxygen. These beneficial training adaptations allow athletes to run faster and for longer before switching to the less sustainable method of anaerobic respiration.

To see the best results, it is important to support your hormone networks by eating the right balance of food types, at the right time, while ensuring good hydration and recovery.

## Medium timescales

Hormone release patterns can fluctuate over weeks or months. These affect the release of hormones, including GH, thyroid hormones and other hormones involved in metabolism and overall health. Fluctuations in female sex steroid hormones during the menstrual cycle impact internal physiology. Women can benefit from synchronising their exercise, nutrition and sleep, with the stages in their cycles. This is discussed in further detail in "Scene 5XX: Of Mice, Men… and Women".

Sports coaches often break down training schedules into micro, meso and macro timescales. These correspond to daily, weekly and season-long training blocks. Training load is a measure that takes account of both intensity and duration of exercise. Periodised training combines different training loads over time, in a structured way. When matched with sufficient sleep and well-timed nutritional intake, hormones are able to drive the desired beneficial adaptations of exercise. For example, a personalised periodised training schedule for an endurance athlete provides the optimal stimuli to hormone-driven adaptations for improved performance of the aerobic system. This type of athlete gains an advantage if a higher level of intensity can be maintained before transitioning from aerobic to anaerobic respiration, as it is only possible to sustain the latter for a limited time.

The cumulative release of hormones, in response to periodised exercise training, directs gene expression to produce proteins to permit a higher level of exercise intensity from the aerobic system. This is achieved by improving the requirements for aerobic respiration: the efficiency of oxygen delivery and induction (production) of the enzymes required for the Kreb's cycle. These physiological adaptations, that occur over a training season, can be measured in the laboratory. For the same exercise test protocol, the athlete shows a right shift the lactate curve. In other words, evidence of a delay in the switch to anaerobic cellular respiration, due to hormone-driven adaptations over several months.

*"Fuel for the work required."*
*Dr Samuel Impey*

In a similar way to periodised exercise, synchronised periodised eating patterns can have beneficial effects on hormone fitness and consequently overall health and performance. The essential premise is that individuals should aim to fuel for the work required[10]. This means eating on a forward-looking schedule so that you have sufficient energy and the right type of energy to perform what you aim to achieve. For example, if you plan to do really demanding intense exercise, you need to take on carbohydrate the night before, so you have well topped up glycogen stores in advance. If the event extends over a long duration with intermittent periods of higher intensity, a well-planned fuelling strategy can ensure that energy stores are topped up before they are depleted. This is why cyclists heading out for several hours of quality training or racing have bottle cages filled with carbohydrate drink and the back pockets of jerseys loaded up with cereal bars and bananas. After taking on an adequate recovery meal, a lighter evening meal would be appropriate ahead of a rest day.

What about tapping into the extensive fat energy reserve? Could periodising intake of fat encourage hormone adaptations to become efficient as using fat as a substrate for cellular respiration? This was found to be the case in a study of athletes. Half the athletes were given a low carbohydrate, high fat "ketogenic" diet. The other participants were given a more usual athlete diet with higher levels of carbohydrate. The good news was that the athletes receiving the high-fat diet did indeed increase fat oxidation. The downside was that they got slower. Although ketogenic diets can be helpful in some medical conditions, like epilepsy, in terms of high-intensity exercise performance, they do not appear to be beneficial[11].

Looking at our teeth confirms that we are omnivores evolved to eat a variety of food types. The timing of when we eat these different food types is key to harnessing our inner hormone fitness, enabling the use of different substrates for cellular respiration. This is known as metabolic flexibility.

This is why it is *not just a question of what, rather when we eat, sleep and exercise.* Harmonising the timing of external behaviours with internal biological clocks supports beneficial adaptation. The aim is for the timing of exercise, nutrition and sleep to hit the resonant frequency of a well-functioning endocrine system.

## Longer timescales

As hormone networks change at different stages of life, so we need to adapt our patterns of exercise, nutrition and sleep. This aspect of hormone timing is covered in detail in Act 2.

## Aligning behaviours with hormone network timing

### *Sleep*

The quantity and quality of sleep have an important bearing on physical and mental health. The timing of sleep impacts our circadian alignment with internal biochronometers and the temporal patterns of hormone release. The old wives' tale advising us to value the hours of sleep before midnight now has the definitive support of a study showing that going to bed after midnight increases the risk of cardiovascular disease. This is most marked in women[12]. The timing of the onset of sleep impacts sleep architecture, a term used to describe the timing and proportions of different types of sleep, such as rapid eye movement (REM) and non-REM stages. Sleep architecture determines when certain hormones are released. Disrupted sleep interferes with the timed neuroendocrine control of energy homeostasis, which includes a reversal of the timing of peak cortisol production from the morning to the evening[13]. You also risk missing out on the benefits of the nocturnal secretion of growth hormone if you go to bed too late. People with good quality and quantity of sleep are more likely to become healthier and fitter.

### *Nutrition*

An evenly distributed intake of food over the day, in terms of food type, frequency and portion size, supports metabolic health and body weight management. This approach to eating works in synchrony with hormone networks, resulting in good insulin sensitivity and a tendency for the body to favour the oxidisation of fat over carbohydrate. The ability to switch between different energy sources of carbohydrate and fat, known as metabolic flexibility, is promoted by regular eating patterns[14]. Optimising the timing of nutrition with sleep has a synergistic effect on weight management and fat loss. Increasing sleep prevents fat gain. Conversely, sleep deprivation favours the oxidation of carbohydrate rather than fat.

The mistiming of food intake, even for the same overall daily energy intake, is bad for health. For example, eating very little or skipping meals during the day and then sitting down for a very large evening meal close to bedtime forces your body to cope with extremes of energy deficit and energy surplus within a 24-hour period. This type of extended fast during the day, with a very restricted time window to eat, can produce modest weight loss. This is comparable to the effect of intermittent fasting, for example, alternate day fasting. However, studies show that this pattern of eating comes with compensatory responses to prevent sustained weight loss. These responses include a different hormone response to meals[15] and behavioural reduction in energy expenditure through exercise[16]. In other words, the endocrine system adapts to maintain homeostasis.

The human brain is an energy-hungry information processing and control centre. Although the brain accounts for only 2% of total body weight, it demands about 20% of total energy intake, largely in the form of glucose. One function of the brain is to control the timing of hormone networks. Large gaps between meals disrupt the timing of hormone networks, especially if energy is expended on exercise during these intervals. For example, performing fasted training, especially in women, disrupts female hormone network timing[17]. This has subsequent adverse effects on female hormone production, metabolic health and body composition in the longer term.

Refuelling promptly with carbohydrate and protein after extended exercise is better for hormone networks. This supports the balance of bone formation over resorption. In summary, optimising the timing of food intake relative to exercise supports both hormone network function and bone health[18]. On the other hand, prolonged low energy availability, in the situation of relative energy deficiency in sport (RED-S) has potentially irreversible adverse effects on multiple hormone biochronometers[8].

## *Exercise*

What is the optimal timing of exercise for improving motivation and fitness? The answer depends on the context and what you are trying to achieve. The best performances in competitive events tend to be in the early evening; a time that matches the most favourable hormonal milieu. Although, in theory, the morning diurnal release of cortisol might be expected to help with exercise, the downside is that it may interfere with blood glucose regulation[19]. On the other hand, intense exercise in the evening has been shown to disrupt sleep patterns[20]. This has an adverse knock-on effect on hormone secretion patterns. A recent study looked at the effects of exercise timing in men and women. It seems that for women there are slightly different health benefits, depending on the time of day. Exercising in the morning helped control the deposition of abdominal fat, while evening exercise was more beneficial for muscular strength in women[21]. However, the overall conclusion was that exercise is good for you whenever you do it, but the time of day to achieve specific outcomes may be different for women and men.

Including bouts of physical activity during the day, to break up a sedentary lifestyle, is also beneficial in supporting metabolic flexibility. This has a positive effect on blood glucose control throughout the day, with lower glucose levels after eating and higher nocturnal fat oxidation compared with those with metabolic insensitivity[22].

On the other hand, although due respect should be paid to our internal biological clocks, becoming too obsessive about sticking to a rigid schedule removes the element of choice. This can have adverse psychological consequences that may negate the expected positive health benefits[23]. Practicality is also a very important consideration. A degree of flexibility is needed when planning the timing of exercise, to fit in with life and work commitments. Be pragmatic, not dogmatic when it comes to the timing of exercise.

## Chronotypes: personal biological clock settings

There is some individual variation in the setting of our biochronometers. Some people are night owls, while others are morning larks: early risers. Some find it a struggle to be as productive in the morning compared with the evening and vice versa. In addition to the central SCN biological clock, individual cells in the body have some say in biological timekeeping. Peripheral clocks in each cell of the body have their own pacemakers to regulate gene expression. These intracellular clocks alter sensitivity to hormone signals. However, the signals of cells marching out of time trigger feedback loops that fine-tune the release of hormones that keep all the internal chronometers in sync[3].

## Circadian entrainment

Some degree of circadian entrainment is possible. In other words, the body has a degree of adaptability to changes in the environment and behaviour patterns.

Altering one's patterns of exercise, eating and sleep affects the time sequence of hormone release, which in turn modifies both central and peripheral biological clocks. For example, getting up for early morning exercise, before school/work, gradually becomes easier. Although, depending on our chronotype, the direction of "phase shifts" in one direction may be easier to cope with than the other[24]. Trying to override personal internal biological clocks, to extremes, does not end well. Circadian misalignment results in a collection of adverse health consequences.

## Circadian misalignment

The importance of maintaining synchronicity between external behavioural patterns and internal physiological rhythms becomes apparent when circadian misalignment occurs. Mistiming of sleep, nutrition and exercise patterns, putting them out of step with internal pacemakers, disrupts hormone networks.

### *Metabolic health*

It is well recognised that shift workers, with disturbed sleep patterns, can experience circadian misalignment, putting them at increased risk of developing cardio-metabolic disease. Circadian misalignment causes a disruption of energy homeostasis and body weight control. This occurs through an accumulative disruptive effect on hormone networks resulting in a positive energy balance, metabolic disturbance and weight gain in the long term. Initially, misalignment interferes with sleep architecture, which disrupts the action of insulin in controlling blood glucose. Cells become less sensitive to insulin and blood glucose runs higher. This has subsequent effects on the hormones controlling appetite: leptin and ghrelin. Furthermore, the hypothalamic adrenal axis and gut hormones get involved[13]. This hormone cascade increases the risk of developing metabolic health problems, grouped together in metabolic syndrome, with a high risk of heart disease and type 2 diabetes.

Circadian misalignment can exacerbate pre-existing metabolic conditions. For example, in women with insulin resistance associated with polycystic ovarian syndrome (PCOS), skipping breakfast can cause increased issues with blood sugar control, high testosterone levels and body composition. Whereas a more even distribution of food intake over the day has a beneficial effect on favourable hormone production, including increased likelihood of ovulation[25]. Anovulation is recognised as a cause of infertility in women with PCOS. So, the timing of lifestyle behaviours has a favourable effect on hormone networks.

## *Bone health*

In men, lack of sleep results in lower levels of testosterone. In a study of young men in their early 20s, sleep restriction to five hours over one week resulted in 15% lower testosterone. This compares with a modest 1–2% age-related decline in testosterone in older men[26]. Low testosterone is well known to have an impact on libido and fatigue. However, testosterone is also important for bone strength, because it is converted to oestradiol, the key hormone for bone health. This is consistent with poor sleep patterns adversely affecting male bone health. A similar situation is found in women with poor sleep, where loss in bone mass has been reported[27,28].

## *Female hormones*

For women, there are complex and fascinating reciprocal relationships between hormone networks and sleep[29]. On the one hand, good sleep patterns keep hormone networks functioning well. On the other, female hormones influence sleep architecture. Some women experience disturbed sleep during the luteal phase of the menstrual cycles. The luteal phase occurs after ovulation and is associated with progesterone levels being higher than at other times in the cycle. This hormone increases metabolic rate and body temperature, which can disrupt sleep. Simple measures to mitigate this effect include sleeping in a well-ventilated room, with a duvet that is not too thick. During pregnancy, high levels of female hormones produced by the placenta, combined with challenges of physically carrying a baby can be problematic for sleep. At the other end of the scale, low levels of ovarian hormones after menopause can also be a factor in sleep disruption. As hormone levels change in the lead-up to menopause, disrupted temperature regulation can impact sleep.

## *Mental health*

Circadian disruption not only impacts physical and metabolic health. Misaligned biochronometers influence mental health. Exposure to artificial light in the evening blurs the boundary between night and day, altering the function of brain regions involved in emotion and mood regulation. This occurs at many levels of biological timekeeping. Light levels are registered by the central SCN clock, altering neuroplasticity and neurotransmission in the brain. Neuroplasticity is the ability of the neural circuits in the brain to rewire and forge new connections. This is particularly important in the developing brain of children, to permit learning. Neurotransmission is the mechanism by which nerve cells, neurons, communicate with each other, using short-range chemical messengers, neurotransmitters. Miscommunication, caused by neuronal "crossed wires", can have adverse effects on brain function, emotion and mood[30].

In conclusion, biological timekeeping is maintained through a variety of mechanisms in which hormone networks play a crucial role. Hormones enable adaptation and entrainment of internal clocks to external changes in behaviours and the external environment. However, circadian misalignment, asynchronicity between the timing of internal and external timing, leads to adverse effects on all aspects of health.

## Strategies to support hormonal alignment

### Sleep "The chief nourisher in life's great feast" Macbeth, Shakespeare

- Consistent sleep patterns keep your biological clocks aligned
- Sleep hygiene strategies can help with attaining good sleep patterns
- If you are still struggling with sleep issues after three months of applying these sleep hygiene strategies, cognitive behavioural therapy (CBT) can be helpful
- Another approach is "sleep scheduling" where you anchor the day with a consistent rising time in the morning and during the night, if you can't sleep, get out of bed into another room and do something until you feel sleepy
- If problems persist, you should discuss with your doctor to exclude medical conditions
- Try to avoid taking sleeping medication

### Nutrition

- Aim for timing of food intake to be consistent with regular eating patterns

- Include a range of food types with energy intake to match personal energy demands for health networks
- Fuel for the work required, in a forward-looking manner

## *Exercise*

- Regular exercise supports metabolic flexibility
- Try to avoid long periods of being sedentary

# Scene 5XY
## Of Mice and Men

*Testosterone rex?*

**Subtitle:** Although the word hormone resembles the name of the Greek goddess of action, the vital importance of hormones is not exclusive to women. For men, hormones play an equally important role in optimising health and performance. Testosterone is the brother of oestradiol. The close relationship between the sex steroid hormones is seen in their similar influences on fertility and other functions.

## Testosterone rex?

Testosterone is the hormone that most readily comes to mind when we are talking about men. This sex steroid hormone underpins the physiological and phenotypic differences between men and women. Post-pubertal men have up to 15 times higher levels of testosterone than women. This accounts for the 8–12% ergometric difference in sports performance[1]. Men are physically stronger due to higher muscle mass and higher levels of haemoglobin, resulting from testosterone's influence on gene expression.

Some men may be surprised to know that their larger body frames are reliant on oestradiol. This is because oestradiol rules supreme when it comes to skeletal bone for both men and women[2]. Oestradiol is the hormone responsible for the closure of the bone growth plates, epiphyses, as puberty progresses. These epiphyses are located at the end of the long bones of the arms and legs. Oestradiol is the key hormone for bone formation and for maintaining the mineral density required for strong bones. In men, testosterone is converted to oestradiol by the process of aromatisation. The close family resemblance between the molecular structures of the two hormones is apparent in Figure 5.1.1. The largest concentrations of the aromatase enzyme are in the testes and in adipose tissue.

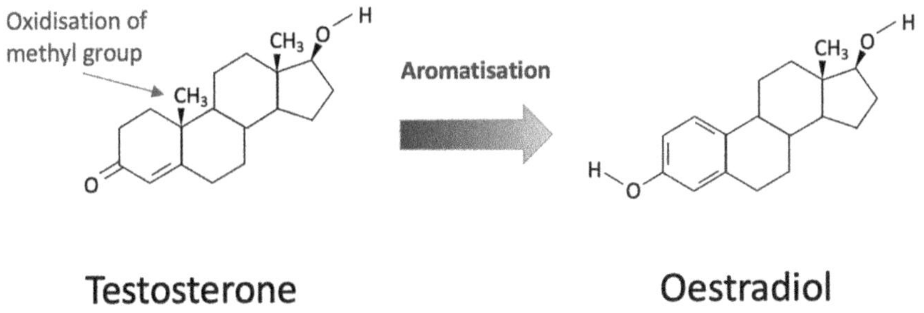

**Figure 5.1.1:** Aromatisation of testosterone to oestradiol

## Male endocrine network

The hormone control network for testosterone production in men follows the same template as the female hormone axis. The hypothalamus, the neuroendocrine gatekeeper located in the brain, produces gonadotrophin-releasing hormone (GnRH), which travels a short distance to the pituitary gland. In turn, the pituitary gland releases follicle-stimulating hormone (FSH) and luteinising hormone (LH). These hormones travel in the bloodstream to the target endocrine organ: in this case, the testes. LH acts on the Leydig cells in the testes to synthesise testosterone. In the absence of any ovarian follicles to stimulate, FSH acts on the testicular Sertoli cells to drive gametogenesis: the production of sperm.

The familiar endocrine leitmotif of a negative feedback loop operates between the control hormones from the hypothalamus and pituitary and the response hormone from the target endocrine gland. Figure 5.1.2 shows how this regulatory control mechanism maintains testosterone levels within range for optimal health.

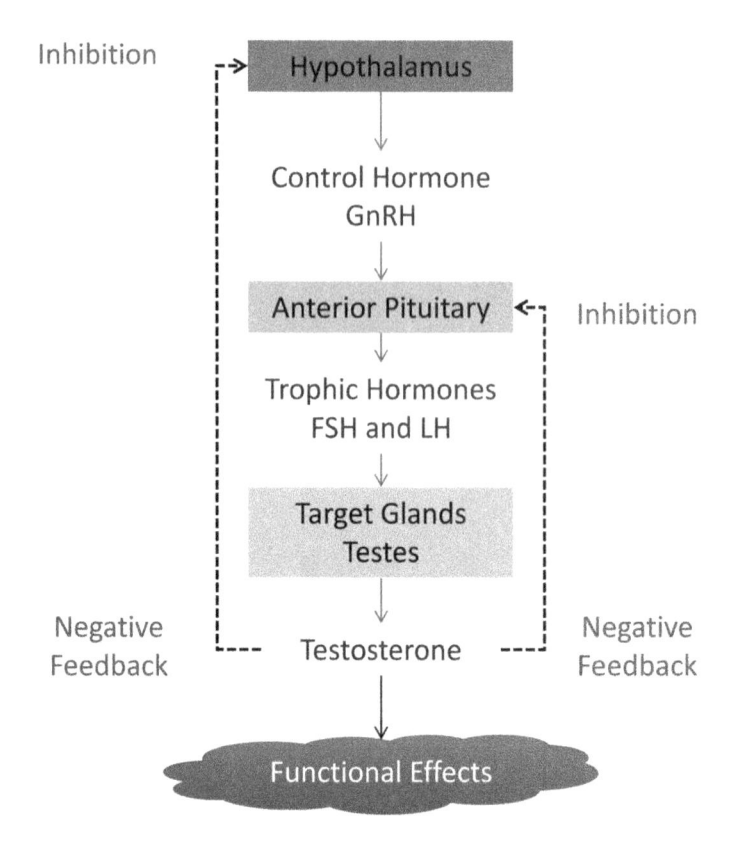

```
           Inhibition  ┌─► ┌─────────────────┐
                       ╎   │  Hypothalamus   │
                       ╎   └─────────────────┘
                       ╎           ↓
                       ╎   Control Hormone
                       ╎        GnRH
                       ╎           ↓
                       ╎   ┌─────────────────┐
                       ╎   │ Anterior Pituitary │ ◄╌╌  Inhibition
                       ╎   └─────────────────┘
                       ╎           ↓
                       ╎    Trophic Hormones
                       ╎      FSH and LH
                       ╎           ↓
                       ╎   ┌─────────────────┐
                       ╎   │  Target Glands  │
                       ╎   │     Testes      │
                       ╎   └─────────────────┘
                       ╎           ↓
    Negative           ╎                         Negative
    Feedback   └╌╌╌╌ Testosterone ╌╌╌╌┘          Feedback
                              ↓
                     Functional Effects
```

**Figure 5.1.2:** Negative feedback control loop of male hormones

The big difference between the female and male reproductive hormone axes is that the male version does not display the periodic variation characteristic of the female menstrual cycle. Instead, the male hormone network runs on a circadian timing, with peak levels of testosterone occurring in the morning. Hence, early morning erections are a good surrogate indicator that testosterone production is following expected physiological variation. In a similar way, regular menstruation in females is a helpful barometer of internal healthy female hormone function. A further contrast exists over a longer timescale. In men, testosterone is produced from puberty through to the end of life, declining only slowly in old age, whereas the female hormone axis goes into retirement when a woman reaches menopause, around the age of 51.

The other important difference between female and male reproductive physiology is that sperm are produced continuously throughout a man's life, whereas a woman's entire lifetime supply of eggs is prepared in utero. Although many eggs are prepared while the female foetus is developing and growing in her mother's womb, a woman's reproductive potential draws to a close at menopause. This is not because she runs out of eggs but rather that the ovulation cycle ceases to function.

Once the testosterone produced by the testes enters the blood circulation, the majority binds with transport proteins, such as albumin and sex hormone-binding globulin (SHGB), leaving about 2–4% biologically active, so-called, free testosterone. This makes free testosterone levels dependent both on testosterone production and on levels of binding proteins. Apart from a few specialised laboratories, free testosterone is not measured directly; rather it is calculated using equations that take account of total testosterone (bound and free) and the concentration of binding proteins.

## Identifying male hormone network issues

The American Association of Clinical Endocrinologists sets out clinical medical guidelines for assessing and treating men whose hormone networks are not functioning well[3]. As male hormones work on the same endocrine principles of control and function found in women, the approach to assessing the sex steroid hormone network is similar.

The clinical presentation of a man with male hormone network issues depends on the exact cause and whether it occurred before or after puberty. Nevertheless, in general terms, lower than expected testosterone can cause fatigue, mood change and reduced libido.

Exactly as in women, in order to address suboptimal sex steroid production, it is important to locate the source of disruption in the reproductive hormone network. To clarify the nomenclature, the gonads are glands where gametes are produced. They are the main production site of sex steroids. In women, the ovaries (gonads) produce eggs (gametes) and oestradiol and progesterone (sex steroid hormones). In men, the testes produce sperm and predominantly testosterone.

There are two possible locations where disruption of the reproductive hormone axis could occur:

- At the level of the gonad: primary hypogonadism; characterised by *raised FSH and LH* and low sex steroid hormones
- At the level of the control centre: secondary hypogonadism; characterised by *low FSH and LH* and low sex steroid hormones

## *Primary hypogonadism*

Primary hypogonadism in men is where the normal production of testosterone in the testes is impaired. The hypothalamus-pituitary control centre reacts to the low level of testosterone by increasing its hormonal signals to the testes. This can be detected in the form of raised FSH and LH.

Primary hypogonadism can be a result of genetic causes, as found in Klinefelter's syndrome, where individuals are born with an XXY karyotype, rather than the typical male XY karyotype. Otherwise, acquired causes of primary hypogonadism include testicular infection (orchiditis) from viruses such as mumps; chemotherapy or radiotherapy for cancer; drugs including excess alcohol consumption; chronic illness or testicular trauma, such as testicular torsion.

If primary hypogonadism occurs before puberty, low levels of testosterone prevent the changes associated with puberty, such as attaining adult-size testes and penis, low pitched voice or growth of facial and body hair. The lack of testosterone results in a lack of oestradiol, which has an impact on bone development. Low oestradiol means that the growth plates do not fuse, so these individuals tend to have proportionately long arms and legs. On the other hand, if primary hypogonadism occurs after the pubertal changes have occurred, the man will have normal skeletal proportions. However, the associated low testosterone and oestradiol increases the risk of osteoporosis in adulthood (weak bones)[4].

## *Secondary hypogonadism*

If the testes have the potential to function as expected, the issue must lie at the control centre of the hypothalamus and pituitary. This is known as secondary hypogonadism, because the problem is not the testes themselves, rather the low levels of testosterone are due to the control centre failing to send a strong signal to the testes. In stark contrast to primary hypogonadism, the hypothalamus-pituitary axis is found to be producing low levels of testes-stimulating hormones (gonadotrophins) FSH and LH. For this reason, secondary hypogonadism is also known as hypogonadotrophic hypogonadism (HH).

Secondary hypogonadism can also have a genetic cause, as found in Kallman's syndrome, where the hypothalamus does not secrete episodic GnRH to entice the pituitary to release LH and FSH for testicular testosterone production. Interestingly these individuals often lack a sense of smell (anosmia), most likely because during foetal development, the location of the hypothalamus-pituitary is quite close to the nerve cells for smell (olfactory nerves).

Otherwise, acquired causes of secondary hypogonadism include situations that disrupt the hypothalamic-pituitary control centre. The most common endocrine cause is an over-secretion of prolactin. Prolactin is made by the pituitary gland and has a down-regulatory effect on the reproductive axis in both men and women. This is why, when assessing possible male hormone network dysfunction, it is always important to measure, as a bare minimum FSH, LH, prolactin and testosterone. Measuring testosterone alone raises questions but does not give answers[4].

Some situations that cause secondary hypogonadism are functional, in other words reversible. These include external stressors, medications, anabolic steroid use and recreational drugs. Imbalances in lifestyle behaviours can have effects that result in HH. This potentially reversible form of secondary hypogonadism is functional hypogonadotrophic hypogonadism (FHH).

## External behavioural influences on male hormone network

An imbalance in lifestyle behaviours can cause functional downregulation of the male hormone network (FHH). Three key areas are exercise, nutrition and sleep. The good news is that by evaluating personal lifestyle factors, in the light of a full range of hormone blood tests (not just testosterone), it is possible to identify modifications of lifestyle choices to help reboot the male hormone axis.

In the discussion on sleep, we saw that restricting the sleep of young men can lower testosterone by 15%, which is a large decline compared with the modest reduction of 1–2% as a result of aging[5]. Other lifestyle factors such as lack of activity and being overweight can cause functional suppression of the hypothalamic-pituitary-testicular axis.

Being sedentary, combined with eating more than your body requires, elevates the production of inflammation mediators and increases insulin resistance, both of which cause a decrease in the production of the testosterone binding protein, SHBG. The consequent increase in free testosterone leads to a temporary increase of oestradiol, because free testosterone is aromatised into its sister hormone. Elevated oestradiol causes an increase in abdominal fat deposition. It also raises the level of the hormone, leptin, produced by adipose tissue, which can lead to leptin resistance. Leptin is a hormone controlling appetite, indicating satiety. Resistance to the effect of leptin can contribute to a tendency to overeat.

The combination of increased levels of oestradiol, leptin and inflammatory mediators causes negative feedback, suppressing the hypothalamus-pituitary axis. The consequent FHH contributes to the further development of metabolic syndrome: disrupted lipid profile, insulin resistance and hypertension, which increases the risk of cardiovascular disease[6]. In other words, a vicious circle ensues between risk factors for developing metabolic syndrome and FHH. The most effective way to break this negative spiral and resolve the situation is by increasing activity levels, reducing excessive calorie intake and improving sleeping patterns[7].

At the other end of the spectrum, we find men who obsessively maintain a high training load that is not balanced by sufficient sleep and/or nutritional intake. This behavioural disequilibrium can also result in suppression of the control centre of the male hormone network. When energy intake fails to meet the energy demand from exercise, the body is put into a state of low energy availability, leading to the syndrome of relative energy deficiency in sports (RED-S)[8]. This includes functional downregulation of the male hormone axis, which, in an attempt to "save energy", shuts down processes that are less essential during a famine, including reproduction. A blood test reveals secondary hypogonadism, characterised by low FSH, LH and testosterone in presence of normal range prolactin.

*Ben is a keen 30-year-old amateur cyclist. He has recently got married and he wants to start a family. This coincided with getting a promotion at work that restricted time to fit in his training. He started getting up early to train before breakfast. But now he is feeling fatigued and reports lack of libido. After a blood test showed testosterone at the lower end of the range, a friend commented that he had heard about men taking external testosterone. Sensibly, Ben sought expert medical advice, as he knew that testosterone was on the World Antidoping Authority (WADA) banned list and potentially he could be excluded from all competitive sports if he were found to be taking a banned substance.*

*Speaking with Ben it transpired that over the last six months, he had not taken a single rest day from training, and he had been getting less sleep due to his early morning starts. He had lost weight, causing his BMI to fall from 21 to 19. A blood test to assess the full range of hormones confirmed functional hypogonadotrophic hypogonadism (FHH): low FSH and LH in the presence of normal level prolactin. The stress response hormone, cortisol, was in the upper end of the range and thyroid function tests, although in range, were all towards the lower end (thyroid-stimulating hormone TSH, thyroxine T4 and triiodothyronine T3).*

*Once Ben understood the message his hormones were telling him, he agreed that he would rebalance his lifestyle choices. He resolved to take at least one rest day per week. He also swapped two of his on-bike sessions for strength sessions. Rather than training fasted every morning before work, he would have breakfast regularly and move training to after work, ensuring a carbohydrate-based snack beforehand and eating dinner within 20 minutes afterwards. Although he was still getting up reasonably early for work, this meant he could be home earlier to get training in the evening. The net result was that he was getting more sleep overall.*

*Three months later he reported feeling less tired and libido had improved. Repeat blood tests showed that the male hormone network had rebooted: with FSH, LH and testosterone now in the normal range. Cortisol was still somewhat elevated, but lower than before. Thyroid function tests were now more comfortably in range.*

## Testosterone replacement therapy

Testosterone Replacement Therapy (TRT) is sometimes known as Androgen Replacement Therapy. There are some medical conditions where TRT is warranted from a health point of view, as outlined in the Endocrine Society Clinical Practice Guideline[11]. These include young men with persistent, permanent low testosterone caused by genetic conditions, medical conditions or medical treatments. This means that, before prescribing TRT, a clinical assessment must first rule out functional, reversible impairments of male hormone network function, such as imbalances in lifestyle behaviours.

In clinically confirmed situations of non-functional, irreversible low testosterone, the aim of TRT is to improve well-being, mood and libido, together with long-term health. This replacement hormone treatment will improve body composition by alleviating depleted muscle mass and function and decreasing fat mass. TRT will also prevent osteoporosis by favouring bone formation via conversion to oestradiol and inhibiting bone loss. The beneficial effects of TRT, as in the case of Hormone Replacement Therapy (HRT) of oestradiol and progesterone for women, will be enhanced by favourable lifestyle factors such as regular resistance exercise, dietary intake to meet personal requirements and good sleep patterns.

There are some contraindications to Androgen Replacement Therapy such as prostate and breast cancer (although rare, breast cancer can occur in men). Clinical monitoring of therapy is also important to pick up any potential side effects on prostate health, excess production of red blood cells (polycythaemia) and disruption of lipid profile, although the effect on long-term cardiovascular health is not known. There are also other reported side effects of external testosterone therapy, including mood swings and fluid retention and gynaecomastia (increased breast tissue as testosterone is converted to oestradiol). In essence, it is not possible to replicate the exquisite control of the male hormone network.

## When is TRT not advisable?

### *Reversible, functional downregulation of male hormone network*

For a man with reversible, functional suppression of the male hormone axis, the priority is to address imbalances in lifestyle behaviours that have caused this situation, not to give external testosterone, which will further suppress internal production. This would apply to men with relative energy deficiency in sport (RED-S). Precisely parallel reasoning explains why the Endocrine Society advises against women with RED-S taking external hormones in the form of the combined oral contraceptive pill. The solution is to redress the balance of lifestyle behaviours[9].

### *Adrenopause(?) v menopause*

From about the age of 40, testosterone levels decline slightly in men. Depending on the laboratory, the typical range shifts from 10–30nmol/L in younger men to 8–29 nmol/L for older men. This is nothing like the precipitous fall in hormone production that women experience at the menopause, when peak levels of oestradiol in the region of 1,000 pmol/L at ovulation drop dramatically to less than 100 pmol/L. It is for this reason that for menopausal women, HRT consisting of physiological doses of female hormones oestradiol and progesterone is recommended for the quality of life and long-term health[10]. In contrast, the Endocrine Society Clinical Practice Guideline[11] recommends that testosterone therapy is not offered to all older men with low testosterone. There can be other reasons why a 51-year-old man is not feeling as sprightly as when 21 years of age, which need to be explored. Concomitant physiological decline of other important hormones, such as growth hormone (GH), is contributing factor. Making modifications to exercise, nutrition and sleep helps mitigate the physiological decline of the whole family of anabolic hormones, including testosterone and GH, which will be explored in Act 2, Scene 5. Furthermore, an increase in SHBG with age can cause a decrease in free, bioavailable testosterone. This means that increasing total testosterone levels with external testosterone may not be particularly helpful, unless modifiable lifestyle factors have been addressed[12].

Nevertheless, the same physiological endocrine mechanisms are at play in both men and women as they get older. Namely that the gonads, the testes and ovaries respectively slow down the production of sex steroids. In the absence of a medical condition, the testes maintain a reasonable production of testosterone and sperm. For women, the ovaries go into retirement at menopause, in terms of both egg and sex steroid hormone production.

## *For fertility*

TRT is not a suitable treatment for men with fertility issues. Taking external testosterone will inhibit the production of FSH and LH from the pituitary, resulting in the reduction of sperm production. For men with secondary hypogonadism, injection with gonadotrophin (e.g. FSH) will stimulate sperm production. For men with primary hypogonadism, who do not respond to this hormone treatment, sperm donation may be required.

## *When replacement is not required*

Taking exogenous testosterone, or other anabolic steroid hormones, is also not advisable in the absence of a clear medical indication for this treatment. Doing so can have adverse health consequences[13]. Furthermore, for those competing in sports events under WADA jurisdiction, any form of anabolic steroid use is banned. Initially, TRT may provide benefits in terms of increased muscle bulk. However, high supraphysiological amounts of testosterone present many problems. In the first place, in an attempt to restore normal order, aromatase enzymes actively convert testosterone to oestradiol. This can cause breast tenderness and gynaecomastia (enlargement of breast tissue in men). The other main issue with high testosterone is that the negative feedback loop of the hypothalamic-pituitary axis goes into full swing. High levels of external testosterone shut down the body's internal production, with the aim of bringing the hormone back into the healthy physiological range. This results in the typical pattern of blood tests where FSH and LH are barely detectable, yet testosterone is sky high.

The concerning unknown is that when external testosterone is discontinued, there is no definitive timeline for when or if full internal production will resume and fertility be recovered. In some cases, long-term low levels of gonadotrophins and endogenously produced testosterone were found more than three years after discontinuing TRT[14].

External testosterone can affect the liver. This is reflected in raised levels of a liver enzyme alanine transferase (ALT), although this could also be partly due to high strength training load. The other adverse effects of external testosterone use are the same as those where there is a medical indication for replacement therapy. However, the negative side effects are amplified. There is disruption of lipid profile, with lower levels of "good" high-density lipoprotein (HDL) cholesterol relative to higher levels of "bad" low-density lipoprotein (LDL). This could be a result of the induction of liver enzymes. Exogenous testosterone also increases red blood cell production and hence haematocrit, where haematocrit is a measure of how tightly packed red blood cells are in the circulation. This combination of adverse lipid profile and raised haematocrit is not ideal for cardiovascular health. High levels of testosterone can also cause mood disturbance. In short, taking external unwarranted testosterone is definitely not the elixir of health or youth.

## Supporting male hormone network function

Some men do require supervised TRT to manage medical conditions causing permanent low levels of testosterone. Conversely, taking unwarranted external testosterone that increases levels above the physiological range has numerous adverse health consequences. Although there is slight, physiological age-related decline in testosterone production from middle age onwards, for all ages there are some practical lifestyle strategies to support male hormone networks.

## Strategies for supporting male hormone network function

### *Exercise*

- Regular activity is beneficial for hormone network function. This helps maintain a healthy weight and relieve stress
- Strength training can be particularly helpful

## Sleep

- Good sleep patterns help maintain the nocturnal episodic release of GnRH for testosterone production
- Ensuring adequate quality and quantity of sleep will also support the alignment of hormone networks, such as diurnal variation of cortisol, that impacts the male hormone axis

## Nutrition

- A varied diet, with energy intake to match personal requirements, helps support healthy male hormone networks

## Other considerations

- Avoiding external anabolic steroid use that is not clinically indicated prevents suppression of internal male hormone networks

# Scene 5XX
## Of Mice and Men . . . and Women!

*Ὁρμή (Horme)*
*Goddess of effort, energy and action*

**Subtitle:** Hormones are key to optimal health. Female hormone networks are the most complex. This presents challenges to studying the effects of female hormones on well-being and quality of life. There has been a tendency to apply the default male physiological model, narrowing research to "mice and men". This scene is dedicated to unravelling the intriguing complexities of the female hormone odyssey.

The word hormone is closely associated with Horme, the Greek goddess of effort, energy and action, reflecting the way that hormones set things in motion. To label someone as "hormonal" should be considered a compliment on that person's ability to get things done. If hormones were merely biological messengers, they might be called "hermenes", after Hermes, the herald of the gods. But a female deity seems more appropriate because they make things happen.

The ancient Greeks postulated that a "wandering uterus" caused women to feel and act differently from men. Today we now know that the uterus stays in place, while hormones travel around the body. The exquisite endocrine choreography underlying the menstrual cycle is comparable to any classical masterpiece. The female hormones rise and fall in a partnership that requires precision and intricate timing. Each hormone plays an essential role that has been finely tuned over the millennia and continues to be passed down the generations.

Yet, despite this well-established and ongoing hormonal choreography, there is surprisingly sparse research on its effects on a woman's quality of life. Rather the default male physiological model is applied, with much research devoted solely to "mice and men". This starts in the laboratory where male cells and male mice are used in medical drug development. This means that potentially effective drugs for women, with distinctive variations in female hormones, are discarded at an early stage and adverse effects in women are not recognised, until too late[1].

The same applies in the clinical medical setting. As medical students (which was a long time ago for me), we were taught that a "heart attack" or myocardial infarction presents with "central crushing chest pain radiating down the left arm and into the jaw" and we were trained to identify characteristic changes on the ECG (electrocardiogram). However, this clinical model was based on males. Women continue to be labelled as presenting with "atypical" symptoms, because they are not typical for a male. This means that the diagnosis of myocardial infarction could be missed in females[2].

The male blueprint is also applied when assessing the many physiological benefits of exercise. Physical activity is well established as a crucial lifestyle factor for harnessing hormones to support all aspects of health. Exercise training drives endocrine adaptations to improve performance in sport and dance. The distinctive sex steroid hormone profiles of males and females affect the endocrine response to exercise[3]. Yet female participants are often excluded from studies to establish the most effective ways to benefit from exercise[4]. This means that there continues to be a lack of evidence-based information and recommendations for women of all ages, who wish to exercise for health and performance[5,6].

What is going on? To some extent, we can understand the desire of researchers to conduct experiments where they can control for variables, such as female hormones, which may have a causal effect on the results. This is a very challenging task, as female hormones have such a complex time signature, which is individual to each woman. This explains the preference for male subjects but leaves a gap in the understanding of female hormonal fluctuations. Getting to grips with these hormonal complexities is not for the faint-hearted. However, doing so is the only way to gain understanding and insights for the benefit of individual women and women's health in general.

## Female motif: menstrual cycles

Typically, a woman experiences menstrual cycles that repeat around every 28 days or so, each starting with a menstrual bleed (period). This characteristic recurring theme of regular menstruation is called eumenorrhoea. The underlying hormonal motif repeats for around half of a woman's life.

Oestrogen is one of the key female hormones produced by the ovary in varying amounts over the menstrual cycle and over the longer timescale of a woman's life. This variation in hormone physiology over the lifespan is shown in Figure 5.2.1.

This illustration shows how oestrogen increases rapidly as menstrual cycles start at the completion of pubertal development. Oestrogen production continues in step with menstrual cycles over a woman's adult life. There may be some brief interludes of these cycles: a steady high level of oestrogen is maintained during pregnancy. Conversely, oestrogen levels are continuously suppressed when taking certain types of hormonal contraception. Oestrogen levels can also be suppressed by imbalances of exercise and nutrition, leading to a lack of menstrual cycles (amenorrhoea).

As a woman enters her 40s, levels of oestrogen start to decline and drop to consistently low levels at menopause (cessation of periods).

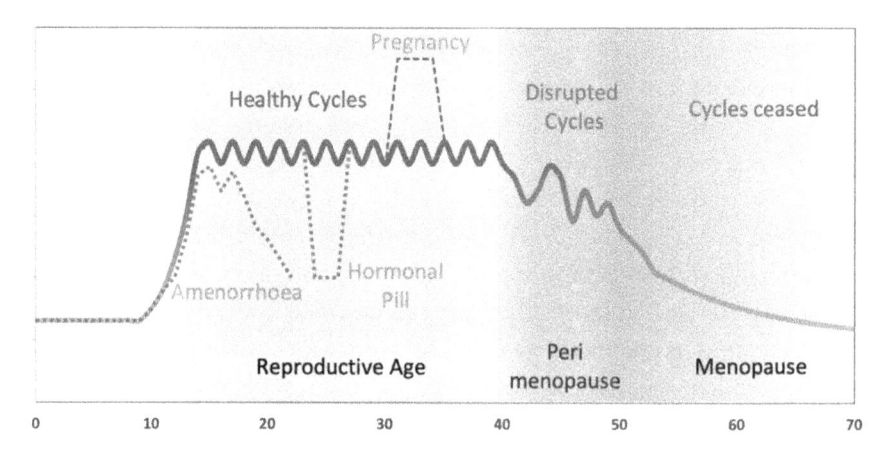

**Figure 5.2.1:** Variation of oestrogen with age.*

The average age for starting menstrual cycles with associated periods (menarche) is 12 years. While there can be some variation on either side of this age, the absence of established menstrual cycles by the expected age of menarche is known as primary amenorrhoea. Lack of periods by age 16 in women with secondary sexual characteristics such as breast development, or by 13 years of age in those with no secondary sexual characteristics, is primary amenorrhoea and requires medical investigation. After menarche, menstrual cycles should continue reasonably regularly, with any pauses in menstruation for more than six consecutive months being known as secondary amenorrhoea[7].

However, as outlined in latest update of the Clinical Knowledge Summaries from National Institute of Health and Care Clinical Excellence (NICE) 2022, there are some iterations on the definitions of amenorrhoea. For example, some experts define primary amenorrhoea as the failure to establish menstruation by 15 years of age in women with normal secondary sexual characteristics, or by 13 years of age in those with no secondary sexual characteristics. Similarly for secondary amenorrhoea, there are some variations in definitions from cessation of menses for 3 or 6 months in women with previously normal menstruation. For women with previous irregular periods (oligomenorrhoea), secondary amenorrhoea can be defined as being where periods have stopped for 6, 9 or 12 months.

Whatever definition is being used, lack of periods is a sign that something may be amiss with female hormone networks. Granted, there are physiological reasons for amenorrhoea, such as pregnancy or breastfeeding. Some medications can cause amenorrhoea, such as certain types of hormonal contraception which prevent ovulation, the event associated with maximal production of oestrogen during the menstrual cycle.

With increasing age, as the production of ovarian hormones starts to falter, periods eventually stop. The average age of menopause is 51. As the average life expectancy of a woman is around 85 years, she may spend about a third of her life in the menopausal state. Each act in this life-long hormonal odyssey can present different challenges, which we discuss, across different age groups, in the second act of this book.

## What's so good about menstrual cycles?

Although having menstrual cycles with a menstrual bleed (period), every lunar month or so, for half your life can be challenging at times, this is normal physiology. Furthermore, regular menstruation is the barometer of healthy internal female hormones. Menstruation is a result of the precise choreography of hormonal fluctuations playing out every menstrual cycle.

Female hormones live up to the eponymous Greek goddess in being instigators of action throughout the body in a range of systems and tissues. This is particularly true of the sex steroid hormones produced in the ovaries: oestrogen and progesterone. Oestradiol, the most active type of oestrogen, plays several important roles. According to the location in the body, there are particular types of receptors for oestradiol to mediate different effects. Alpha receptors for oestradiol are found in the female reproductive tract, while beta receptors for oestradiol are found in other tissues including bone, the cardiovascular and the neurological system. So oestradiol can exert different effects according to the site of action. Although the primary evolutionary purpose of menstrual cycles is reproduction, actually the ovarian hormones are essential for overall health and well-being.

## *Bare bones*

Make no bones about it; oestradiol is essential for the bone health of both men and women. In men, testosterone is converted to its sister hormone, oestradiol, by a process known as aromatisation. It is often oestradiol that determines the beneficial health effects, including bone health[8]. In young exercising men and women with low levels of testosterone and oestradiol respectively, there is a big increase in the risk of stress fractures[9]. For older women, the cessation of oestradiol production by the ovaries at menopause is directly linked with loss of bone mineral density and potentially the development of osteoporosis "brittle bone disease"[10]. It is no coincidence that the change in oestrogen over the lifespan of a woman traces the same path as the variation in bone mineral density, discussed further in "Scene 7: Bare Bones". Oestrogen is the hormone elixir of bone health.

Although oestrogen is often in the spotlight, progesterone has important health effects over the menstrual cycle. There is evidence that progesterone also has a part to play in bone health and in soft tissue injury. Among women with subclinical ovulatory disturbances and associated low levels of progesterone, there is evidence of a negative impact on bone health[11]. When it comes to soft tissue injury (muscle, ligaments, tendons), initially it was proposed that increased levels of oestrogen before ovulation could increase the risk of anterior cruciate ligament injury in the knee. However, recent evidence suggests that low levels of progesterone could be a factor when it comes to soft tissue injury[12].

## *Cardiovascular health*

Oestrogen is crucial to cardiovascular health[13]. It plays an important part in supporting a good balance of cholesterol ratios and maintains the reactivity of the endothelium: the lining of the artery walls. Furthermore, oestrogen plays a role in so-called autonomic neurological control of heart rate and blood pressure[14]. This is another reason why amenorrhoea should be addressed for health reasons, not just from a fertility point of view. Once again progesterone also has a part to play. Subclinical ovulatory disturbances of menstrual cycles, where progesterone levels are low, impact cardiovascular health[15].

Physiological decline in oestrogen levels with menopause, just as with bone health, impacts cardiovascular health. Younger women are at less risk of cardiovascular disease than men, but this risk rises to match that of men once the cardioprotective effect of oestrogen dwindles after menopause[16].

## *Neurological health*

Neurological function is influenced by variations in oestrogen and progesterone over a woman's lifespan[17]. There are many receptors for oestrogen and progesterone in the brain. These hormones exert an influence on the physical structure of the brain including the complex wiring of the neuronal (nerve cell) connections. These interconnections are important for cognitive function. Female hormones also interact with their short-range chemical messenger counterparts: neurotransmitters, such as serotonin and dopamine. These "feel good" neurotransmitters impact mood. So, it is no coincidence that alteration in mood can occur during changes in female hormone levels, for women at pre-menstrual or post-partum stages. As with bone mineral density, the prevalence of depression in women follows that of the trajectory of oestrogen variation over the lifespan[18].

For young exercising women whose periods have stopped (amenorrhoea), consequential lower-than-expected oestrogen levels for their age have been shown to have an adverse effect on neuromuscular function[19]. In other words, low oestrogen levels mean a less effective and efficient connection between nerves and muscles. This results in these women having poorer reaction times, balance and awareness of body position in space, known as proprioception. Bearing in mind that low oestrogen is not good for bone health, this is a bad combination. Consider a gymnast balancing on a beam only 10 cm wide and over a metre off the ground. Low oestrogen levels would make her more likely to lose balance and fall off, landing on fragile bones: a perfect storm for a bone injury. The same applies to a female cyclist negotiating a corner at speed on two wheels.

## *Sleep*

Sleep, "the great nourisher in life's great feast", is affected by ovarian hormones. The variation of oestrogen production over a woman's lifespan impacts the quality, structure and timing of sleep. Oestrogen levels determine sleep architecture and the brain's neural control of circadian rhythm[20].

Considering a selection of biological systems in the body, it becomes clear that having regular menstrual cycles is very beneficial for many aspects of physical and mental health, thanks to the ovarian hormones. Variations in these hormones over the lifespan of a woman impact the dependent biological systems.

## Precision choreography of menstrual cycle hormones

The variations in female hormones over the menstrual cycle are an example of an infradian biochronometer, where the periodicity is around a lunar month or 28 days. The characteristics of hormonal cycles change over the lifespan of a woman.

Initially, as a young girl, all the female hormones are quiescent. As the dormant endocrine control system for female hormones wakes up and stirs the ovaries into action, menstrual cycles and menstruation start: the onset of menarche. The repeating precision choreography of fluctuating female hormones each menstrual cycle continues until the ovaries become less responsive to the conductors of the endocrine orchestra. Eventually the ovaries stop responding, despite entreaties by the hypothalamus and pituitary, resulting in very low levels of ovarian hormones after menopause.

## The interplay between endocrine conductors and performers

To understand the choreography of the female hormones in the menstrual cycle, we need to look at the hormone feedback control loops involved shown in Figure 5.2.2.

The conductors of the endocrine orchestra are located in the brain. They are the hypothalamus and pituitary glands, which produce the control hormones and monitor the response. The performers are the ovaries, which react by producing the response hormones oestradiol and progestogen.

The hypothalamus secretes gonadotrophin-releasing hormone (GnRH), which makes the short journey to the anterior pituitary gland, which in turn releases the control hormones, luteinising hormone (LH) and follicle-stimulating hormone (FSH). The precise instruction from GnRH secretion is encoded in an analogue code: the frequency and amplitude of the signal determine whether the pituitary releases FSH or LH.

## Scene 5XX: Of Mice and Men... and Women!

FSH and LH released by the pituitary travel in the bloodstream to the ovaries, which release oestradiol and progesterone in response. These response hormones have effects on the tissues of the female reproductive tract and throughout the body. In common with all endocrine axes, a negative feedback system is in operation. Increased levels of the ovarian hormones are recognised by the hypothalamus and pituitary, which in turn reduce the release of the FSH and LH control hormones. This reduction in stimulus maintains levels of the ovarian response hormones within physiological ranges. However, if this negative feedback system were the only hormonal choreography occurring, then there would be no large fluctuations in female hormone levels seen in the menstrual cycle. What is the missing mechanism?

Positive feedback is the rare and significant extra dimension of the endocrine control system arising in females. At the beginning of a menstrual cycle, there is a competition between the ovarian follicles (immature eggs) for the leading role. After all, these follicles have been waiting to perform since being formed in the foetus before birth. The follicle that produces the most oestradiol becomes the chosen one for ovulation. The more oestradiol produced in response to FSH, the hungrier this follicle becomes for FSH. This dominant follicle corners the market for FSH by producing more receptors than any other competing follicle. Ultimately this dominant follicle, gorging on FSH, produces a high concentration of oestradiol, in the region tenfold higher than just 12 days or so earlier. While this has the expected negative feedback effect of reducing the production of FSH, something else happens. These high oestradiol levels alter the sensitivity of the pituitary to the coded signals from the hypothalamus. The pituitary now interprets the GnRH signals from the hypothalamus as a positive signal to release significantly more LH. The result of this unusual positive feedback is a sharp surge of LH, triggering ovulation[21]. Once set in motion, this part of the late follicular phase follows a sequence of events from the oestrogen peak to trigger the LH surge (around 24 hours) to ovulation (around 12 hours).

After the positive feedback phase in the menstrual cycle, normal service resumes in terms of negative feedback for hormones and LH drops back down. However, an amazing metamorphosis occurs. The remnants of the dominant follicle transform into the corpus luteum. These cells that were once so responsive to FSH now change their allegiance to responding to LH and switch production principally to progesterone, which is the predominant ovarian hormone in the luteal phase of the cycle after ovulation has occurred.

*Hormones, Health and Human Potential*

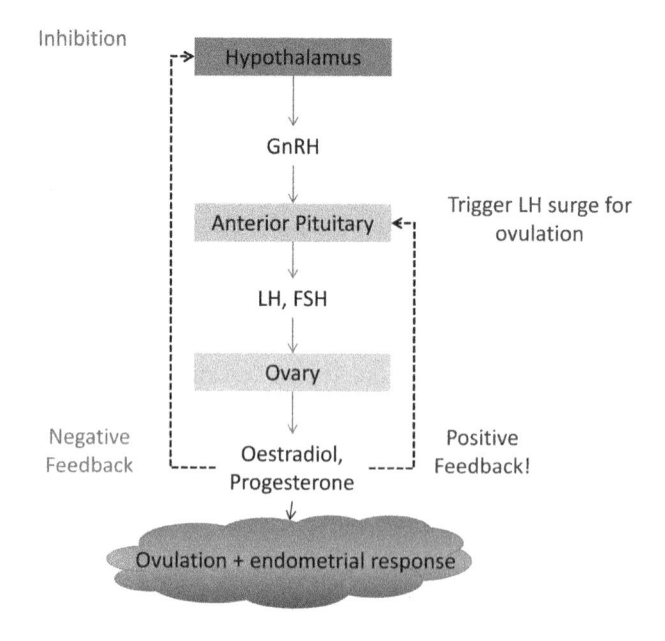

**Figure 5.2.2:** Menstrual cycle feedback control loops: hypothalamic-pituitary-ovarian axis

## Menstrual cycle

The cycle length, from the start of one period to the start of the next, can vary between 22 and 35 days. However, all ovulatory menstrual cycles have two phases determined by distinctive hormone patterns, illustrated in Figure 5.2.3.

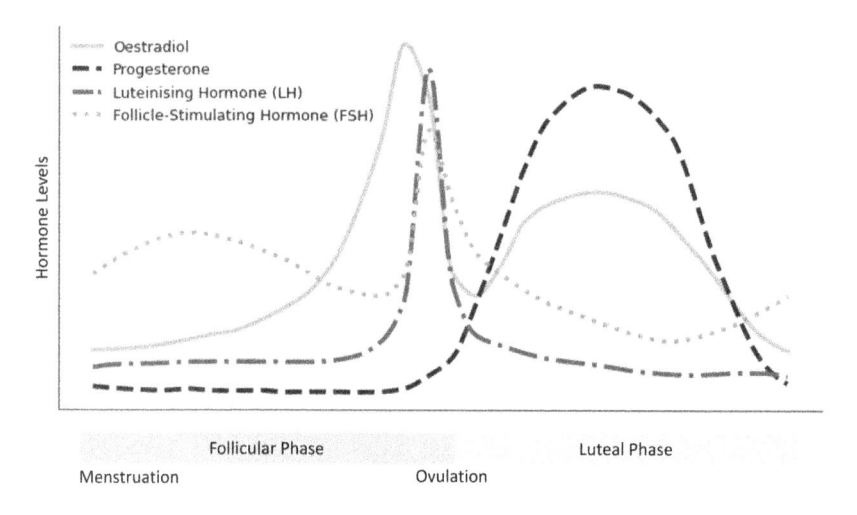

**Figure 5.2.3:** Female hormone variations over the menstrual cycle

## Scene 1 of the menstrual cycle: follicular phase

The starting point of the menstrual cycle on day 1 is the onset of menstruation, a period. This menstrual bleed is the shedding of the endometrial lining (inner lining of the uterus). Typically, this lasts around five days. From a hormone point of view, the nature of this bleed, in terms of heaviness and duration is to some extent determined by oestradiol levels in the preceding cycle. Oestradiol causes thickening of the endometrium. So higher levels of oestradiol produced during the preceding cycle mean more endometrial lining to be shed and lower levels may be followed by a lighter period.

From the start of the current follicular phase up to ovulation, oestradiol levels increase dramatically, up to tenfold. As discussed above, the endometrial lining thickens in anticipation of the LH surge that triggers ovulation. Ovulation is the release of the dominant follicle from the ovary to wend its way down the Fallopian tube, wafted on its journey by cilia, to arrive at the uterus.

## Scene 2 of the menstrual cycle: luteal phase

Once ovulation has occurred, typically mid-cycle, the remainder of the cycle until the onset of the next menstrual period is called the luteal phase. This phase is so named due to the formation of the corpus luteum from the remnants of the dominant follicle. The corpus luteum produces the predominant hormone of this phase: progesterone. Progesterone is derived from "pro" and "gestation". In other words, the effect of progesterone is to prepare the body for a fertilised egg. At the endometrial level, this means maintaining the thickness and changing the nature of the lining into a potentially welcoming "nest" for a fertilised egg. Just as oestradiol levels in the follicular phase of the cycle influence the nature of the menstrual bleed at the start of the next cycle, progesterone in the luteal phase also has an effect.

However, not every menstrual cycle goes exactly to plan. Experiencing shorter cycles, where the gap between periods is less than 21 days, is known as polymenorrhoea (literally many periods). This contrasts with oligomenorrhoea (few periods) where fewer than nine periods occur per calendar year. In some situations, even in eumenorrhea where cycle lengths fall between 22 and 35 days, there can be associated mistimings of menstrual hormone choreography. For example, disruption of the positive feedback required for ovulation may result in no ovulation, no corpus luteum and no progesterone.

There can also be situations of "luteal phase deficits" or subclinical ovulatory disturbance. This means that although the ovary tried to ovulate, the expected levels of progesterone were not attained. Low levels of progesterone during the luteal phase lead to an earlier than expected menstrual bleed. There is no "incentive" for endometrium to hang around. Occasionally these subclinical ovulatory disturbances might not shorten a cycle length, yet due to the adverse health consequences of low levels of progesterone, it is important to identify this situation[22]. This is where blood samples and more sophisticated analytical techniques are required to identify these subtle, yet crucial variations on a theme. This topic is discussed in detail in "Scene 6: Hormone Supermodels".

There are also other systemic effects of progesterone and oestradiol that we discuss next.

## Female hormones in harmony

You could consider oestrogen and progesterone as complementary dance partners. Oestrogen tends to be anabolic (favouring building up of tissue) whereas progesterone is catabolic (favouring the breakdown of tissue), so at any point in the menstrual cycle considering the ratio of these two ovarian hormones can help inform which hormone is leading the dance in terms of physiological effects[23]. Fluctuations in ovarian hormones affect metabolism and physiology, having a bearing on exercise performance and in disease prevention[24].

In terms of metabolism, oestrogen favours the use of fat as a substrate or fuel source. In theory, this could be very helpful if you want to run a marathon. Fat is a very energy-dense fuel source, so oestrogen could help you get over the finishing line of a long endurance event. Oestrogen facilitates the efficient use of glucose and the storage of carbohydrate in the form of glycogen in fast-twitch muscles, which could help with strength work, like weightlifting[25].

Conversely, progesterone tends to have opposite effects. Progesterone tends to favour deposition of fat rather than fat breakdown and utilisation as a fuel source. In terms of carbohydrate as a substrate, progesterone tends to favour the use of glucose as a short-term fuel, rather than supporting storage in muscles in the form of glycogen. In other words, progesterone is doing its "pro gestation" job, preparing the body for supporting a fertilised egg. On the other hand, this might not be so helpful if you want to run a marathon or lift weights.

However, before female readers rush off to plan their exercise according to the hormones of their menstrual cycles, there are several caveats. The first is that this theoretical model only works if you do know accurately the levels of your ovarian hormones throughout the menstrual cycle. Other considerations include underlying diet, fitness and fuelling during activity. Simply lining up at the start of an endurance race with a favourable oestradiol/progesterone ratio does not guarantee a good performance. A well-planned diet, training and race fuelling strategy are all essential. Even then, other practical constraints, not least that races and training schedules, may not align with personal hormone ratios.

Nevertheless, tuning into female hormone harmony can be helpful for women. If ovulation has occurred, then progesterone is the dominant dance partner to oestrogen in the luteal phase. The catabolic action of progesterone is reflected in an increase in resting metabolic rate, in other words the rate at which fuel is used. This results in a slight increase in body temperature after ovulation[26]. See Figure 5.2.4.

This means that increasing protein and spreading out carbohydrate intake over the day can be helpful during this phase of the menstrual cycle. A recent study showed that by maintaining a consistent intake of glucose can mitigate the metabolic effects of varying ratios of oestradiol and progesterone over the menstrual cycle[27]. In other words, exercising fasted and/or without fuelling during the exercise of long duration and/or high intensity is especially problematic if you are a woman with menstrual cycles.

There are some downsides when progesterone takes the lead. This hormone can have a direct impact on sleep, not just due to increased body temperature which can disturb sleep[20]. Progesterone can also impact mood: it is no coincidence that pre-menstrual syndrome occurs in the two weeks before menstruation[28].

Although progesterone tends to get more of a bad press than oestradiol, low levels of progesterone relative to oestradiol can cause issues in the clinical context. For example, although anovulatory cycles of women with polycystic ovary syndrome (PCOS) have fertility implications, they may also experience metabolic issues due to lower levels of progesterone. The lack of catabolic, metabolic rate boosting progesterone has been proposed as contributing factor in weight gain and insulin insensitivity found in women with PCOS[29]. Another example of the importance of oestrogen and progesterone working in harmony is illustrated by subclinical ovulatory disturbances, where low levels of progesterone can have adverse effects on cardiovascular and bone health[30]. So, while the evolutionary purpose of menstrual cycles is reproduction, focusing solely on fertility can, quite literally, be bad for a woman's health.

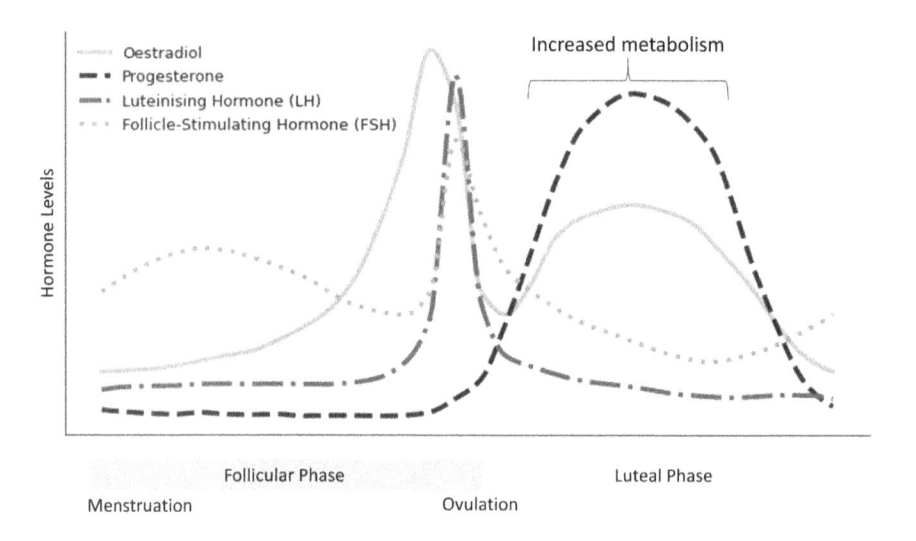

**Figure 5.2.4:** Physiological impact of fluctuating hormones

## Variations on a theme

Given that the variations in ovarian hormones have distinctive impacts on physiology over the course of the menstrual cycle, it comes as no surprise that, in a large study of women, effects were reported on physical and mental well-being together with work and exercise performance[31]. In another in-depth study, 93% of women reported that their menstrual cycle impacted how they felt and their exercise performance[32]. Therefore, what is surprising, and a first glance incomprehensible, is that a paper that performed meta-analysis of many studies found no significant effects of menstrual cycle phase on exercise performance[33]. This is an example of statistical significance not being synonymous with clinical significance. In any case, the difference between winning a gold or silver medal can be hundredths of a second: very fine margins.

It transpires that the problem is the timing: hormone timing. A "textbook" menstrual cycle of 28 days lends itself to very neat maths, with the mid-point of ovulation at day 14 conveniently dividing the cycle into follicular and luteal phases. However, as noted earlier, a cycle can vary in length from around 22 to 35 days. Given that cycle length varies between women and between the cycles for an individual woman, then rather than mean cycle length it would be more informative to consider the distribution of cycle lengths[34]. Indeed, ovulation itself is not fixed exactly at mid-cycle, whatever the cycle length[35]. This is why it becomes very difficult to compare results from different studies where there is variability in methodology of determining the menstrual cycle phase.

That is not to say that some women do indeed feel very different according to the phase of their menstrual cycle, whereas others may not experience any differences in well-being over the course of the menstrual cycle. However, this becomes obscured if like is not compared with like, in terms of menstrual phase[36]. To this end, standardisation of measurement of the menstrual cycle is an important starting point[37].

## Hormones are the key (again)

There are other variables to contend with, even employing a standardised methodology to identify phases of the menstrual cycle, based on the time of ovulation: specifically, the fine detail of menstrual hormones in terms of precise timings and concentrations. Periods are a good surrogate indicator of internal hormone fluctuations: the barometer of internal healthy female hormones. However, it is important to note that the terms eumenorrhoea, polymenorrhoea, oligomenorrhoea and amenorrhoea all refer to the frequency of periods. These terms do not refer to how female hormones are fluctuating, either in terms of timing or levels. Even eumenorrhoeic women, with regular periods, differ in the details of the exact network effects and concentrations of female hormones over each cycle. For example, over an apparently normal cycle, slightly suppressed levels of progesterone, suggestive of subclinical ovulatory disturbance, can have health implications beyond fertility in terms of bone and cardiovascular health[30].

In addition to the variations between women, every individual woman observes variation from cycle to cycle in terms of timing and hormone concentrations. Finally and perhaps most important of all is that the response of an individual to exactly the same timing and concentration of menstrual hormones may be different from one month to the next. For this reason, generalisations on how a woman should or shouldn't feel during the menstrual cycle can be irritating at best. Generic advice is not always helpful. Rather an individual, personalised approach for each woman is more appropriate and desirable. A good starting point is menstrual tracking and matching up with well-being. This approach was found to be very helpful in our study including female professional dancers where a tracking system was set up with input from dancers[38]. How to address the important topic of individual menstrual cycle hormone variation is discussed in "Scene 6: Hormone Supermodels".

## Coda of menstrual cycle hormone choreography

The timing of menstrual cycle hormone choreography becomes even more challenging to pin down as ovarian responsiveness reduces from around the age of 40 years. The ovaries start to approach retirement during perimenopause, until eventually at menopause (average age of 51 years) the ovaries become unresponsive to the control hormones FSH and LH. The characteristic hormone signature of menopause is continuously high levels of FSH and LH together with low levels of oestradiol and progesterone, as shown in Figure 5.2.5. The unvarying levels of hormones involving the hypothalamic-pituitary-ovarian axis indicate that the expected feedback loops are no longer in operation. The fact that the control pituitary hormones are constantly high and the ovarian response hormones are continually low, identifies that the breakdown of the feedback circuit is at the level of the ovaries.

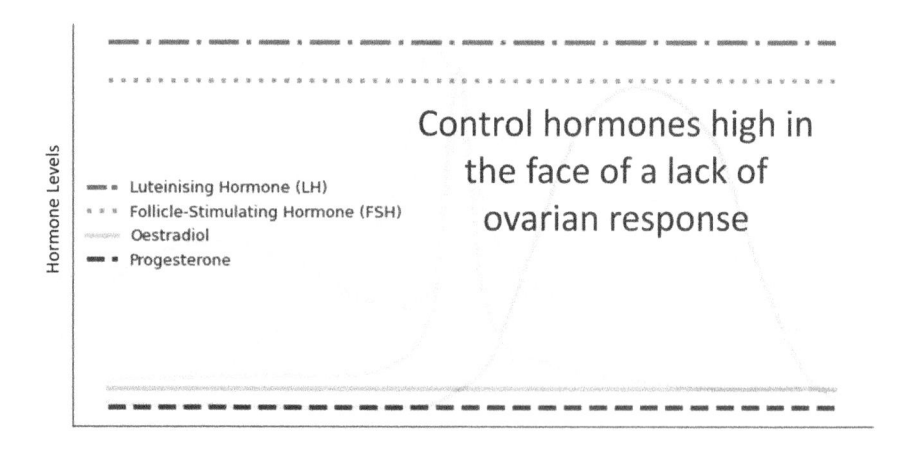

**Figure 5.2.5:** Hormones after menopause

This progression of ovarian retirement is more of an intermittent fault than a smooth trajectory. This situation reflects how a woman feels during the coda of menstrual cycles. Unpredictable hormone choreography can produce changes in the nature of menstrual periods: faltering timing of an ageing biochronometer. Variable ratios of oestradiol and progesterone produce sometimes heavy or light menstrual bleeds. Uncoordinated hormones can impact physical and psychological well-being. The perimenopause is discussed in more detail in Act 2 "Scene 5: Middle Age".

In a twist of fate, lacking the benefit of their ovarian hormones brings women level to men, at least in terms of an increase to the equivalent male risk of cardiovascular disease after menopause. Ironically, perhaps once her ovarian hormones have dwindled a woman might be labelled as presenting with "typical" myocardial ischaemia.

## When will I reach the menopause?

The typical age of menopause is on average 51, with a range from 45 to 55 years. About 1% of women experience primary premature ovarian insufficiency (POI), which means reduced ovarian function before the age of 40. For 0.1% of women, this occurs under the age of 30. POI may lead to early menopause, occurring between 40 and 45, or premature menopause occurring before 40 years of age. It is important to identify POI promptly, as a drop in ovarian hormones increases the risk of cardiovascular disease, osteoporosis and decline in cognitive function. Replacing ovarian hormones through hormone replacement therapy (HRT) is important for long-term health, especially for women with POI[39]. Fertility may also be compromised, although the British Menopause Society stresses that it is only when menopause is reached that ovarian function completely stops.

### *What determines the age of menopause?*

As with the timing of many physiological processes, the natural age of menopause is thought to be determined by both genetic and environmental factors. A paper published in Nature[40] describes how clusters of genes can be used to provide a polygenetic score (PGS) which accounts for 10% of the variation in the age of natural menopause (as opposed to medically induced menopause). The impact of each genetic variant ranged from 3.5 weeks to 1.5 years. While the PGS accounted for a very modest 10% variation in natural age of menopause, the top 1% of the PGS range corresponded to a fivefold increase in POI compared with women with mid-range scores. The authors themselves urge caution in the clinical application of this multigenetic test approach for predicting natural age of menopause, even in those families with a family history of POI.

The PGS as an indicator of increased risk of POI is not the novel finding of this paper. The authors state that this result is the same as that obtained through a current single gene test. The most interesting part of the research was **how** these genes influence the age of menopause. These specific genes code for the DNA repair system for the eggs in the ovary.

Incredibly all the eggs in the ovary are "prepared" while the female foetus is in the mother's uterus during pregnancy. The double-stranded DNA in each egg unwinds and is partially split, leaving it literally in suspended animation. These eggs have to wait for another 15 to 50 years before being called upon to complete the halving of double-stranded DNA. Ultimately an egg has one DNA strand when ovulated during the menstrual cycle, ready to be united with a matching single strand from a sperm. Some eggs never make the cut for ovulation.

As all the eggs were prepared in the ovaries of the female foetus, they all have the same "shelf life". Over adult life, the shelf on which the eggs are resting metaphorically starts to tip. The DNA repair mechanisms try to keep the shelf level. However, inevitably the shelf tips over at menopause. This shelf life of eggs contrasts with sperm in men, which are made continuously throughout adult life.

From an evolutionary perspective having a shelf life on eggs and reaching menopause is probably for the benefit of the mother and the potential baby. Although life expectancy has increased, the ageing process is something that none of us can avoid. Pregnancy, childbirth and raising a child are demanding, even more so beyond middle age. From the baby's point of view, it is well documented that increasing maternal age increases the risk of genetic issues for the embryo. This is where genetic repair mechanisms outlined in the research paper become really important. As the DNA in the eggs in the foetal ovaries are in suspended animation, in a delicate state for the rest of the woman's life, the DNA repair enzymes need to be on high alert to keep the eggs "fresh" and ready for ovulation.

In experiments on female mice, manipulating the two genes for DNA repair did prolong fertility and one of these genes also bolstered the ovarian response to hormone stimulation. However, the downside is that in the latter case this could also increase the risk of cancer. Furthermore, we do not know how manipulating maternal genetics would translate to the genetics of the offspring, nor how this genetic manipulation translates from mice to women.

Ideally it would be helpful to keep a watching brief on all factors contributing to egg health.

## *The missing link: female hormone networks*

The authors state that their paper focused on genetics and did not consider the other key influencers of female health, fertility and definition of menopause, namely, hormones[41]. If genetic factors account for 10% of the variation in the age of menopause, that leaves 90% unexplained. A significant proportion of the variation is likely to be due to environmental factors. Lifestyle and behavioural choices influence hormones, and it is hormones that regulate gene expression in DNA.

This means that, whatever your genetic endowment, making good lifestyle choices on nutrition, exercise and sleep, while avoiding negative choices like smoking, certainly helps hormone networks and therefore impacts gene expression.

Ideally a measure of dynamic hormone function would be more informative about transition to menopause. Such an approach is now possible, by combining medical and mathematical expertise through artificial intelligence techniques[42]. Quantifying ovarian responsiveness with a scoring system of female hormone network function gives a real-time watching brief on female health[43]. Chronological monitoring can track any decline suggesting a transition to menopause.

### *What can we conclude about the age of menopause?*

- Menopause is a significant physical and psychological event in a woman's life. Declining ovarian hormones pose challenges for long-term health.
- Average age of natural menopause is 51 (range 45–55 years). Early menopause occurs between 40 and 45 years of age and premature menopause under 40. Primary ovarian insufficiency (POI) is where the ovaries start to lose responsiveness before the age of 40.
- The age of menopause is determined through a combination of genetic and environmental factors. A research genetic test combining various genes could predict up to 10% of the variation in the natural age of menopause, leaving 90% determined by non-genetic factors. In 1% of the outlying genetic scores, this corresponded to an increased likelihood of premature ovarian insufficiency, the same as the current single gene test.
- The authors of the research urged cation that these multiple gene tests are not a suitable clinical test for women, even for those with a family history of POI. Nevertheless, this research sheds light on the DNA repair mechanisms that play a part in determining fertility.
- This paper focused on genetics and did not discuss the hormone networks. Menopause is defined as no further menstruation when the ovaries stop producing hormones.

## Practical take-home points

- You can obtain a free genetic test by asking your female family members about their age of menopause. This also opens up conversations about menopause.
- Premature ovarian insufficiency does not definitively exclude the possibility of pregnancy.
- For all women, ovarian responsiveness and fertility decline after 40 years, at a variable rate.
- Female hormone networks should be considered and assessed as part of the assessment of ovarian function, because hormones determine genetic expression.

It is important for women to be aware of their personal female physiology. Genes are passed down through the generations, but the expression of those genes is determined by hormone networks. Since lifestyle choices affect hormones, they determine to a large extent how your personal story unfolds.

## Female hormone odyssey

The goddess, Horme, awakes at menarche, followed by regular performances of menstrual cycle hormone choreography, with a fitful coda before finally retiring and falling into slumber.

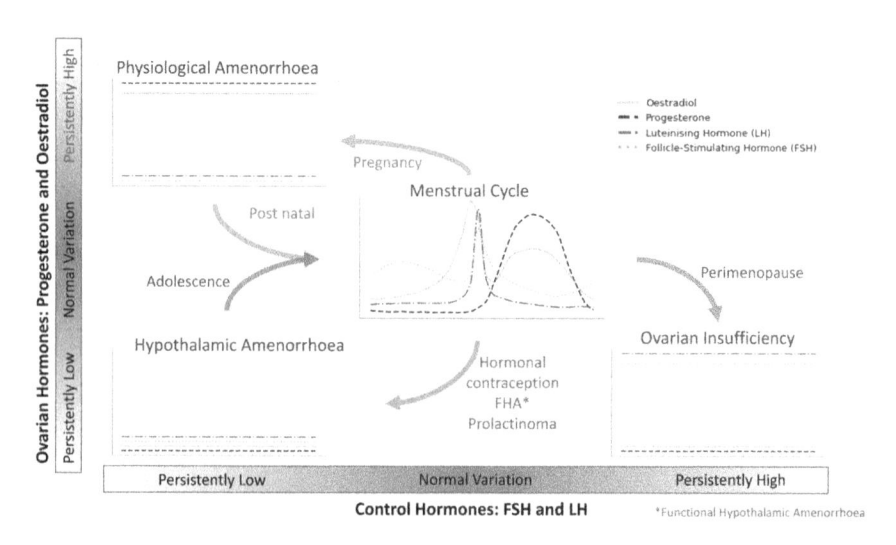

**Figure 5.2.6:** Female hormone odyssey

Figure 5.2.6 shows the epic journey that all women travel over their life. Staring in the bottom left corner of this diagram, a young girl begins her journey with all her female menstrual cycle hormones lying dormant. Gradually, at the completion of puberty the female hormones settle into their characteristic cyclical choreography shown in the central panel. This variation of hormones continues throughout her adult life, with possible excursions to the top left of the figure, presented by pregnancy. During pregnancy ovarian hormones are high and control hormones low: a state of physiological amenorrhoea. Menopause, shown in the lower right, is the mirror image of pregnancy, namely high control hormones and low ovarian hormones, due to a lack of ovarian responsiveness. Certain situations cause backtracking to low levels of all female hormones in the bottom left corner. These include functional hypothalamic amenorrhoea or contraceptive hormone induced amenorrhoea.

The physiological odyssey of hormone variation follows an arc: from prepubescent hormonal hibernation, to repeating menstrual cycles, eventually reaching the natural coda of menopause.

## Strategies for female hormone health over the odyssey

### *Menstrual cycles*

- Menstrual cycles provide a barometer of healthy internal female hormones. Female hormones are important for many aspects of health, not limited to reproduction.
    - If a woman's periods have not established by 16 years of age (primary amenorrhoea), then medical advice should be sought
    - Once periods have started, if they become irregular (oligomenorrhoea) or stop for more than 6 months (secondary amenorrhoea), medical input is needed
- How a woman experiences her menstrual cycle is personal to her, coinciding with individual female hormone variations and subjective biological responses.
    - Tracking menstrual cycles, in alignment with subjective well-being, can be a good starting point to tune into how the body responds to your personal hormone choreography
    - Being aware of the effects of female hormones makes it easier to adapt behaviours and raise awareness to any changes that occur over the female hormone odyssey

# Scene 6
## Hormone Supermodels

> *"The practice of medicine is an art."*
> Sir William Osler

**Subtitle:** Personalised female hormone intelligence is at our fingertips. Combining deep medical and mathematical understanding with personal hormone data through the application of artificial intelligence techniques offers personalisation of female hormone health.

Sketching out the curves illustrating the variations in menstrual cycle hormones, a few years ago, I imagined how valuable it would be for individual women to know their personalised hormone variations. To empower each woman with her own signature hormone data was my goal. However, I had a big problem. Precisely because each woman is an individual, how could I achieve this goal bearing in mind that daily blood tests are not an option?

Fortunately, my husband loves solving complex mathematical problems. He was also one of the pioneers in the use of neural networks in business. So, when I presented my concept to him, he immersed himself in the challenge of cracking this seemingly impossible hormone mathematical modelling challenge. Here is an allegory of the background behind the quest for hormone intelligence.

***Clemency*** had been a ballet critic for a leading newspaper for many years. On her way to a preview of a performance of The Nutcracker, she became stuck in a huge traffic jam of Christmas shoppers. When she finally arrived at the theatre, the first act had already started. No sooner had she taken her seat and begun to take in the scene with her expert eye, identifying the performers on stage and the conductor in charge of the orchestra, when she received an urgent text message from her husband, asking her to call back immediately.

*Somewhat reluctantly, she slipped out of the auditorium to find out what crisis had occurred at home. Her husband was worried because their young daughter had been feeling ill and a long discussion ensued over what they should do. By the time Clemency was able to return to her seat, the performance was already well into the second act. Thanks to her familiarity with the ballet, she recognised the point the plot had reached, noting that this particular performance must have skipped one or two of the standard segments of choreography.*

*Then another buzzing message popped up on her phone: her husband had managed to lock himself outside the front door and could she please come home straight away. Clemency resigned herself to the fact that she would have to write a review of the ballet, based only on short snapshots from the two acts of the ballet. Nevertheless, she felt confident that by combining her knowledge of the ballet and the performers with the small parts she had seen, she had a pretty good idea of how the whole performance had gone.*

Clemency faced a problem similar to one I encounter as a medical doctor, seeking to understand the personal hormonal choreography of a female patient. For me, the performers are the female hormones and the specific ballet is clearly recognisable as the menstrual cycle. Just as every ballet company has its own take on a ballet and every performance is slightly different, I know that every woman is an individual and every cycle is unique. And just as Clemency would have preferred to watch the whole performance, I would love to be able to monitor a woman's personal hormone levels continuously throughout her cycle. But, in practice, I might only have access to a limited number of blood samples. By adopting Clemency's strategy of cleverly combining my background knowledge with the available observations, I am able to gain a very good idea of how an individual woman's hormones performed over her cycle. This allows me to write a personalised hormone medical review. In the world of artificial intelligence, computers can help augment medical expertise.

## Monitoring menstrual cycle hormones

The finely balanced hormonal networks driving the menstrual cycle are affected by internal and external factors. The levels of hormones produced during the cycle have consequential effects on the body. A woman possessing a detailed knowledge of her hormone profile can better understand her current state of health and the way she feels during her cycles. Charting female hormones through time would provide her with a valuable barometer of health, helping her track changes linked to important life events.

Some relatively simple, indirect methods of monitoring female hormone health are available. Recording menstrual cycle length, by noting when periods occur, is a good starting point. Annotating the cycle can be helpful, using surrogate indicators of ovarian hormone actions, such as ovulation temperature readings and cervical mucous changes. It is also possible to measure a limited number of hormones and their metabolites in the urine. Ovulation strips measuring luteinising hormone (LH) try to pin down the timing of the LH surge associated with ovulation. Saliva sampling can be used for measuring steroid-based hormones oestradiol and progesterone. These approaches shed a narrow beam of light on some parts of the overall network of feedback mechanisms. This means that if any advice is offered, it tends to be generic rather than personalised.

While some hormones can be detected in the urine and saliva, the more accurate "gold standard" method is to measure the serum levels of hormones directly in a blood sample. However, in clinical practice, female hormone blood tests are usually confined to sampling three hormones: follicle-stimulating hormone (FSH), LH and oestradiol, on day three of the menstrual cycle. This practice avoids the complication of individual menstrual cycle hormone timing beyond the first few days of the cycle. However, a test conducted on day three provides very little useful information for a pre-menopausal woman, because all the measured hormones are at their lowest levels at this stage of the cycle. This is equivalent to a cursory look at the ballet stage, just after the curtain has opened. This may confirm that the expected performance will probably start but gives no further information about how it might progress, nor how the audience might react. Even a woman with functional hypothalamic amenorrhoea (FHA) may have hormones falling into the expected ranges at this early stage in the cycle. Many women whose periods have stopped come to see me, perplexed at having been told that their day three female hormones are "normal". However, a sample taken on day three obviously cannot register the fact that a woman's hormones failed to rise during the month, in the expected fashion associated with a menstrual cycle.

The other time point in the cycle, where blood levels of progesterone are conventionally measured to indicate ovulation, is "day 21" or 7 days before menstruation starts. However, due to the personal timing of events in the menstrual cycle and variation from cycle to cycle of an individual woman, this approach can be somewhat hit or miss.

To gain a complete picture and more useful insights, we would ideally measure the "full house" of the control hormones: FSH and LH, and the ovarian response hormones: oestradiol and progesterone. Daily measurements throughout a cycle would provide an assessment of the entire performance of the conductor, orchestra and dancers in the full hormonal ballet. The pituitary gland is the conductor, setting the tempo for the endocrine orchestra of control hormones, which evoke the dance of the ovarian response hormones.

The only problem is that it is not practical to take a blood sample every day. Given this constraint, would it be feasible to model the overall profile of a woman's hormones based on fewer blood samples during a cycle? Looking at Figure 6.1, it is clear that the most action is happening around ovulation and when progesterone peaks in the luteal phase.

## Machine learning for personalised health

*"Medicine is a science of uncertainty and an art of probability."*

Sir William Osler

Combining the attributes of deep medical understanding with individual characteristics through machine learning is an exciting field that is revolutionising healthcare. This is explored in "Machine Learning for Individualised Medicine", a report by the UK Chief Medical Officer[1]. Applying mathematical techniques, to make sense of large amounts of data, has the potential to transform medicine and healthcare. Machine learning can direct integrated, precision medicine at all stages of clinical practice through prevention, screening, diagnosis, treatment and monitoring. This offers the prospect of valuable scientific insights into the art of medicine and enables the personalisation of health[2].

## From generic to personalised menstrual hormone choreography

Interpretation of an individual's blood samples needs to be set in the clinical context of our medical knowledge of the endocrine system itself and studies of the variability in the timing and levels of hormones over the menstrual cycle.

The predictable sequence of hormone fluctuations is coordinated by interrelated networks. Each of the key hormones needs to attain levels that are sufficiently high, or low, to trigger the next phase of the performance. These levels vary between women and are affected by other factors. The normal menstrual cycle length is confined to a range (around 22 to 35 days), because it takes time for the control hormones to induce responses in the ovarian hormones and then for these response hormones to complete the feedback loop to influence the control hormones. Some sections of hormone choreography are performed at fast allegro, like the LH surge to induce ovulation. Other segments, such as the rise and fall of progesterone in the luteal phase, follow a steadier tempo. Biological limits determine how much the hormones change and how fast or slow the menstrual hormones can complete a full cycle.

## Menstrual cycle hormone supermodels

Bayesian inference is an artificial intelligence technique, used widely in social sciences, ecology and medicine[3]. The approach provides a way to draw conclusions from observed data, in the context of background knowledge, making it particularly useful in this context. In the case of modelling menstrual cycles, we can imagine building a library containing a huge range of possible cyclical variations. Taking data drawn from scientific studies, one can attach

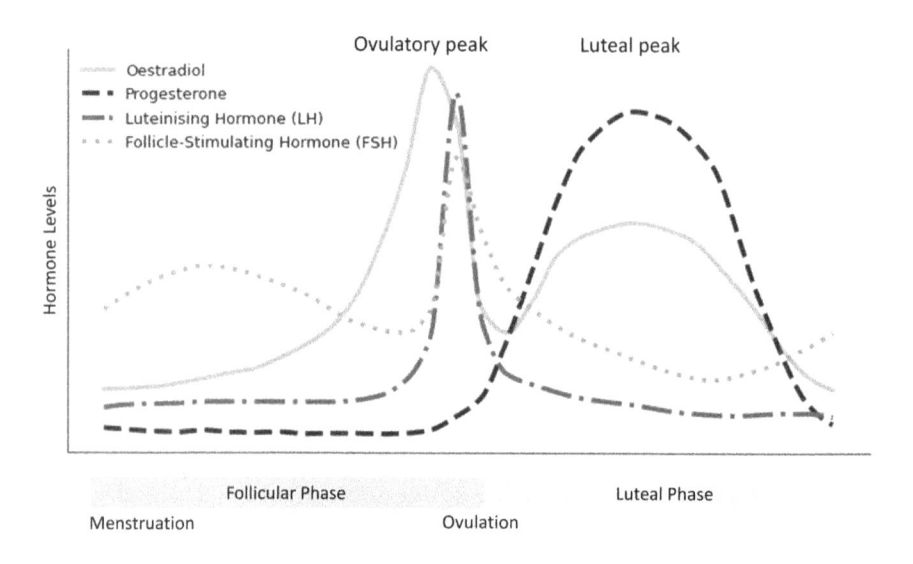

**Figure 6.1:** When to test female hormones?

to each cycle in the library the probability of seeing this sequence of events in a normal healthy woman This approach facilitates selection of the most likely hormone cycle to fit a limited number of data samples.

Of course, turning this into a practical tool involves dealing with many more subtleties, such as personal menstrual variability and the specific timing of obtaining blood samples. These can be resolved mathematically, in a manner that maximises the amount of information drawn from the samples provided.

## Hormone intelligence

Techniques such as this allow a woman to identify the most likely set of personalised curves showing the evolution of each hormone during her cycle. Machine learning approaches can improve as they accrue more data.

Returning to the analogy of reviewing a performance of The Nutcracker based on one observation in each act. This type of menstrual cycle hormone modelling takes account of the understanding of the progression of a typical hormone performance, the set sequence of hormone choreography. The blood samples provide details of the nuances of that performance, in the context of the individual's previous hormone performances. It is beneficial to have samples at key moments to gain a snapshot of the menstrual cycle hormone performance, based on our knowledge of the set running order.

Artificial intelligence[4] also provides a framework for generating expert medical reports that relate a woman's hormones to the way she feels and for creating new metrics that can be tracked over time.

## Personalised hormone health reports

> *"Medical expertise, filed systematically in a vast library of possible clinical interpretations and health reports can be retrieved by the most effective librarian: an expert report system. This enables many women to access their personalised female hormone health report."*

It is all very well using cutting-edge artificial intelligence techniques, but what benefit does this bring to an individual woman? How can a personalised hormone health report help? In broader terms, what is the potential clinical impact on women's health?

For the past 30 years, I have been working with women asking me questions about their female hormone health. These are some of the questions often asked.

> Am I entering the perimenopause? Should I consider hormone replacement therapy (HRT)?
> Am I making the best lifestyle choices for my personal hormone health?
> How can I better understand the interaction between my hormones and my sports performance?

Women are absolutely right to be asking these important questions to optimise physical and mental health. Women are also aware that lifestyle choices influence health. The mediators between our behaviours and health are hormones.

Figure 6.2 illustrates one of the central messages of this book. External factors impact hormones; hormones networks have effects throughout the body; these internal consequences feed back to the hormones; completing the loop, hormones determine our ability to be effective in the world. This means that our hormones explain why external behaviours ultimately determine how effective we are as human beings. The work of a medical doctor with experience in endocrinology is to distinguish which external actions feed back in a positive sense to improve performance and well-being.

What is my approach to answer these questions about female hormone health?

I start by asking a woman for some background details, specifically, her age, her menstrual history, her lifestyle and her well-being. Next, we look over her hormone blood results, and I explain what these numbers mean. When I look at a set of hormone blood results, I scan for patterns and biological meaning. This is a bit like translating a complex piece of prose written in a foreign language. The language of hormones has its own grammar and subtle nuances.

After explaining the hormone patterns, we discuss how personal lifestyle patterns tie into well-being and what would be the best course of action to optimise hormone health through lifestyle changes and sometimes medication where clinically indicated. After our discussion, my summary letter includes an

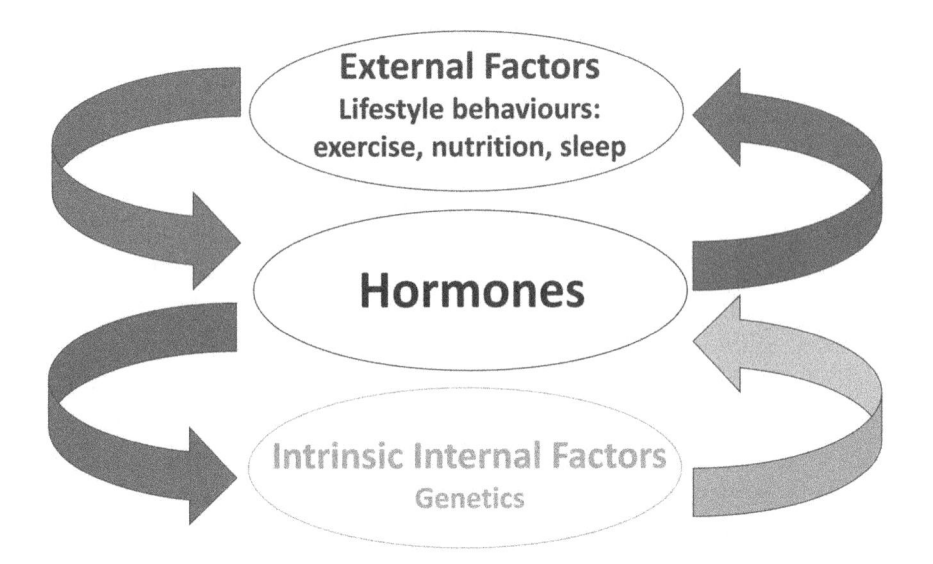

**Figure 6.2:** Feedback between external and internal factors mediated by hormones

evidence-based action plan. An AI system that speeds up the process of delivering a personalised hormone health report would allow me to support more women with hormone health questions.

## The process of making an expert report library

In my brain, I have stored a vast library of clinic letters covering diverse hormone network results for women over a range of ages and activity levels. An expert system is an artificial intelligence system that replicates the decisions or actions of an expert. I sat for hours, days and months "downloading my brain" into such a system, encompassing my 30 years of medical experience as if I had a "real" woman sitting in front of me with particular personal characteristics and results. The contents of these medical summaries and the evidence-based advice were definitely not generated by "artificial" intelligence, rather the expert system acts as a very efficient librarian. Presented with the request for a particular book and a specific page in the chapter, the expert librarian retrieves the exact page required that has been written by the author of all the books in this hormone library.

## Individual response to menstrual cycle choreography

*"If it were not for the great variability between individuals medicine might as well be a science and not an art."*

*Sir William Osler*

The equivalent of the audience reaction to a ballet performance is the response of the body to fluctuations in female hormones over the menstrual cycle. Having a tool that more accurately assesses the personal timing and levels of hormonal fluctuations shines a new light on historical generalisations and null results. It is a bit like setting sail with a Harrison clock on board aligned to Greenwich mean time, thereby avoiding the inaccuracies in calculating longitude that had resulted in many ships going off course and being unaware of their position in time and space, sometimes ending in shipwreck.

*"He who studies medicine without books sails an uncharted sea, but he who studies medicine without patients does not go to sea at all."*

*Sir William Osler*

A more reliable way of calculating the personal hormone levels over a cycle means less reliance on "dead reckoning". AI-based approaches allow a more accurate and reliable link to be made between the exact stage in the menstrual cycle and the woman's sense of well-being. By repeating this type of clinical evaluation over several menstrual cycles, a woman can gain further insights into the link between her hormone timing and the way she feels. By gathering this information, a woman can better understand her own body: computerised machine learning can inspire personal human learning. Figure 6.3 shows the concept of hormone intelligence at your fingertips.

## Injured hormone cast members in menstrual cycle hormone performance

Menstrual hormones are very sensitive to stress: emotional, physical, exercise and nutritional. As menstrual periods are the barometer of hormone health, the cessation of periods (amenorrhoea) is a clear warning sign that something is not right. However, a more subtle spectrum of hormone dysfunction, where the precise timing of hormones may not be synchronised correctly, cannot be identified by tracking menstrual periods alone, or by measuring hormones in a single time point blood sample. However, identifying subtle issues in menstrual hormone choreography is crucial as any small deficits can have implications for female health[5]. The ability to model hormone variation over the entire cycle increases the chances of identifying this situation without having to perform daily blood tests.

These types of clinical tools can be highly personalised training metrics for athletes and dancers. Early warning signs of individual hormone disruption caused by imbalances in exercise training, nutrition and recovery can be promptly detected and swiftly addressed. Implementing this strategy with professional female dancers in a ballet company, can help ensure that each dancer is ready to perform at her best throughout her menstrual cycle, over the entire performance season[6]. This approach has also proved helpful for professional female football players[7].

*Isabella is a 24-year-old dancer. When it was not possible to practice in the studio due to the COVID pandemic, she started doing lots of online Zoom ballet classes. Being anxious not to lose fitness, she also found extra online exercise classes. Although her menstrual cycles remained regular, she noticed that she was feeling more fatigued than usual and mentioned that she was not taking a rest day. I suspected that she may well have subclinical low energy availability as she was not eating sufficiently for her level of exercise.*

*Evaluation of Isabella's hormones revealed that her oestradiol was somewhat low over the cycle and her peak progesterone suggested that ovulation had not occurred. In other words, the results indicated subclinical anovulatory cycle. When we discussed these finding, she realised that she wasn't getting the benefits she had expected from dancing more than usual, rather this was disrupting her hormone networks. So, she agreed to moderate the number of classes and have a rest day. Re-testing of her hormone networks after a few months indicated that by rebalancing her behaviours, her hormones were now performing their full repertoire and Isabella reported feeling better. This averted the potential progression to downregulation of the hormone network and functional hypothalamic amenorrhoea (FHA).*

## The road to hormone network restoration

Monitoring the restoration of fully functioning hormone networks in recovery from low energy availability is a valuable clinical tool. Generally, my advice would be to wait for three regular periods, before increasing the training load. Without further testing, it is not possible to be certain that hormone networks are fully restored. Artificial intelligence techniques now make it possible to quantify the improvements in menstrual hormone function. This evidence can be helpful to guide the female exerciser.

*Alexandra is a 21-year-old triathlete. A high training load with insufficient energy intake has left her with low energy availability and functional hypothalamic amenorrhoea (no periods for more than 6 months). Alexandra had also experienced a bone stress fracture. I explained that it was important to increase energy intake and temporarily reduce training load, in order to reboot her hormone network.*

*Alexandra agreed and a few months later she had a period. Although she was eager to increase her training load, I suggested that we confirm that the menstrual cycle hormones were back to full function. After evaluating her hormones, we found that her next cycle was anovulatory with low oestradiol. The predicted shorter cycle length with a light period ensued. As athletes like data, Alexandra was able to see that it had been too soon to increase training. After reverting to a lower training load, I am pleased to report that subsequently Alexandra went on to have ovulatory cycles. This demonstrates that if we had relied on having a period as evidence of full resumption of hormone network function, Alexandra potentially would have increased training load too soon and may have reverted to FHA and increased risk of injuries.*

## Further performances of menstrual cycle hormone supermodels

Imagine the same cast and audience were involved in continuous performances of The Nutcracker over many seasons and many years. Gradually, the nature of the performance would change. With increasing age, the dancers would not be able to jump so high, nor respond with the same alacrity and precision to the pace set by the conductor as when in their prime. The audience response would become more subdued.

The perimenopause is the period of change and uncertainty for a woman, when knowledge of the status of her female hormones can be valuable. The problem is that ovarian responsiveness is not an on/off switch; it is more of an intermittent fault. So, doing a one-off blood test on the standard day three of the menstrual cycle is not a reliable way of determining where a woman is on her journey towards menopause.

Modelling the fluctuations of menstrual hormones over successive cycles during perimenopause might be valuable as a monitoring tool. This could help a woman chart and navigate the decline in ovarian function, in relation to perimenopausal symptoms. This approach could prove valuable for women to reduce uncertainty. For female masters athletes, this has the potential for a practical way to distinguish between the effects of low energy availability and perimenopause[8].

***Isadora*** *is a masters athlete in cycling, aged 49. She is experiencing irregular periods, feeling generally fatigued and struggling to train well. She explains that recently she had increased her training load, without increasing energy intake. From this history it could be that low carbohydrate availability is causing her symptoms. On the other hand, given her age it could be that she is experiencing perimenopause. Doing a day three female hormone blood test is unlikely to be able to distinguish between these situations. Therefore, we evaluated Isadora's hormones. This showed that her ovaries were lacking in responsiveness, indicated by low oestradiol and progesterone, in presence of consistently raised FSH and LH, over the full cycle. This made perimenopause the more likely diagnosis. We discussed better periodisation of training and nutrition and considering HRT (hormone replacement therapy) as an option to improve quality of life in the long term (for further discussion of HRT see Act 2 scene 5).*

## Clinical applications of hormone intelligence

Having wrestled with the challenge of unlocking female hormone intelligence, further research will provide further insights and clinical validation of similar tools. Most important of all, supermodels of menstrual hormone cycles make an important contribution to female personal well-being. Artificial intelligence to enable hormone intelligence is an important step for personalised female health[9].

Every woman is different, but all share the need for personalised female healthcare.

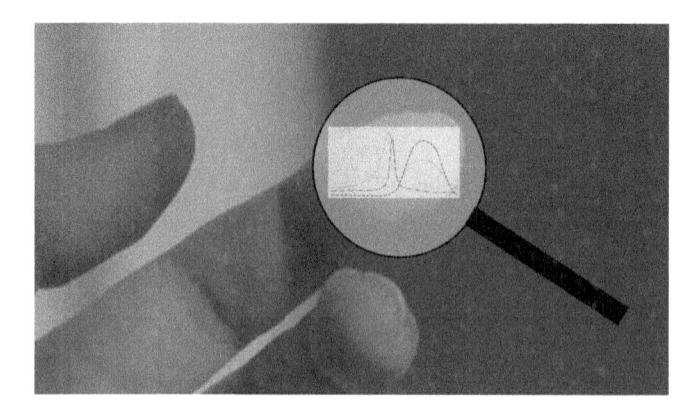

**Figure 6.3:** Hormone intelligence at your fingertips.*

# Scene 7
# Bare Bones

*"Make no bones about it."*

**Subtitle:** In addition to providing protection for the body, bones form the internal scaffolding that enables our muscles to create movement. But the skeleton is much more than just a fixed framework. Bone is a dynamic tissue, whose structure is influenced by hormone networks throughout our lives. Lifestyle factors, including exercise, nutrition and sleep, affect these hormone controllers, with consequences for bone health.

Bone, being both light and strong, is the ideal material for the internal scaffolding of our body. The skeletal system has many functions, with movement being top of the list. The skeleton is subdivided into units of bone, with joints as the interface between different units: we have an articulated internal skeleton. The skeletal muscle forms an overlay on the bones, acting across these joints to enable movement. For example, to walk, the hip flexor muscles acting across the hip joint cause the thigh bone, femur, to move upwards. Once these muscles relax, and our foot strikes the floor, the muscles at the back of the leg and pelvis contract causing extension at the hip joint and backward movement of the femur: one small step for man.

In addition to movement, the skeleton protects the internal organs: for example, the ribcage encloses the heart and lungs, and the skull safeguards the brain. Some bones, such as the ribs, spine and pelvis also act as sites for blood cell production: red blood cells for transporting oxygen, white cells for fighting infection and platelets for blood clotting. Blood cells are produced in the spongy internal bone marrow. The production of these blood cells is under the control of the hormone erythropoietin. This hormone is produced by the kidney and secreted according to the oxygen saturation of the blood. The renal artery is one of the first branches of the descending aorta, so the kidney is ideally positioned to monitor blood oxygen saturation. Furthermore, all the bones of the skeleton also act as an important mineral store, particularly for calcium. Calcium is important for both bone strength and contraction of muscle. Calcium homeostasis is under hormone control which is described shortly.

Bone is a composite material, made of a combination of protein and minerals. Collagen is the type of protein the body uses for many soft tissues, like tendons (connections between muscle and bone for movement) and ligaments (connections from bone to bone for the stabilisation of joints). Collagen is the protein component of bone on which mineral is deposited. The bone mineral is hydroxyapatite, containing calcium and phosphorous. It is this mineralisation of collagen that transforms bendy collagen into the formidable tissue that is bone.

Take away either component of bone and it becomes either bendy or brittle. You may be familiar with the "kitchen science" experiment demonstrating this composite nature of bone. Vinegar (an organic acid) dissolves the mineralised component of bone, leaving the collagen part: a bending bone. In practical terms, it has been found that cola carbonated drink intake is associated with lower bone mineral density (BMD) measurements[1]. It may be that the acidic nature of many carbonated, sugary drinks impairs the absorption of calcium, which is as important for bone mineralisation[2] as it is for the sustenance of coral reefs! The caffeine content of many sugary carbonated drinks has also been proposed as a cause of the adverse effect on bone. Another factor is that these types of drinks may displace other dairy-based drinks which provide important minerals and protein for bone health.

Conversely, if the bone is devoid of protein, only the mineral crystal remains, rendering the bone very brittle, like the desiccated skeletons found in deserts. The combination of collagen and mineral crystal makes bone a uniquely strong tissue.

All the bone of the skeleton is strong; however, at the microscopic level the structure of bone material takes two main forms. Trabecular bone (from the Latin, trabecula, meaning small strut), also known as cancellous bone, has a characteristic internal structure with cross struts of mineralised bone, giving the appearance of a honeycomb. This spongy structure is ideal for its function of shock absorption. Trabecular-rich bone is found in the vertebrae of the spine, the pelvis and heel (calcaneus). The loss of internal cross struts and the integrity of the honeycomb structure leave trabecular bone looking more like Edam cheese, with big spaces in the internal structure. This is characteristic of osteoporosis. Lack of internal structure means that osteoporotic bone is less able to withstand compression forces. Rather than acting as a shock absorber, osteoporotic trabecular bone becomes a crumple zone.

In contrast to trabecular bone, cortical bone (from the Latin, cortex, meaning shell or bark) is more compact. Cortical bone provides a protective surface around trabecular bone. Cortical bone thickness is increased in areas of the skeleton requiring robustness and mechanical leverage, such as the longer bones in the arms and legs, and in areas where strength is important, like the neck of the femur. As we discuss later, trabecular and cortical bones are also different in their sensitivity to hormones.

## Measuring bone health

DXA stands for dual X-ray absorptiometry. This is the gold standard way of assessing BMD. A very low dose X-ray is used to assess BMD, typically at two sites in the skeleton: lumbar spine as a representative of trabecular-rich bone and the femoral neck of the hip reflecting cortical rich bone. The measurement of BMD can be represented in two ways, known as the T-score and the Z-score. Both of these metrics take account of the fact that men tend to have higher bone density than women, due to their stature.

The T-score expresses the result in terms of standard deviations, which is the number of units above or below the average BMD of a healthy young person. The risk of breaking a bone increases with age. A negative T-score provides an assessment of how far BMD lies below its expected peak level.

The T-score from a DXA scan is used in the World Health Organisation (WHO) definition of osteoporosis. A T-score between −1 and −2.5 is defined as osteopenia: a notable loss of BMD. A T-score of −2.5 or below indicates osteoporosis. To assess the risk of osteoporotic fracture, there is questionnaire for those over 40 years, to which T-score can be added to provide extra detail. This is known as the Fracture Risk Assessment Tool (FRAX) questionnaire. As we discuss later, young active populations can also be at risk of poor bone health and in this case other approaches in terms of questionnaire and interpretation of DXA need to be applied.

The Z-score compares the result with the BMD of people of the same age. This age-adjusted assessment takes account of the changes in BMD over the lifespan. Healthy active adults who experience a slower decline in BMD are likely to see a positive Z-score, whereas people with an imbalance between diet and exercise may have negative Z-scores.

In addition to assessing bone health through BMD measurement, it is important to bear in mind that the microarchitecture and protein content of bone contribute to overall bone health and strength. Assessing bone microarchitecture requires higher radiation levels. Peripheral quantitative computed tomography (pQCT) is limited to peripheral sites of the skeleton, not the crucial trabecular bone of the spine. A potential solution to this challenge is to use a special type of ultrasound, called Radiofrequency Echographic Multi Spectrometry (R.E.M.S.), which does not involve ionising radiation and has the possibility to assess both BMD and bone structure at the lumbar spine. This has shown early promise in a study we conducted, with the added benefit of being a portable device, compared with a DXA scanner, which is a large static piece of equipment found in hospitals and universities[3].

Although DXA measurement of BMD is the gold standard in assessing bone health and defining osteoporosis, there is a move to recognise the combined factors that contribute to bone health and, importantly, to link bone strength to the clinical outcome of fracture risk. This is reflected in the National Institute of Health (NIH) consensus conference where the following statement was made "osteoporosis defined as a skeletal disorder characterised by compromised bone strength predisposing to an increased risk of fracture".

Putting this information into a practical setting, elderly people are warned of the risk of hip fractures of the neck of femur that occur as a consequence of low bone strength. However, the fracture risk of *all* bones in the skeleton increases with age. My mother used to be taller than me, but by the time she was 70, she had become shorter than me. This is not because I was growing, rather she was shrinking. Loss of height occurs as the trabecular bone of the vertebrae develops wedge compression fractures, especially in the thoracic spine. This is due to a crumbling of the internal honeycomb structure. As this occurs particularly after the menopause, the resulting hunched posture is known as a "dowager's hump". In the case of lumbar vertebral compression fractures, DXA results can be misleading, as the compressed vertebrae can give an apparently high BMD reading.

The fact that bone health deteriorates most markedly after the menopause in women, when oestrogen production in the ovaries takes a nosedive, indicates the vital role of this hormone on bone health.

## Hormones at work

Why are we talking about bone in a book about hormones? Hormone networks are key to bone health over your lifespan. Although bone health is to a certain extent genetically determined, gene expression is directed by hormones. In turn, hormones are influenced by environmental factors, particularly lifestyle choices of nutrition, exercise and sleep. Making the right choices can support good bone health and mitigate the increasing risk of osteoporosis.

Bone is an active tissue, which is dependent on a nurturing hormone milieu. About 10% of the skeleton is remodelled annually. This means that the whole skeleton is "recycled" every 10 years or so. If you tagged all the bones of your skeleton, it will all have vanished in a decade, replaced by a whole new skeleton. At the microscopic level, a remodelling cycle consists of breaking down bone, resorption, and then replacing it by building bone, formation. Bone turnover reflects the balance between bone resorption, performed by specialised bone cells called osteoclasts and bone formation, performed by another type of specialised bone cells called osteoblasts. The osteoclasts and osteoblasts act as a tag team. The osteoclast team kicks down the bone and the osteoblast team builds it up again.

Figure 7.1 shows how the relative strengths of these teams shift with age. The male hormones that tend to make men larger and more muscular than women result in greater mechanical forces acting on the bones. This explains why average BMD is greater in men than in women of the same age.

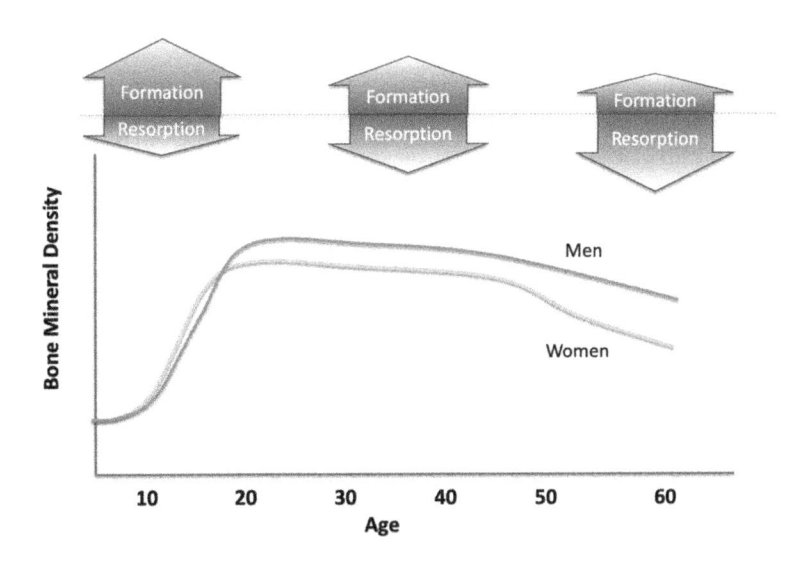

**Figure 7.1:** Bone turnover in men and women

What is the purpose of this seemingly Sisyphean task? Bone remodelling is very important for repair and adaptation of bone, together with calcium regulation. Initially in the repair of a fractured bone, there is often an increase in the gap between the broken ends as some tidying up with resorption occurs, then bone formation swings into action. On an X-ray you often see what is described as callous formation: an initial rather messy repair which then smooths out over time with further remodelling cycles. The speed and successful repair of bone depend on favourable hormone networks.

Adaptation of bone depends on remodelling. Osteocytes are a specialised type of bone cell that sense mechanical strain: mechanoreceptors[4]. The detection mechanism has been proposed to be through the generation of miniature electrical circuits via the piezoelectric effect. Strain picked up by this mechanotransduction system promotes orientation of the trabeculae to deal with this loading pattern and in the longer term promotes the bone formation side of the equation, resulting in increased BMD and potential thickening of the cortical shell, depending on the skeletal site. Adaptation of bone to changing mechanical forces is important so that the newly formed parts of the skeleton can deal with changes in loading patterns, for example, after repair of a fracture, joint replacement or starting a particular type of exercise.

Calcium homeostasis is maintained by hormones that control the balance of bone turnover. Parathyroid hormone (PTH) is produced by the four parathyroid glands nestled next to the thyroid gland in the neck. When circulating calcium is low, PTH is released to mobilise bone resorption and release calcium ions into the circulation. Stable calcium levels are essential for muscle contraction (skeletal and cardiac). Hyperparathyroidism, where there is an inappropriately high level of PTH, leads to excessive bone resorption and high levels of blood calcium ions.

It is possible to assess bone turnover balance by measuring factors associated with formation, such as the bone-specific version of the enzyme alkaline phosphatase. It is not surprising to see a high level of this enzyme during growth in children, mirrored by a high level of growth hormone (GH). However, high levels of alkaline phosphatase in adult life could indicate an underlying bone metabolism issue. Other markers of bone formation include fragments of Type 1 collagen, released when it is laid down as the bone matrix. Conversely, makers of bone resorption include collagen cross links. In practice, these indicators of bone turnover are mainly used in research. For example, when I was working on an international medical team to establish an anti-doping test for athletes misusing GH, measuring GH directly was not an option as GH is a peptide hormone with a short half-life and, in any case, the injected, exogenous form is virtually indistinguishable from endogenous, internally produced GH. Nevertheless, GH is a potent stimulator of bone turnover, so measuring bone markers provided an indirect, surrogate indicator of GH abuse.

## Which hormones are linked to bone health?

Bone is not just an active tissue with a mechanical function. Bone itself has an endocrine function per se. The hormones produced by bone have local autocrine and paracrine effects on bone, together with systemic effects. For example, osteocalcin is a peptide hormone produced by bone which acts locally on osteoblasts to support bone formation. However, osteocalcin also has a role in metabolism, specifically in blood glucose control, through insulin release and sensitivity. Bone fibroblast growth factor plays a role in the regulation of phosphate, which is part of the mineralised component of bone.

There is a suite of hormones produced in endocrine glands distant from bone tissue which play a part in bone health. These include calcitonin produced by the parafollicular C cells of the thyroid, which influence the activity of osteoblasts. There are also gut hormones that play a role in calcium absorption and bone turnover. These esoteric hormones currently lie more in the realms of research.

The main hormone protagonists for bone health include thyroxine, cortisol, PTH and GH, with the stars of the show being the sex steroids, particularly oestradiol. High levels of thyroxine, due to an overactive thyroid or overtreatment with external thyroxine, can harm bone health, by effectively speeding up bone turnover, favouring the resorption side of the equation. Conversely, low thyroxine, resulting from a global downregulation of hormone networks in low energy availability, can also have a negative effect on bone health, which is discussed shortly. Regarding cortisol, sustained high levels found in the medical condition of Cushing's disease can push the bone turnover balance in favour of resorption. The same applies to PTH where overproduction in hyperparathyroidism revs up bone turnover. As mentioned above, GH and its derivative IGF-1 (insulin-like growth factor 1) speed up bone turnover[5]. Being a peptide hormone, GH docks on the outside of a cell and exerts its effect on gene expression through a second messenger molecule. Through this mechanism, GH boosts both bone resorption and formation. Although, in the presence of oestradiol, this peptide and steroid hormone combination tends to favour the bone formation side of the equation. GH also favours bone formation indirectly by its anabolic effect on skeletal muscle. Stronger, larger muscles pulling on bone have a positive effect on bone.

## Oestradiol rules

Oestradiol is the sex steroid hormone that rules supreme when it comes to bone health, in both men and women. In men the sex steroid hormone, testosterone, is converted through aromatisation to its sister sex steroid hormone, oestradiol, which acts on bone. There is a specific type of alpha receptor for oestradiol found in the skeletal system. Through these bone-specific oestradiol receptors, this sex steroid hormone exerts its effect by regulating gene expression to inhibit bone resorption and favour bone formation. It is therefore no surprise that changes in BMD over the lifetime mirror the changes in oestradiol levels. See Figure 7.2.

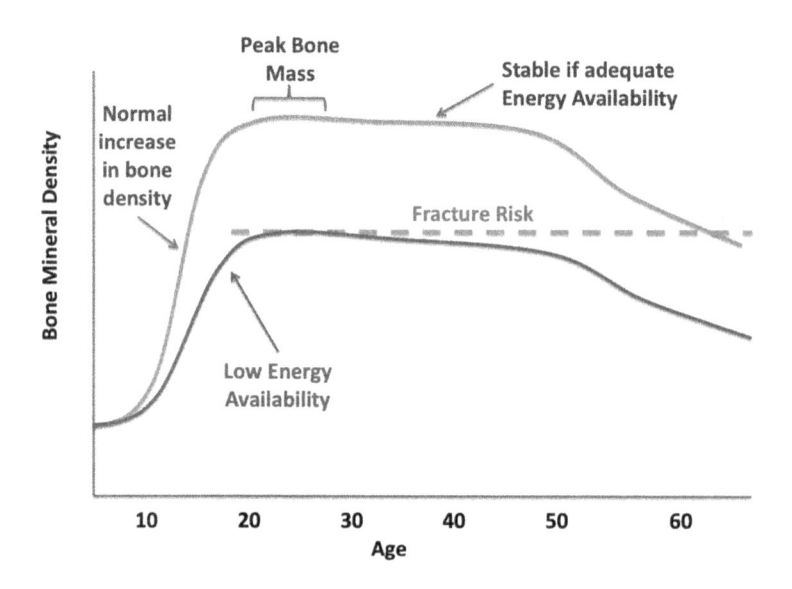

**Figure 7.2:** Bone mineral density variation over lifespan

## Early start for bone health: increase of bone mineral density

The most rapid increase in BMD occurs during the teenage years, when puberty occurs, and the sex steroid hormones increase dramatically. The bone mineral density accrual increases rapidly to attain peak bone mass (PBM) by the early 20s. Although there may be small increases into later 20s, especially for men who have later puberty than women, the most significant gains are in the teenage years when sex steroid hormones are in most rapid flux, en route to attaining adult levels and adult patterns in the case of the menstrual cycle.

Attainment of PBM is crucial for adult bone health[6]. A 10% increase in peak bone mass is estimated to reduce the risk of an osteoporotic fracture in adult life by 50%. Conversely, delayed puberty with delayed production of adult levels of sex steroids has an adverse effect on bone health and attainment of optimal PBM. Delayed puberty can be caused by imbalances in energy intake and expenditure leading to low energy availability. This is shown by the lower curve in Figure 7.2, where low energy availability limits bone mineral density accrual. This was the finding in my study that followed 87 prepubescent and adolescent female dancers over three years, comparing those in vocational training against a control group at a non-vocational dance school[7]. The youngsters in dance training had a high energy demand from exercise, on top of the high demand for growth and development. If this total high energy demand was not met through food intake, then a physiological "energy saving mode" delayed the onset of periods (menarche). Furthermore, once periods did start, they were less frequent than the regular periods in the control group. The net result was that low energy availability depressed the levels of oestradiol, which resulted in lower BMD particularly the trabecular bone in the spine. BMD was adjusted for bone size to provide a volumetric measurement to reflect biological age, rather than chronological age. This takes into account that growth affects bone size and that the timing of growth varies between individuals of the same age.

Although genetics plays a part in determining bone health, modifiable lifestyle factors impact hormones, which in turn influence gene expression. This was demonstrated by two pairs of identical twins in this bone health study. Fortunately for the study, in each twin pair, one was in ballet dance training and the other in a non-dance school. So, they had identical genes, but different gene expressions due to external factors of exercise and energy availability. The ballet dancer of each twin pair had lower BMD of the lumbar spine than her non-dance twin. This is not to say that dancing per se is bad for bone health. More a question of balancing exercise and nutrition for healthy hormones and bones. On a positive note, the best BMD of the lumbar spine was found in the girls in the musical theatre dance stream who reported regular periods. These pupils were exercising less than the ballet dancer stream, but more than the control pupils. So, a good balance of exercise and nutrition supports healthy hormones and good accrual of bone health in the teenage years[8].

Evidence of the importance of optimising peak bone mass for bone health in adulthood comes from our other study of 47 older, pre-menopausal retired female dancers[9]. Differences in BMD were explained by the independent variables of the age of menarche, duration of any amenorrhoea (lack of periods for more than 6 months) and lowest body weight for height during their dance career. In other words, dancers who had any issues with female hormones due to an imbalance of training load and nutrition as youngsters carried evidence of this in their bone health into adulthood. Entering menopause with already low BMD is not ideal.

## Stabilisation of bone mineral density

Returning to the graph of BMD against age, bone health should remain relatively stable during adulthood, reflecting adult levels and patterns of sex steroids. As hormones continue to influence bone health, any imbalances in lifestyle choices adversely impacting hormones have a knock-on effect on bone health. For example, if high energy demand from exercise is not matched by sufficient energy intake, the resulting low energy availability causes downregulation of hormones, which has a negative effect on bone health in women[10]. This also applies to situations of subtle dysfunction of female hormones[11]. Bone health in men can also be affected by imbalances in exercise and nutrition, which cause low testosterone levels. The ensuing low oestradiol impairs bone health, particularly for parts of the skeleton rich in trabecular bone[12].

At the other end of the spectrum, excessive energy intake with low levels of activity, coupled with poor sleep disrupts hormone networks, particularly the hormone axis of hypothalamus-pituitary-gonads (testes or ovaries) involved in oestradiol production. This pattern of unbalanced lifestyle behaviours also has adverse effects on hormone networks and consequently bone health[13].

Conversely, physiologically high levels of oestradiol that occur during pregnancy act as a boost for bone health. Consequently, women without children (nulliparity) have an increased risk of low BMD.

## Decline of bone mineral density

Increasing life expectancy is challenging for hormones and bone health. From the age of 40, hormone production starts to decline gradually, particularly the sex steroids and GH, which are the key players in bone health. This results in a 0.5% annual loss of BMD. Then for women after menopause (average age of 51 years), this loss increases to 5% annually. This sharp drop-off relative to men is shown in Figure 7.1. Women experiencing an earlier decline in female hormones associated with early menopause (40–45 years of age) or premature ovarian insufficiency (POI) before 40 years of age, are at increased risk of low BMD. This is a compelling reason for these women to start hormone replacement therapy (HRT) with immediate effect, at very least until the average age of menopause, to bring female hormones up to levels of their contemporaries and mitigate the effects of bone loss[14].

What about men? GH declines with age in a similar pattern to women; however, the drop in oestradiol, the most potent hormone for bone health, is much less dramatic. In men, oestradiol is produced from the aromatisation of testosterone, which declines only gradually with age. This explains the gentler fall in male BMD in contrast with women shown in Figure 7.1.

## Building bone

How can you optimise the accrual of peak bone mass, maintain bone strength through adult life and mitigate bone loss in later life? This comes down to mechanically loading this dynamic tissue and supporting bone-boosting hormone networks through lifestyle choices.

## Loading bone

Exercise has an osteogenic, bone-building effect[15]. Movement involving changes of direction is particularly useful in promoting the remodelling of bone in a positive way. Strength work has a beneficial effect on bone health, as skeletal muscle attachments pull on the bone to stimulate formation. The positive mechanical effect on bone is reinforced by hormones, such as GH, produced in response to exercise. The ideal combination for bone health is exercise that involves both changes in direction and strength work.

Figure 7.3 shows the effects of different types of sport on BMD. Rugby comes out on top for bone. On the other hand, the amount of multidirectional exercise for positive effects on bone health is dependent on age. A mechanical training overload can be detrimental for young athletes[16].

## Feeding bone

There is a paradoxical effect of exercise on bone. More is not better. If high training load is not matched by sufficient energy intake, there is not sufficient energy available to derive a positive hormone response to support bone formation. In this situation, despite high bone loading, bone health deteriorates. Continued high loading patterns on weakening bone can lead to bone stress responses and ultimately stress fractures, which occur because of repetitive loading.

Not all bone is equally susceptible to low energy availability and the consequences of bone weakness and stress fractures. Figure 7.3 shows the site-specific effects on BMD of various sports. Along the horizontal axis is the BMD of the lumbar spine, trabecular bone, which is particularly sensitive to hormone and nutritional factors. The BMD of the femoral neck, predominately cortical bone, is shown on the vertical axis, which is more responsive to mechanical loading[17]. Rugby ranks well on all skeletal sites. Although long-distance running provides mechanical loading for the femoral neck, unintentional or intentional low energy availability can slightly compromise BMD of the lumbar spine. Conversely, in lightweight rowing, mechanical loading of the lumbar spine can mitigate the negative effects of low energy availability on trabecular bone[18]. As it happens, I was one of the dancer subjects in this study at the British Olympic Medical Centre when I was working as a junior doctor in A&E at Northwick Park Hospital. This investigation sparked my interest in pursuing my own research into bone health in dancers and athletes.

Although swimming does not load the skeleton, it involves the whole body with muscle pulling on the bone to help with bone strength. It is a disadvantage to have low body fat as this reduces buoyancy. Therefore, swimming is not the best for bone health, nor is it the worst.

Road cycling is excellent for cardiovascular fitness. However, this form of exercise does not load the skeleton and tends to involve the legs predominately. In contrast to track cycling where the main challenge is overcoming air resistance; road cycling, especially up inclines, involves overcoming gravity. This can lead some road cyclists, especially those of amateur level without a medical support team, to reduce body weight intentionally, in the belief this will confer a performance advantage. If this comes at the expense of compromising hormone networks, poor bone health follows and performance may be impaired. This is what we found in a study of male cyclists. Those identified, through a sport-specific questionnaire and interview (SEAQ-I), as having insufficient energy intake to cover the energy demands of training had low BMD at the lumbar spine[19]. Furthermore, over 6 months of the race season, persisting in pursuing low body weight resulted in the loss of BMD to the same extent as an astronaut on the internal space station, where there is no gravity[20]; a good reason why cyclists should speak to astronauts[21]. What about improved performance? Sadly, this did not materialise as this group of cyclists underperformed compared to those in the study who paid attention to fuelling and did regular off-bike exercise for bone health.

Trabecular bone, found in the spine, is more sensitive to hormones, whereas cortical bone, found in the femoral neck, reacts to mechanical loading. This is reflected in the recommendation from the International Olympic Committee, that when assessing bone health in exercisers it is most informative to compare the Z-score (age-matched) of the lumbar spine to the femoral neck. You would expect that the Z-score would be similar at both sites. However, where the Z-score of the lumbar spine is below $-1$, this indicates compromised bone health due to low energy availability, especially if Z-score of the femoral neck is not so negative[22].

However, the detrimental effect of low energy availability on bone health is not restricted to elite or professional athletes[23]. Recreational exercisers can also be at risk of compromising bone health through imbalances in training and nutrition impacting hormone networks. We have developed a bone health questionnaire for active populations which can identify those potentially at risk[3]. Restoring bone health requires a combination of nutritional and bone loading strategies[24].

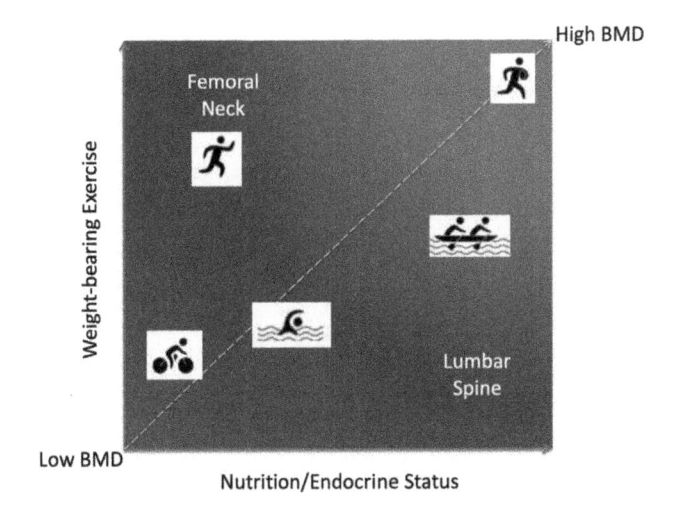

**Figure 7.3:** The effect of different sports on bone mineral density.*

## Solar powered hormone: vitamin D

Vitamin D is unique in many respects[25]. Firstly, vitamin D is a hormone. Its molecule includes a tell-tale ring of five carbon atoms that is typical of the steroid hormone family. Furthermore, the mechanism of action, as with all hormones, is to direct gene expression. There is a receptor on DNA specific for vitamin D. The other unique and fascinating aspect about vitamin D is that its production is solar powered.

The action of ultraviolet B (UVB) light on the skin results in the production of a low activity version of vitamin D. After some modifications by the liver and kidney, the activated vitamin D is ready to get to work. This bioactive metabolite interacts with the vitamin D receptor (VDR) in bone and muscle tissue to modulate gene expression, in keeping with how hormones exert their effects on DNA[26].

There are dietary sources of vitamin D such as dairy products or oily fish. However, even if you are an avid consumer of these foods, you cannot gain sufficient vitamin D, all year round, from diet alone.

The downside of being a solar-powered hormone is that production is dependent on sunlight. This is a particular challenge for those of us living in northern or southern latitudes. Even if you were to walk around naked all winter in the UK, you still would not be able to produce sufficient levels of vitamin D for health. So, this is not recommended as a vitamin D boosting strategy. Public Health England advises all of us to take supplementation, especially over the winter months.

What is so good about being replete in vitamin D? Figure 7.4 shows the Greek sun god Helios in his chariot pulling the sun across the sky, powering the main actions of vitamin D.

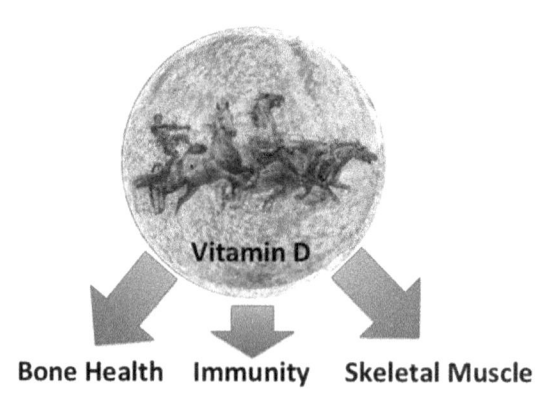

**Figure 7.4:** The actions of vitamin D.*

## Bone health

Vitamin D is essential for bone health at all ages, but especially for the young and old. Rickets, bendy bones, is a condition seen in children with insufficient vitamin D. Such was the public health issue that, before vitamin D supplementation, the Royal National Orthopaedic Hospital installed curious-looking rooms, with walls on three sides, that rotated so the children could gain benefit from the sun as it moved across the sky. Like sunflowers, they followed the path traced by Helios from sunrise to sunset. In a study of active adolescent girls, those with good levels of vitamin D had a lower stress fracture risk than those with lower vitamin D[27]. In adult females undertaking exercise training, the same effect of vitamin D on bone health was found. Those taking vitamin D supplementation sustained a lower number of stress fractures than those not taking vitamin D[28].

For older people who tend to spend less time outside, resultant low levels of vitamin D can contribute to poor bone health: osteomalacia. This can be compounded by declining sex steroid hormones, specifically oestradiol, which results in osteoporosis.

In adults, even if sex steroid hormones are in the expected healthy range, low vitamin D can have a detrimental effect on bone health. This was the finding in our study of male road cyclists[19] Although road cyclists spend time outside in the sun, much of their skin is covered with cycling attire and as mentioned above, depending on where you live, the sun might not be enough[29].

In men and women oestradiol is the chief bone health sex steroid hormone, acting in synergy with vitamin D. Optimal bone health depends on having healthy levels of both oestradiol and vitamin D. This means that even if you are replete in vitamin D, low levels of oestradiol are detrimental to bone health. In a study, male and female athletes with low range levels of testosterone (and therefore oestradiol) and oestradiol respectively had a far higher lifetime risk of stress fracture than those with normal steroid hormone levels[30].

## Skeletal muscle

Vitamin D is also important for soft tissue, including skeletal muscle attached to bone. Since dance studios and theatres are mainly indoor venues, lacking direct sunlight, dancers can be low in vitamin D, especially over the winter months[31]. In a study, dancers who received winter supplementation had increased muscle strength, which translated to larger jump heights. These dancers also suffered fewer soft tissue injuries[32].

For athletes seeking marginal gains, vitamin D supplementation is a totally legal and healthy performance enhancer. Conversely, low levels of vitamin D are a well-recognised cause of muscle weakness, lack of energy and general malaise.

## *Immunity*

There is a reason why sanatoriums are often in sunny places like the south of France. Before vaccination, tuberculosis (TB) was a widespread, potentially fatal condition. Although starting in the lung, the slow-growing bacterium responsible for TB spread throughout the body causing "consumption" and ultimately death, as dramatised in La Traviata. The tell-tale sign of TB was coughing up blood. As TB presented as a pulmonary condition, the rationale was that fresh air could help. As it turns out, sunshine was probably the main factor. More contemporary evidence for the beneficial effect of vitamin D on immunity comes from studies where people who are replete in vitamin D, especially over the winter, were less likely to develop upper respiratory conditions or viral infections[33]. This was a very relevant consideration during the COVID-19 pandemic. Reduced viral illness in athletes over the winter has been associated with higher levels of vitamin D[34].

## Bare bones of bone health

The cumulative effect of challenges to bone health determines the state of our bones as we enter middle age. The situation becomes more challenging in later life, where declining hormone levels, in particular oestradiol, have an adverse effect on bone health. This applies for both men and women, although the risk of osteoporosis is higher for women, who have a lower peak bone mass than men as a starting point. In men, testosterone, and hence oestradiol, declines gradually from middle age onwards, accompanied by a gradual loss of bone mineral density. This contrasts with women reaching the menopause, where the ovaries stop oestradiol production, resulting in a particularly rapid loss in bone mineral density the year before and for two years after menopause where up to 5% of bone mass can be lost annually.

Although oestradiol is the key hormone for bone health, the reduction in testosterone and GH in both men and women with advancing age plays a part in bone loss both directly and indirectly. Reduction in these anabolic (bone and muscle building) hormones results in a reduction of both bone formation and muscle strength and function: sarcopenia. This means less mechanical force is being exerted on bones to stimulate bone formation. The combination of reduced hormone and mechanical stimulation with age contributes to an increased risk of poor bone health and fragility fractures.

A fragility fracture is the result of a low trauma event, such as a fall from no more than standing height. A Colles' fracture is a broken wrist, often resulting from a fall onto an outstretched hand. Fractures of the spine and hip have the most impact from a personal and health economic standpoint. Osteoporotic fragility fractures in these areas of the skeleton lead to loss of independence, disability and reduced life expectancy. Compression fractures of the spine result in difficulty breathing and loss of height. For the elderly, those sustaining a hip fracture, 20% die within one month, 30% within a year and 50% can no longer live independently. Osteoporosis is described as the silent killer. One in two women and one in five men over 50 will sustain an osteoporotic fracture[14].

Although poor bone health in older people is most likely due to declining hormones, it is important to consider and exclude other secondary causes of osteoporosis. For example, other causes of amenorrhoea in women apart from menopause such as prolactinoma (over production of prolactin in the pituitary) or functional hypothalamic amenorrhoea FHA (due to an imbalance in lifestyle choices). Certain endocrine conditions adversely impact bone health in men and women, such as Cushing's (overproduction of cortisol), hyperparathyroidism (over production of PTH) and hyperthyroidism. Gut issues causing malabsorption can impact bone health, alongside autoimmune inflammatory conditions such as rheumatoid arthritis. Some medications impact bone health. Malignancy (cancer) can adversely affect bone health and cause pathological fractures.

Primary osteoporosis is where poor bone health is a result of the physiological decline in bone-promoting hormones. Secondary osteoporosis occurs as a result of medical conditions (e.g. rheumatoid arthritis) and/or medication (e.g. steroids). Unfortunately for bone, often these two scenarios co-exist: steroids are used to manage flare-ups of rheumatoid arthritis. Furthermore, women are more susceptible to autoimmune diseases like rheumatoid arthritis. What are the treatment options for primary osteoporosis? For women, HRT is the most effective treatment for supporting bone formation[14] The primary reason for a woman starting HRT in her late perimenopause and early menopause is to combat challenges to quality of life, particularly "vasomotor" symptoms, such as temperature regulation issues, the cause of hot flushes. HRT is also very effective in supporting bone health. As the most rapid time for bone loss is around the menopause, it is better to start taking HRT sooner than later. The same applies for women who experience premature ovarian insufficiency and those with FHA, the aim being to restore female hormones to pre-menopausal levels for bone protection.

Another treatment for osteoporosis which is licensed for older men and women is a group of medications known as bisphosphonates. These act by shutting down bone turnover, in contrast to HRT which promotes bone formation. Although bisphosphonates are very cost effective, the downside is that this family of medications has some unwelcome side effects on the gastrointestinal system. More recent hormonal treatments include PTH and an interesting group of medications going by the name of SERMS. Selective oestrogen receptor modulators (SERMS) have a positive oestrogenic effect on bone, but not on breast tissue or the endometrium (uterine lining). On the downside, potential side effects of hot flushes and joint aches make this option less attractive if you are already experiencing these due to the menopause. An exciting new medication is a monoclonal antibody targeted to act on bone to prevent bone resorption, which is administered as a six-monthly subcutaneous injection.

## Lifestyle choices for bone health

Although bone health is partly genetically determined, environmental and lifestyle choices influence bone health through the action of hormones. Hormones respond to exercise and nutrition, ultimately determining gene expression. This enables us to influence our bone health in a positive way to support maximal peak bone mass accrual and maintain bone health during adulthood.

The good news is that it is never too late to do exercise that supports bone health. Those with osteoporosis, especially in advanced years, understandably can be slightly nervous about being active, fearing fracture. However, there is evidence that weight-bearing exercise and/or resistance exercise can maintain and, in some cases, even improve bone health[35]. Where possible exercise that includes changes in the direction of travel or loading of bone is particularly beneficial. Of course, exercises should be carefully chosen for the individual and supervised where indicated.

The other aspect of reducing the risk of fracture is looking at ways to prevent or least mitigate risk of falls by working on balance and posture. This is the essence of the information provided in the excellent resource provided by the Royal Osteoporosis Society "Strong, Straight, Steady"[36]. The "strong" aspect covers activity and exercise modalities to maintain and promote bone health. "Straight" refers to maintaining good posture by engaging the back muscles.

Most of everyday life involves forward flexion of the spine: sitting leaning slightly forward over a computer, eating food, riding a bike. Vertebral wedge compression fractures exaggerate this forward flexed posture. To counteract this, engaging the back muscles encourages back extension, in other words a straight, more upright posture. This facilitates easier breathing and contributes to better balance with the centre of gravity of the (heavy) head and skull, over the base of support.

"Steady" encompasses the balance element of reducing fracture risk. With increasing years, balance, reaction time and proprioception (awareness of where your body is in space) can be challenged. Blood pressure control may not be optimal anymore and some conditions like Parkinson's disease cause issues with balance. Medications, including those used to treat hypertension and Parkinson's can also contribute themselves to unsteadiness. So simple exercises to re-equilibrate balance control can be helpful, especially when combined with the strong and straight elements for reducing fragility fracture risk.

In summary, bone health is another important aspect that is dependent on the action of hormone networks. Harnessing hormones, through positive lifestyle choices, helps support good bone health throughout life.

## Strategies for bone health

### Exercise

- Take regular weight-bearing and strength exercise to mechanically support bone health

### Nutrition

- Ensure a diet with sufficient energy for personal requirements to avoid situations of low energy availability which negatively impact hormones and bone health
- Include adequate protein and calcium dietary intake

### Other considerations

- Ensure vitamin D supplementation, at very least over winter, for those living in northern/southern latitudes where there is less sun
- Limit intake of drinks and activities known to impair bone health, such as caffeine, alcohol and smoking

# Scene 8
## Mind the Gut

*"Let food be thy medicine and medicine be thy food."*

*Hippocrates*

**Subtitle:** Hormone networks influence many aspects of brain function, including behaviours and emotional well-being, reflected in mental health. Hormones are also involved in the function of the gastrointestinal system and energy homeostasis, as part of physical health. There is a bidirectional interaction between the gut and brain, mediated largely by neuroendocrine interactions. The influence of the gut microbiome is emerging as a key player in the gut-brain axis, impacting many physiological processes. This supports Hippocrates' view that food and the gut are major determinants of mental and physical health and disease. He had recognised the gut-brain-body axis.

## Endocrine and mind interactions

Hormone networks are crucial to brain function and mental health. Mental health includes cognition, behaviour and emotional well-being. Mental health has an interactive effect on how we handle life stresses, our relationships and our physical health. The communication between hormones and the mind starts in utero, where the hormonal milieu affects neurodevelopment. Puberty is another time when fluctuations in hormones produce significant behavioural transformations, in addition to physical change and development. Later in life at menopause, dramatic adjustments in female hormones, particularly the drop in ovarian hormones, the protagonist being oestradiol, can have a significant impact on mental health. For example, in menopause, issues manifest as anxiety and low mood, together with labile emotions and "brain fog" reflecting some cognitive impairment, especially short-term memory.

Areas of the brain can be identified as having a particular specialised function such as cognition, motor and sensory control, memory storage and the seat of emotion. However, the same system of communication exists throughout the brain via nerve cells, neurons. Messaging between neurons is achieved via neurotransmitters that act as very short-range hormones. Neuronal connectivity, mediated by neurotransmitters, is important for mental health. Treatments for psychological conditions, such as depression, include medication that boosts neurotransmitters. For example, selective serotonin reuptake inhibitors (SSRIs) limit the reabsorption of the neurotransmitter, serotonin, leaving more of this messenger molecule available to facilitate neuronal crosstalk, thereby improving symptoms of depression.

In the endocrine hierarchy of control, systemic hormones, circulating in the bloodstream, influence our mental health in terms of mood and emotion. The psychological sequelae of endocrine disease states are well documented. For example, in Cushing's syndrome, characterised by an overproduction of cortisol by the adrenal glands, elevated cortisol levels lacking in diurnal variation are associated with depression. The symptoms of hyperparathyroidism, where there is an overproduction of parathyroid hormone, are summarised in the medical student mnemonic as "painful bones, renal stones, abdominal groans and psychiatric moans". Many endocrine conditions have both physical and mental effects.

*"If you are in a bad mood go for a walk.*
*If you are still in a bad mood, go for another walk."*

*Hippocrates*

Hippocrates recognised the link between mood and behaviour, in this case the behaviour being exercise. However, he was not aware that hormones provide the link between physical activity and the mind. The neuroendocrine hormone control centre, which includes the hypothalamus and pituitary, is located deep in brain, where it is ideally situated to receive and process both internal and external signals. This provides the mechanism for the fascinating connection between mental and hormone health.

Furthermore, how you think directly impacts your hormones. In our study of female dancers, those who were anxious about missing exercise training and reported anxiety about controlling food, body weight and shape experienced more menstrual disruption than their more relaxed counterparts[1]. An emotional "drive for thinness" has been found to be linked with a reduction of thyroid hormone triiodothyronine (T3) and menstrual hormone disruption[2]. Similarly in men, cognitive (intentional) restraint of eating has been associated with hormone signs of low energy availability[3].

There is a reciprocal relationship between behaviours and hormones. Although Hippocrates advocates going for several walks to improve mood, excessive exercise has a negative effect on mental health. This is the consequence of hormones attempting to bring the body back into equilibrium. Exercise dependence, also known as exercise addiction, is where an obsession with sticking rigidly to an exercise schedule negatively impacts mental health[4]. If high levels of exercise are not matched by sufficient energy intake, this results in low energy availability. This, in turn, causes downregulation of thyroid and reproductive hormone axes and upregulation of stress hormones such as cortisol, in an attempt to maintain energy homeostasis. This disruption of hormone networks has adverse psychological effects[5]. For example, women in low energy availability can experience menstrual hormone disruption, with consequential psychological effects, such as low mood and possible withdrawal from social interaction. This is thought to be due to reductions of both oestradiol and the brain neurotransmitter, serotonin. The topic of relative energy deficiency in sport (RED-S) is discussed in further detail in "Scene 10: In the Red". Suffice to say that an imbalance in behaviours, for whatever reason, has an adverse knock-on effect on hormone health and consequently on mental health.

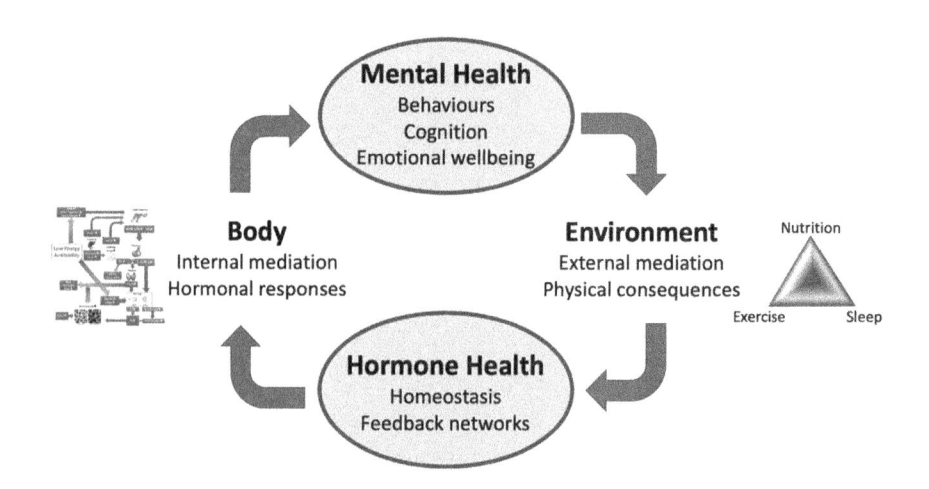

**Figure 8.1:** Mental-hormone health

Figure 8.1 summarises the interactions between hormones and mental health. Hormone networks maintain internal homeostasis and respond to external challenges. Hormones signal to the brain, influencing cognition, emotional well-being and behaviours. This alters the ways we interact with our environment, in terms of our decisions to take exercise, our choice of food and ensuring we have sufficient sleep. The physical consequences of our behaviours influence our internal hormone networks, which complete the feedback loop by affecting mental health.

## Food for thought

How do hormones influence eating patterns to maintain internal energy homeostasis? This balancing act is achieved by two-way neuroendocrine communication between the hypothalamic/pituitary complex in the brain and the peripheral hormone-producing tissues of the gut and adipose tissue.

Looking in the detail at this interaction between hormones and behaviour reveals one of the largest endocrine systems in the body. The enteroendocrine cells, located in the gut, secrete hormones, including cholecystokinin (CCK), glucagon-like peptide-1 (GLP-1), oxyntomodulin and peptide YY (PYY). Among these, PYY is an anorexigenic hormone (a signal to stop eating) that is secreted by the small intestine in response to calorie intake. PYY acts on the hypothalamus to halt feeding behaviour. Obese individuals tend to secrete less PYY, so are more likely to continue eating. The counterpart to PYY is ghrelin, the "hungry hormone", which is an orexigenic peptide (promoting eating behaviour). Ghrelin, secreted by the stomach, acts on the hypothalamus to direct our behaviour to seek out food.

The adipokines form another group of hormones that interact with the hypothalamic-pituitary axis to control eating behaviours and regulate energy status. The adipo- prefix indicates the origin of these hormones: adipose tissue (fat). Discovered in 1994, leptin is an anorexigenic hormone which signals the hypothalamus to stop eating. Leptin shows a diurnal pattern of release to regulate eating patterns. If there is a fault in leptin production, or the brain is insensitive to leptin, the lack of a signal to stop eating can be a cause of obesity. In those with low body fat, such as some athletes, a shortage of adipose tissue causes leptin levels to be continuously low. However, these individuals may be intentionally or unintentionally restricting food intake, leaving them less dependent on a hormonal signal to stop eating. Continuously low leptin acts as a signal to "save energy". This includes hypothalamic suppression of female hormones in women, resulting in menstrual disruption[6]. Other actions of low leptin with sustained, cumulative low energy intake include a downregulation of the thyroid hormone axis at the hypothalamic level to lower metabolic rate[7].

Adiponectin is another anorexigenic hormone derived from adipose tissue. Like leptin, this adipokine influences the hypothalamic-pituitary axis. The gut is also a source of precursor molecules for brain neurotransmitters, such as serotonin, which influence behaviour and emotion.

Cardiovascular disease reduces the quality of life and is a major cause of death. The importance of hormones in regulating energy homeostasis was demonstrated in a large study investigating the possible origin of risk factors emerging in childhood, linked with eating behaviours and weight control. Levels of adiponectin and leptin, reflecting energy status, were linked to heart rate variability, which is an indicator of cardiovascular health[8].

## The gut microbiome

You may be wondering why a book about hormones should discuss micro-organisms in the gut. It turns out that microbes use our hormones to influence both physical and mental health.

In the past, the mention of micro-organisms in the gut has tended to have negative associations with problems like infective gastroenteritis. However, improved understanding of the gut microbiome has highlighted the numerous "good" gut microbes that have beneficial effects on many aspects of health, such as regulation of energy metabolism, immunity and inflammation[9]. Conversely, a scarcity of "good" gut microbes can lead to diseases such as obesity, diabetes mellitus, autoimmune and cardiovascular disease[10]. Somewhat surprisingly, gut micro-organisms also affect appetite and eating behaviours. How can gut micro-organisms have such a powerful influence on our physical and mental health?

Microbiota is the term used to describe a community of micro-organisms. The microbiome is the sum of the genetic material of all the microbes in a particular environment. The microbiome in a human outnumbers the human genome. However, it is the metabolites that the gut microbiota produce (metabolome) that influence the health of the individual.

Gut microbiota ferment dietary fibre in the colon, producing short-chain fatty acid (SCFA) metabolites, including butyrate, acetate and propionate. Butyrate has an important local effect in causing cell death (apoptosis) of colon cancer cells and providing an energy source to maintain good proportions of health-promoting microbiota. Propionate and acetate are transported away in the bloodstream to act on other tissues and organs.

The "hot line" from the gut to the liver is the hepatic portal vein. From here the combination of absorbed food molecules and gut microbiome metabolites can exert systemic effects on health through a variety of mechanisms. This can be mediated via the enteroendocrine system, described below. Epigenetic effects influence DNA expression and the production of proteins, without changing the structure of DNA. This is a mechanism by which the microbiome can direct the production of proteins, playing roles in hormone production, immune regulation, metabolism and brain function[11].

Furthermore, the diurnal rhythmic movement of the gut microbiota has been shown to regulate the circadian epigenetic, transcriptional and metabolite oscillations of the "host"[12]. This adds another level of biological time keeping: a microbiome biochronometer that could impact "host" physiology, disease susceptibility and potential response to medications.

## Hormone gut-brain axis

The gut-brain axis describes a two-way communication channel, mediated by the neuroendocrine system. The combined effects of the nervous and endocrine systems influence our behaviours and mental and physical health.

Metabolites of gut microbiota (the gut metabolome) have an impact on local hormone production, such as serotonin which has short-range, paracrine effects and potentially longer-range effects on brain neurotransmitters. The influence of the gut metabolome on the hormone secretion of the enteroendocrine cells provides the established mechanism of hormone gut-brain communication[13]. Evidence for the gut microbiome influencing the gut-brain hormone axis comes from obese individuals treated with bariatric surgery. Part of the gut is removed which reduces the amount of gut available for absorption of digested food and impacts the gut hormones that control appetite in the brain and subsequent feeding behaviours. Furthermore, there is some evidence that weight loss following this procedure may be mediated through a change in the gut microbiome[14].

The prenatal and post-natal period offer a window of opportunity in neurodevelopment for the foetus and baby. This is discussed in detail in Act 2, Scene 1. Emerging evidence suggests that maternal and environmental factors impacting the offspring's gut can influence the development of the brain. Transfer of hormones and metabolites from mother to foetus occurs via the placenta. The mode of birth and feeding are routes of transfer of the microbiome from mother to baby, especially in the case of vaginal birth and breastfeeding. Early breast milk, colostrum, impacts the immune gut health of the baby and some studies have reported a higher intellectual quotient in breast-fed children[15].

Figure 8.2 shows how the food molecules and gut metabolome can influence the brain via hormones of the enteroendocrine system, which in turn regulates brain neuroendocrine signals directing feeding behaviours.

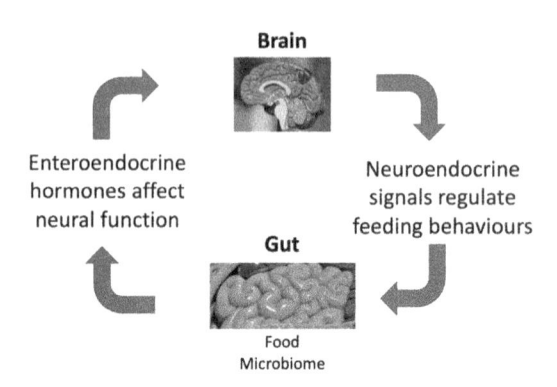

**Figure 8.2:** Gut-brain hormone axis

## "Gut feeling"

The neuroendocrine system maintains energy homeostasis by modulating metabolism through insulin sensitivity and lipid usage. Metabolic flexibility, the ability to change the use of fuel sources according to demand, is advantageous in matching external and internal stimuli. This adaptive ability is mediated via hormone networks[16]. Furthermore, hormones are the protagonists in central appetite regulation. The "gut feelings" relating to eating behaviours could be better described as "hormone feelings".

A key aspect of metabolism is the conversion of energy from food into internal energy to support physiological processes. This occurs in the mitochondria, the "powerhouse" organelles found in cells throughout the body. Emerging evidence shows that the gut metabolome influences both the effectiveness of energy production by mitochondria and the output of potentially harmful by-products like reactive oxygen species (ROS). In turn, the mitochondria modulate the effects of gut microbiota on gut immune function. This crosstalk between gut microbiota and mitochondria is achieved by a variety of short-range hormones[17]. Figure 8.3 illustrates this bidirectional mode of communication via messenger molecules.

*Scene 8: Mind the Gut*

**Mitochondria**

Metabolites

Regulatory factors

**Microbiota**

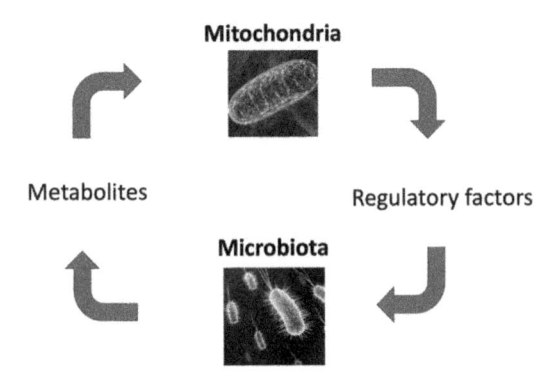

**Figure 8.3:** Interactive feedback: gut microbiota and mitochondria

Athletes have been found to have particularly healthy gut microbiota, which support effective energy production[18]. It remains uncertain whether this is a consequence of an athlete's exercise and diet or whether a healthy gut microbiome helps you become a good athlete. Nevertheless, however you arrive there, having an "athletic" microbiome is good news for health and performance.

On the other hand, some endurance athletes are known to be prone to a "leaky gut". When exercising, the body diverts blood away from the gut, preferentially to meet the demand of the muscles. On stopping exercise, the return of blood flow to the gut can cause a reperfusion injury resulting in a "leaky gut". The cells lining the intestinal tube form a very tight seal that controls absorption into the bloodstream. It acts as a screening system, allowing passage of digested food of certain molecular types and sizes, while keeping out molecules or micro-organisms that could cause harm. If the tight junctions between the gut lining cells lose their integrity, the permeability of the gut wall changes, allowing unwanted microbiota and molecules to move out of the gut. This can cause gut microbiota dysbiosis: an imbalance in healthy/less healthy gut microbiota. The net effect is compromised absorption of required nutrients and initiation of local and systemic inflammatory responses. Although some degree of inflammatory response to exercise helps beneficial hormone-driven adaptations to exercise, excessive systemic inflammatory response is counterproductive[19]. The consequences of these changes in gut wall permeability and gut microbiota dysbiosis can not only disrupt effective hormone-driven adaptation to exercise[20] but have a further negative impact on health and contribute to disease states.

*"All disease begins in the gut."*

*Hippocrates*

Identical twins sharing the same DNA and brought up in the same environment would be expected to show similar disease patterns. However, this is not the case. Research has sought to explain these discrepancies by studying the role of the gut microbiome, which carries its own source of genetic material. It turns out that the diversity of the gut microbiome is a better disease predictor and indeed a better indicator of developing autoimmune conditions (such as inflammatory bowel disease and rheumatoid arthritis) and metabolic conditions (such as obesity and diabetes mellitus) than our own DNA.

### *Autoimmune disease*

Autoimmune disease results from an overactive immune system. The immune system effectively turns against its own host, causing damage to tissues. Autoimmune damage to gut tissues causes inflammatory bowel disease. Autoimmune activity against the beta cells of the Islets of Langerhans in the pancreas results in low insulin production and type 1 diabetes (T1D). Autoimmune harm to synovium lining joints causes rheumatoid arthritis. The problem with any autoimmune disease goes beyond the damage done to a particular tissue. The increased level of inflammation has a knock-on effect on other aspects of health, both physical and mental. For example, elevated systemic inflammation leads to an increased risk of cardiovascular disease and reduced healthy life expectancy.

There is a genetic propensity to autoimmune disease. However, the trigger could come from the gut microbiome. There is increasing evidence that gut microbes have a dynamic interaction with the immune system[21], through a variety of mechanisms. For example, "good" gut microbiota can exert a beneficial regulatory role on "rogue" immune responses. This may involve the gut version of the hormone serotonin, which has an immune regulatory role as well as a link with the gut microbiota. Tantalisingly, serotonin is also a brain neurotransmitter and low levels are known to cause low mood, often associated with chronic autoimmune disease[11]. On the other hand, "bad" gut microbiota can stir up an inflammatory response. "Leaky gut" and the consequences on gut microbiota balance and inflammation have been described as a potential contributing factor in the development of autoimmune diseases[22].

The crosstalk between the gut microbiome and immune function also has therapeutic implications. Improving the health of the gut microbiome may help as an adjunct to disease modifying medication and improve the response.

## *Cardiometabolic disease*

Cardiometabolic disease includes cardiovascular disease and insulin resistance associated with poor blood glucose control. Disrupted metabolism and inflammation are intertwined as underlying aetiological factors. Lack of gut microbiome diversity has been reported in obesity, which stirs up systemic inflammation[11] Exercise in obese children has been shown to improve gut microbiota and inflammatory signalling[23]. Gut dysbiosis has been implicated in other associated maladies, such as non-alcoholic fatty liver disease, chronic kidney disease and endocrine dysfunction including thyroid networks, polycystic ovarian syndrome (PCOS) and growth hormone deficiency[24].

# Feeding the mind and gut

An important starting point in seeking to improve gut health is to consider what you eat as well as your eating patterns. I have avoided using the word "diet" because this can be misconstrued to mean a restrictive way of eating over a short period of time, often with the objective of weight loss. More correctly, a diet should provide nutrition, for life.

Popular restrictive "diets" such as strict vegan diets, raw food or "clean eating" diets can have adverse effects on gut health. Although plants-based foods provide many beneficial effects for supporting a healthy gut microbiome, restrictive diets do not appear to provide additional health benefits. For example, after accounting for confounding healthy lifestyle factors apart from diet, a large Australian study of men and women found no additional health benefit on mortality in those following diets restricted to certain food types[25]. Some types of restrictive diet are prescribed by doctors to treat medical conditions. For example, gluten-free diets are used to treat the relatively rare autoimmune gut condition of coeliac disease and the low FODMAP (fermentable oligosaccharides, disaccharides, monosaccharides and polyols) diet is used to alleviate the symptoms of irritable bowel syndrome. Nevertheless, following these types of restrictive diet when a medical condition is not present has been shown to have more of a negative than positive effect on health by reducing microbiome diversity[10].

Consistent eating patterns are needed to provide sufficient energy, with a range of food types and covering essential micronutrients, vitamins and minerals. Your diet needs to meet your personal requirements to nourish your hormones and consequently your mind and gut.

A diet "for life" is one that supports all aspects of health, including mental health over your lifespan[26]. Micronutrients should not be overlooked, for example, the vitamin B family plays an important role in neurological function and mental health. Lack of thiamine (vitamin B1) causes the brain disorder, Wernicke–Korsakoff syndrome. Low thiamine can result from excessive alcohol intake or other causes of malnutrition/malabsorption, resulting in damage to certain areas in the brain. This can present as Wernicke's encephalopathy where the patient is confused, unsteady and has eye movement problems. As a young hospital doctor, I remember injecting a sticky, yellow substance containing thiamine into patients presenting like this. Prompt treatment is important to prevent progression to Korsakoff's syndrome where there is more permanent damage to the brain, associated with memory loss. Typically, the patient can remember what happened 20 years ago, but not what they ate for breakfast. There is a tendency to confabulate. For example, a patient in hospital reporting having a marvellous silver service breakfast with smoked salmon and quails' eggs would elicit a high index of suspicion of confabulation.

Vitamin D affects well-being. It is unique among vitamins, being a steroid hormone, whose main source is the action of sunlight on skin. Like other hormones, vitamin D acts by influencing gene expression[27].

Many highly processed foods contain synthetic additives to make them palatable after the flavours and benefits of the ingredients have been destroyed during manufacture. Limiting the consumption of highly processed foods helps minimise the intake of synthetic molecules that can potentially disrupt both hormones and the gut microbiome. For example, artificial sweeteners are linked to an overgrowth of more harmful gut microbiota and increased insulin resistance[28]. Ironically, these synthetic molecules, consumed with the aim of controlling weight, might actually have the opposite effect.

## The constant gardener

There are some general principles in feeding the gut microbiota to ensure a healthy gut-brain-body hormone axis. Promoting the diversity of the gut microbiota is a bit like gardening. Examples of each food type are provided below.

The first step is to prepare the gut by eating prebiotic fibrous food. These can be divided into two types of plant-based food: those that the gut microbiota cannot ferment and those it can. The cellulose, found in the cell walls of plants, cannot be fermented, but it helps to keep the gut moving. This prevents the slow transit of digested food, which may encourage "unfriendly" gut microbiota to proliferate.

Fermentable fibrous foods provide fuel for the "friendly" gut microbiota[29]. There is some truth in the saying "an apple a day keeps the doctor away", as apples contain pectin which is a fermentable type of carbohydrate. Long-chain inulin, found in a diversity of fibrous foods, such as wheat, onion and bananas, is particularly effective as a prebiotic. The long-chain makes it more likely to remain reasonably intact until it reaches the colon, the lower part of the gut, where the majority of the good gut microbiota reside. The downside of some of these fibrous foods is that fermentation produces by-products in the form of methane and even alcohol.

Once you have prepared your gut with prebiotics, you can proceed to "fertilisation" of the gut microbiota with probiotics found in fermented foods. Duplibiotic is a term that has been suggested for dietary elements high in polyphenols, which appear to act as both prebiotic and probiotic. These may prevent gut dysbiosis and have been linked to a reduced risk of markers for cardiometabolic disease[30].

> Prebiotic foods: non-fermentable fibre of cellulose, for example, bran and dark-green leafy vegetables and fermentable fibre found in fruit and vegetables, for example, garlic, onion, leeks, chickpeas, beans, lentils, artichoke and asparagus
> Probiotic foods: sourdough bread, yogurt, kefir (similar to yogurt), sauerkraut, kimchi (Korean fermented vegetables), tempeh and miso (fermented soya products) and kombucha (fermented teas)
> Duplibiotic foods with polyphenols: berries, green tea, coffee, black tea, red wine, dark chocolate and apples

## Gut-brain-body hormone axis

*"Let food be thy medicine and medicine be thy food."*

*Hippocrates*

Including a variety of plant nutrients (phytonutrients) and fibre types in your diet, "eating the rainbow", promotes the diversity of the gut microbiota. A diverse gut microbiome supports the production of short-chain fatty acids, which have far-reaching influences on epigenetic regulation and the healthy function of many organs and systems in the body, often mediated by hormones. This feedback network is shown in Figure 8.4.

Your diet determines the diversity of your gut microbiome. The gut microbes have a local effect on gut health, ensuring the integrity of the selective intestinal barrier and maintaining appropriate levels of immune and inflammation activities. This is mediated by short-range metabolites and hormones.

The systemic effects of diet and the gut microbiome are often mediated by longer-range hormones. For example, food and the gut microbiome influence gut hormones and hormones, such as insulin, which regulate metabolism and body weight control. Regulation of systemic immune and inflammatory responses through these pathways contributes to overall cardiometabolic health. There is also evidence that the diet and gut microbiome are factors in kidney and musculoskeletal health and the endocrine system itself.

Aside from the interplay with physical health, the diet and gut microbiome play roles in mental health via the bidirectional gut-brain axis. In particular, the diet and gut microbiome impact our neurobehavioral traits, specifically our feeding behaviours, which brings us back full circle to diet.

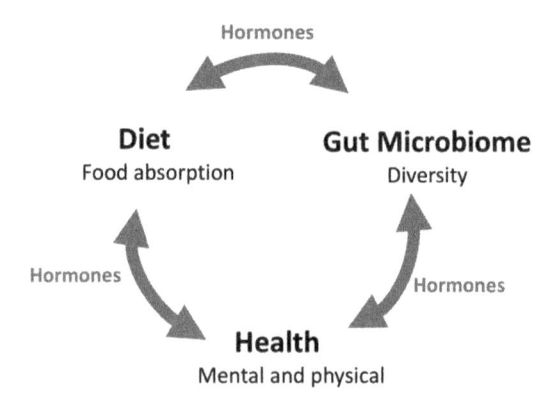

**Figure 8.4:** Diet-gut-health triad

Ultimately a personalised approach to nutrition is best for brain-gut-body health[31] bearing in mind Hippocrates' comment that *"Let food be thy medicine and medicine be thy food"*.

# Strategies for healthy gut-brain-body hormone axis

## *Nutrition*

- Adopt eating patterns that provide sufficient energy and a range of food types and micronutrients
- Avoid highly processed foods
- Avoid very restrictive diets that are limited in energy intake and/or food types
- Aim to maintain good intake of prebiotic foods
- Aim to maintain good intake of probiotic foods

## *Other considerations*

- Avoid, unless absolutely necessary, medications that adversely impact gut microbiome diversity (e.g. antibiotics and proton pump inhibitors)

# Scene 9
# A Balancing Act

> *"All parts of the body which have a function, if used in moderation and exercised in labours in which each is accustomed, become thereby healthy, well developed and age more slowly, but if unused they become liable to disease, defective in growth and age quickly."*
>
> *Hippocrates*

**Subtitle:** Balancing exercise, nutrition and recovery optimises hormone health. Conversely, imbalances in these behaviours can compromise hormone health. Hormone dysfunction can arise as a result of mistiming between external behaviours and internal biological clocks: circadian misalignment. This mistiming, together with a sedentary lifestyle, can lead to metabolic syndrome. Although exercise is beneficial for hormone health, too much of a good thing can be problematic. Exercise, with insufficient recovery time, can lead to maladaptation over different time scales from shorter-term non-functional overreaching (NFOR) to overtraining syndrome (OTS) in the longer term. Psychological dependence on exercise can have adverse health effects.

Hippocrates sums up the situation of balanced behaviours favouring good health very succinctly. As discussed in Act 1, "Scene 3: Harnessing Hormones", balancing exercise, nutrition and recovery favours optimal hormone function and responsiveness. Exercise causes a certain level of "stress" and inflammation, which act as a trigger to stimulating hormone responses. These include setting in motion anabolic pathways to gain the adaptive benefits of exercise across the body with improvement in metabolic, cardiovascular, musculoskeletal and mental health. This in turn supports reaching your personal full potential. This is the internal biological mechanism by which your lifestyle choices impact your health. The triangular interaction between lifestyle choices and health is shown in Figure 9.1.

*Scene 9: A Balancing Act*

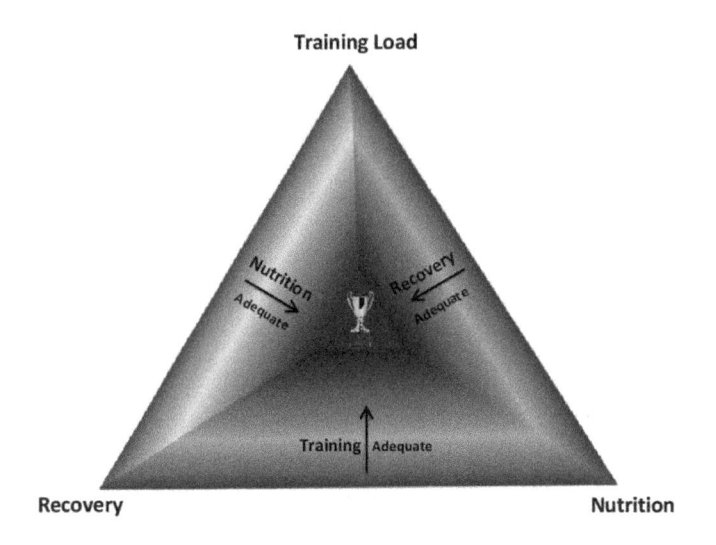

**Figure 9.1:** Behavioural triumvirate of health

However, what happens when behaviours become unbalanced? What are the consequences in terms of hormone dysfunction and effects on health?

## Circadian misalignment

Circadian alignment describes the synchronisation of sleep, eating patterns and physical activity with internal biological clocks. As discussed in Act 1, "Scene 4: It's all in the Timing", misalignment of external behaviours and internal pacemakers can lead to endocrine network dysfunction and numerous consequential health problems[1].

In a large international study, long working hours were found to increase the risk of cardiovascular disease and cerebrovascular disease, stroke[2]. Long working hours, regardless of age, trigger physiological responses, including the activation of hormonal stress pathways. Furthermore, less time remains available for behaviours favourable for circadian alignment and health, in terms of nutrition, exercise and sleep. Rather there may be a tendency towards unhealthy behaviours such as smoking, drinking alcohol, inactivity, unhealthy eating behaviours and reduced sleep.

Unbalanced lifestyle choices, such as poor sleep, overeating and a sedentary lifestyle, can become a self-perpetuating vicious cycle. This cumulative disruption of the endocrine system has adverse health consequences. Metabolic syndrome[3] includes a constellation of outcomes: weight control issues leading to abdominal obesity, insulin resistance and ultimately type 2 diabetes mellitus. Other complications include raised blood pressure, adverse lipid profile, inflammatory state and non-alcoholic fatty liver disease which are all recognised risk factors for cardiovascular and cerebrovascular disease. Optimising lifestyle choices is important in both prevention and management.

## Too much of a good thing?

Hippocrates warned against too little exercise, but can too much of a good thing be a problem for our hormones and our health? After all, physical exercise is effective in supporting health and well-being, by challenging the endocrine networks to be responsive. We exercise in the hope and expectation that our hormones will drive the adaptive changes we seek to become citius, altius, fortius. Or at the very least, we aim to support our overall physical and mental well-being.

## How much exercise?

In the ideal scenario, exercise elicits a hormone response that drives positive adaptation resulting in increased fitness, known as supercompensation. All forms of exercise put the body under stress, to a greater or lesser degree. This causes the hormones to respond, but it is not until exercise ceases that they work their magic. You become fitter when you are resting, after exercise.

For this sequence of events to result in positive change, you need to provide just the right amount of training stimulus and just the right amount of recovery in terms of rest, sleep and nutrition. Supercompensation describes the body's ability to rebound to a higher level of fitness than the previous base line, so that when you next exercise you are on the next step upwards on the path to improved fitness. The exact recipe of how much exercise and recovery depends on your starting point in terms of fitness and age. The process of supercompensation is shown in Figure 9.2.

*Scene 9: A Balancing Act*

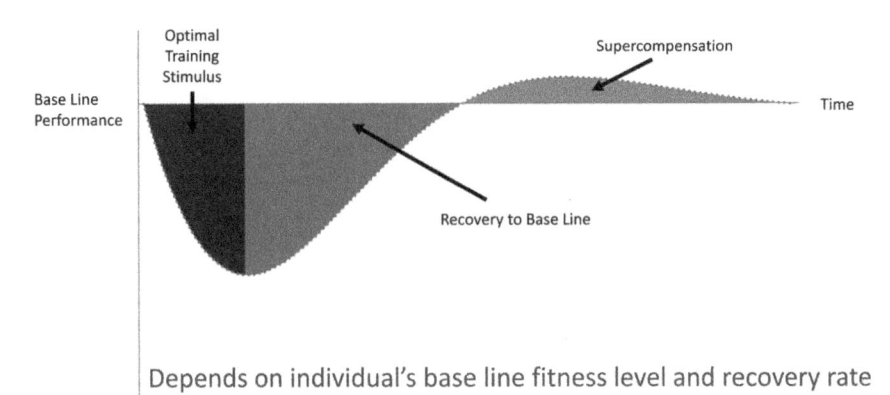

**Figure 9.2:** Optimal training stimulus

This may appear straightforward: exercise, recover and repeat. However, the first challenge is determining how much training stimulus and how long a recovery you need to gain maximal positive adaptations. Too little training stimulus with too much recovery means you won't gain the benefits of exercise. For example, exercising once a week at a very easy level for your age and ability might maintain a degree of fitness, but it is unlikely to improve. The hormonal response is insufficient to cause supercompensation, as shown in Figure 9.3.

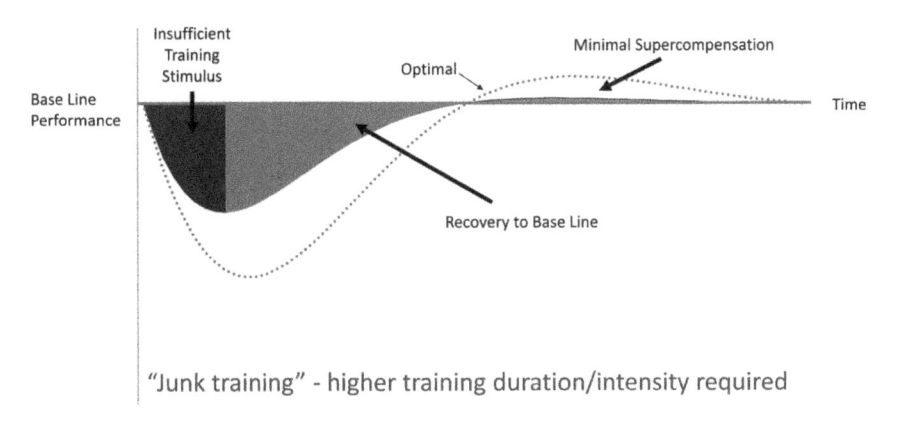

**Figure 9.3:** Insufficient training stimulus

On the other hand, training excessively, with insufficient recovery for your age and ability, also means you cannot gain the full benefits of exercise. The full hormonal response is required simply to return to base line fitness, as shown in Figure 9.4.

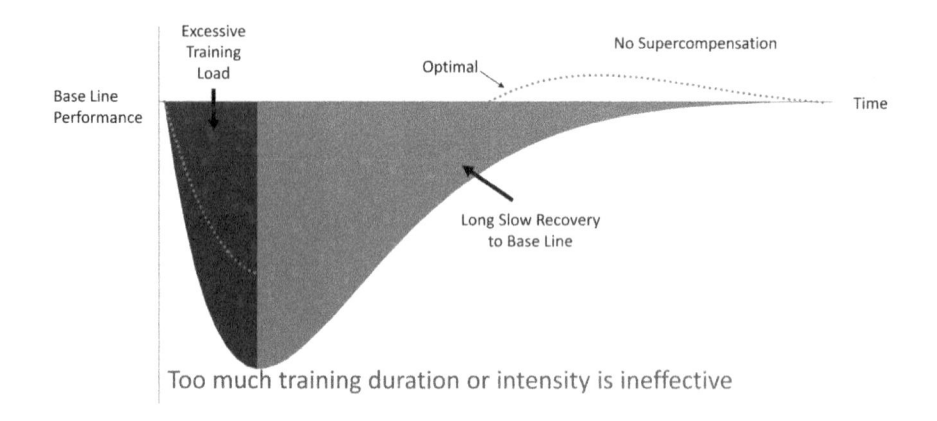

**Figure 9.4:** Excessive training load

## How much recovery?

The next challenge comes when considering recovery after exercise. Why is recovery such a crucial component of getting fitter and not simply an optional extra? The period of rest and recovery, in particular during sleep, is when your hormones spring into action to drive positive adaptive changes. To benefit from exercise, you need to rest afterwards, just the right amount to match the amount of exercise you have done.

## Getting the timing right

Furthermore, you need to time your next exercise session for when you are fully recovered and, ideally, in a peak supercompensated state. If you try to exercise again before you have fully recovered, or wait too long, you do not gain the full benefit from your physical activity. This key timing that harmonises exercise and recovery is known as periodisation.

Periodisation can be considered over a range of time scales: over a week, a month or over a year and beyond. After successive hard training days, an athlete should take a rest day. A coach would typically include one lighter week in a monthly training block, often timed as to allow supercompensation to peak at the season's target events.

Periodisation, over all time scales, varies according to the individual and their objectives, so it is a question of getting to know your own body. A guide to the ideal timing of periodisation is shown in Figure 9.5. The zone on the far left, represents the stress imposed on the body by exercise or training, which is the product of duration and intensity. The central zone shows the process of recovery has begun, but training again during this period is suboptimal, because it does not give the body enough time to recover back to base line. The best timing for the next training session or for competition is the peak of the zone on the right, when the body has achieved the maximum state of supercompensation.

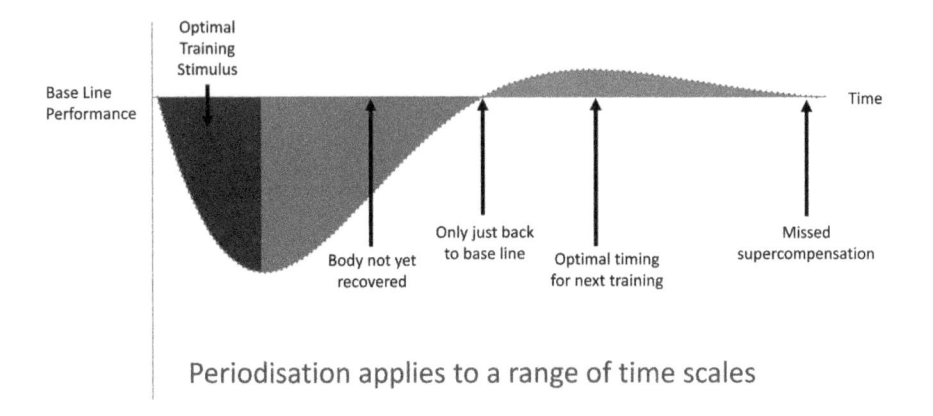

**Figure 9.5:** Periodisation

## Long-term balance

If you are successful in periodisation of the amount and timing of exercise and recovery, you benefit from cumulative supercompensation. Harmonising the amount and timing of exercise with optimal recovery favours the internal responsiveness and action of anabolic hormones, such as the sex steroids (testosterone, oestrogen and progesterone) and insulin-like growth factor 1 (IGF-1). Concurrently, as long as this process of adaptation does not cause excessive internal stress, the physiological diurnal variation of cortisol is not disrupted. Over time your health and fitness improve, and you gain the full health benefits of exercise. Figure 9.6 shows the beneficial process of cumulative, stepwise, positive adaptation, driven by an effective anabolic hormone response, known as functional overreaching (FOR)[4].

*Hormones, Health and Human Potential*

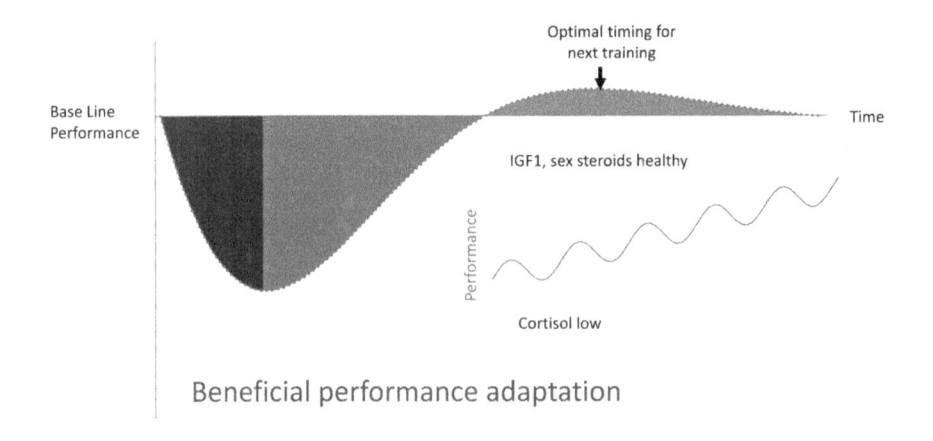

**Figure 9.6:** Functional overreaching (FOR)

On the other hand, poor periodisation of training and recovery can lead to the situation of non-functional overreaching (NFOR). An imbalance or mistiming of exercise and recovery can impair the beneficial adaptive response. In practical terms, this results in the stagnation in performance shown in Figure 9.7. Hormonal warning signs that the body is feeling the strain may be seen in reduced diurnal variation of cortisol and lower than expected levels of sex steroids.

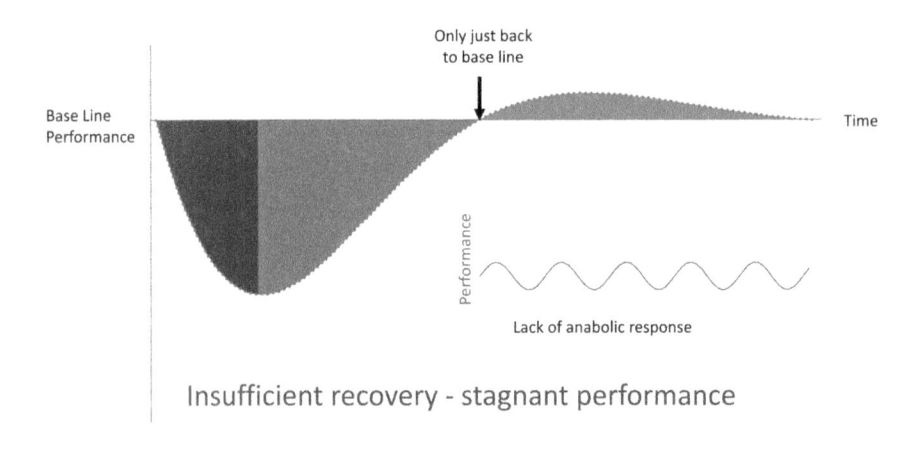

**Figure 9.7:** Non-functional overreaching (NFOR)

If an athlete or exerciser continues in this situation of NFOR over months, with insufficient recovery relative to training load, this can progress to overtraining syndrome (OTS) and deterioration in performance[4]. This is often accompanied by reduced levels of anabolic hormones and increased levels of stress-response hormones (eg. prolactin) and markers (CK creatinine kinase is the break down product of muscle). The consequences of continually exercising without sufficient recovery are apparent in Figure 9.8.

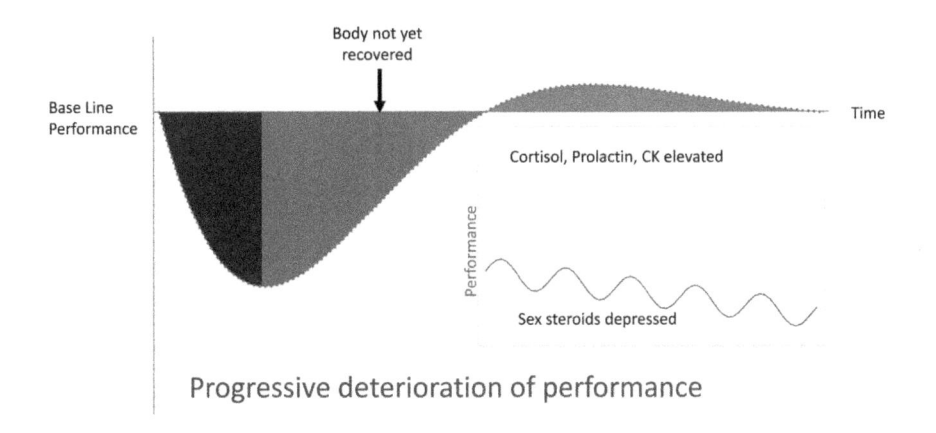

**Figure 9.8:** Overtraining syndrome (OTS)

The consequences of FOR, NFOR and OTS act over different time scales. Your performance level declines during hard exercise: you are unlikely to achieve a personal best over the last 100 metres of a tough cross-country run, but you might be able to do a quick sprint after a day or two of recovery. Repeatedly exercising with insufficient recovery over several days/weeks results in NFOR and a stagnation in performance. Potentially NFOR is a recoverable situation: all it requires is for the athlete to adapt training to include sufficient rest to return to a fully recovered state. However, those who progress to OTS by continuing to push on with exercise without sufficient recovery, month after month, may face a longer road to recovery. In other words, if you dig yourself into a deeper and deeper hole, it becomes increasingly harder to climb out[5]. These different time scales are shown in Figure 9.9.

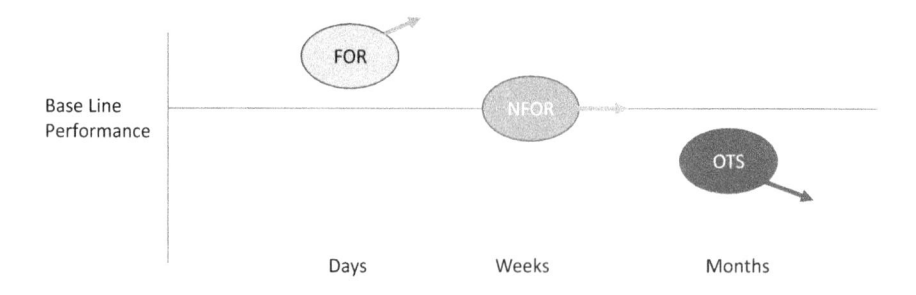

```
                    FOR
Base Line  ─────────────NFOR─────────────
Performance
                                    OTS

        Days        Weeks        Months
```

Time since last in a fully recovered state
Resolution dependent on duration of problem

**Figure 9.9:** Long-term consequences

## What are the candidate hormones to detect imbalances in behaviours?

In the short term, a good indicator of recovery state from training load in men is the testosterone (anabolic) to cortisol (catabolic) ratio[6]. The ratio of testosterone to cortisol has been reported to be of practical value in male soccer players[7]. A decrease in this ratio shows that full internal recovery from exercise has not yet occurred. In females, the equivalent outcome of increased internal stress levels in NFOR can reveal itself in subtle changes in menstrual cycle, such as subclinical ovulatory issues discussed previously (see Act 1, "Scene 5XX: Of Mice and Men . . . and Women"), which have health consequences[8]. Prolactin, another hormone that is sensitive to increased stressor levels, can be used to indicate NFOR[9].

Although the purpose of exercise is to produce some increase in stress levels to spur the endocrine system into actions that initiate adaptation, excessive exercise-induced "stress" can be detrimental to this process. High levels of microtrauma to tissues and systemic inflammation from high training loads can increase inflammatory markers, such as cytokines. So theoretically these could be used as markers of NFOR[10]. Insulin-like growth factor 1 (IGF-1) is an important hormone with anabolic effects. Exercise and sleep favour its production and drive adaptations[11]. So, measuring levels of IGF-1 can be an indicator of good balance between training load and recovery, conversely falling levels of this hormone could indicate NFOR.

Another approach to assess hormone responsiveness is in a dynamic test. A two-bout exercise hormone test has been shown to identify OTS. In those with OTS repeating an exercise test in short succession resulted in a lack of hormone response in terms of "the usual suspects" of growth hormone, prolactin, cortisol, ACTH (adrenocorticotrophic hormone) and testosterone[12]. Of particular note is that lack of response of ACTH, the control hormone for cortisol release from the adrenals. This indicates that the issue of overtraining causes downregulation from the top level of the hormone control system: the hypothalamus. Although these studies give important insights into the biological mechanisms by which imbalanced behaviours impact endocrine networks, the types of protocols employed are not practical outside of the research setting.

Another approach is to focus on other indicators of imbalances in behaviours that reflect underlying hormone dysregulation. For example, low mood is linked with hypothalamic-pituitary axis dysfunction and disrupted hormone networks in those with OTS[13].

## Heart rate variability

A different type of indicator of an impending disequilibrium between training load and rest could be the balance between the sympathetic and parasympathetic branches of the autonomic nervous system. The sympathetic branch is associated with "fight or flight" response, or a very hard training session. The parasympathetic branch is associated with "rest and digest", which predominates when you are resting or fully recovered from exercise.

Both these branches of the autonomic nervous system act on the rate of heart contraction. Specifically, the variability of your heart rate from beat to beat reflects the push and pull of autonomic nervous system. This is known as heart rate variability (HRV). High HRV reflects a good balance of sympathetic and parasympathetic input, in other words you have recovered from the previous exercise and you are ready to train again. On the other hand, low HRV would suggest that the sympathetic nervous system is winning against the parasympathetic and you are not fully recovered. Although this can be helpful in deciding whether you are ready to exercise again, it has been shown that HRV does not distinguish between FOR, NFOR and OTS[5]. Furthermore, HRV variability does not distinguish between "stress" from exercise or other things happening in your life, like meeting the deadline for writing a book. Combining all the indicators of well-being gives a more comprehensive picture[14].

## Not so fast!

You might think that is straightforward to assess if you are on the verge of NFOR. However, there are several caveats when it comes to detecting the warning signs of NFOR and OTS. The first consideration is that we are all individuals, and we respond to exercise in different ways. This could be partly down to other factors, such as poor nutrition adding "stress" to our physiological systems. The hypothalamus summates all sources of internal and external stressors in its regulation of hormone response and output. So, if you have an imbalance in training and recovery, this may well include insufficient nutrition for recovery. There is evidence of additive effects of NFOR and low carbohydrate intake in the downregulation of hormones in both males[15] and females[16]. We return shortly to the discussion of overtraining and underfuelling being different facets of imbalanced behaviours, resulting in similar patterns of endocrine dysfunction.

Ultimately, whatever combination of objective and subjective parameters are used to assess the optimal balance of exercise and recovery, it is important to bear in mind that NFOR and OTS are diagnoses of exclusion. In other words, you need to be certain that there is no underlying "medical" reason why you are feeling subpar and not getting the full benefits from exercise. For example, low-grade viral infections such as "glandular fever" Epstein Barr virus or other inflammatory or endocrine conditions per se may have a bearing.

If you think that too little recovery is only an issue for elite, professional athletes, then think again. Amateur athletes and exercisers have to fit in exercise around work and family commitments. Some underestimate energy expenditure by not considering walking or cycling to work to be "real" exercise training. This situation can erode recovery time and potentially lead to suboptimal benefits from exercise.

Making a schedule can be helpful, but if sticking to it rigidly becomes the overarching objective, with exercise as the priority, then this could be a warning sign of exercise dependence[17]. This is when you become anxious if you are not sticking precisely to the exercise plan you have set yourself. Your focus on exercise overrides social interactions and commitments. You feel obliged to exercise even if you are ill or injured. Being committed to an objective is laudable, but in the situation of exercise dependence, too much of a good thing can become unhealthy.

Figure 9.10 shows the two types of exercise dependence. Primary exercise addiction is when a person sticks rigidly to an exercise regime, without sufficient recovery, showing the characteristics of NFOR and OTS. Secondary exercise addiction is when, in addition to high levels of exercise, energy intake is intentionally restricted. This results in a situation of low energy availability and adverse effects on many hormones networks, encompassed in the clinical syndrome of relative energy deficiency in sports (RED-S) which will be discussed in detail in the next scene.

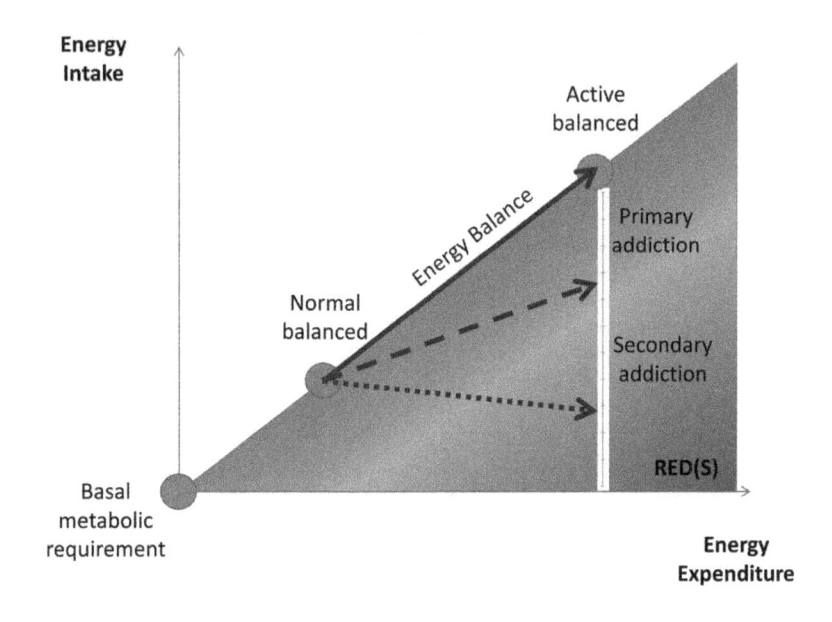

**Figure 9.10:** Exercise dependence and relative energy deficiency in sport (RED-S).*

## Conclusions

Hippocrates was correct that the "labours" of exercise are important for health. We now understand the key roles of hormone networks. Insufficient activity does not provide the required stimulus for positive adaptation. Conversely, excessive exercise, without sufficient nutrition and recovery for hormones to drive positive change, results in no advantage: a null outcome. Sustained excessive exercise relative to recovery can be detrimental to health.

# Strategies for balancing lifestyle choices for hormone health

## *Exercise*

- Regular exercise is important for hormone health. However, avoid the extremes of inactivity or excess exercise
- Ensure that you are sufficiently recovered before your next exercise session. This will help avoid the situations of non-functional overreaching (NFOR) and overtraining syndrome (OTS)
- Adaptable approach to exercise: don't exercise if you are fatigued, ill or injured. This will help avert developing exercise dependence

## *Nutrition*

- Try to match energy intake with energy expenditure

## *Sleep*

- Sleep is essential to gain the hormone-driven benefits of exercise.
- Good sleep patterns help avert circadian misalignment

# Scene 10
## In the Red

> *"Before you heal someone, ask him if he's willing to give up the things that make him sick."*
>
> *Hippocrates*

**Subtitle:** Imbalances in lifestyle behaviours can lead to hormone dysregulation. Mismatch between food intake and energy expenditure can result in a surplus or a deficiency of energy availability. Sustained low energy availability can lead to an adaptive, functional downregulation of hormone networks and consequent adverse effects on health. Originally described in the female athlete triad, low energy availability is now recognised to occur in males and females of all ages and all levels of exercise. Relative energy deficiency in sport (RED-S) describes the negative clinical health and performance consequences. We discuss the underlying causes, identification, consequences and restoration of hormone network function.

## Too little of a good thing?

Even when exercise and recovery are matched, inadequate nutrition can impact hormones and impair the positive adaptive responses to exercise in the long term. Although a tripod is a very stable structure, if you alter the height of any of the supports, things fall out of equilibrium.

When food intake is insufficient to meet the demands of exercise and health, hormonal dysfunction can ensue. First described in female athletes back in the 1990s, this is now recognised to be an increasing problem that can impact males and females of all ages and at all levels of exercise. If you take regular exercises, keep reading!

Returning to the triumvirate of behaviours shown in Figure 10.1, the optimal balance of exercise, recovery and nutrition is the central zone. It is possible to fall into the peripheral danger zone in two ways. An unhealthy excess of exercise, nutrition or recovery leads to one of the points in the triangle, whereas a deficiency in any of these three is described on the opposite edge. While insufficient exercise results in undertraining, insufficient recovery leads to non-functional overreaching and progression to over-training syndrome.

Our focus is on the third axis, where insufficient food intake for training load results in low energy availability. This issue tends to arise in the more athletic segment of the population, where a high level of performance is often a key objective.

We take a deep dive into a whole range of hormone networks that become disrupted, including the reproductive axis. These effects may have evolved to cope with famine conditions, illustrating how the interconnected elements of the endocrine system are the key link between the environment and internal health.

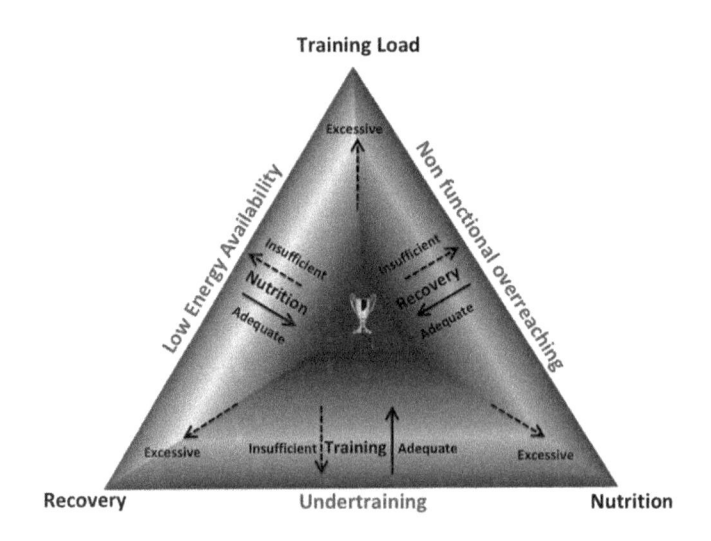

**Figure 10.1:** Behavioural triumvirate of imbalances

## Low energy availability

A minimum level of energy is required to power the basic metabolism that maintains life. This energy comes in the form of food. A variety of life processes require energy, including growth, reproduction, cellular respiration (conversion of food to energy), excretion, movement, reaction to stimuli and assimilation of food (digestion). Even lying totally still in bed all day requires a significant amount of energy. The housekeeping tasks of breathing, maintaining blood circulation and brain function all require energy. As mammals, we also need a fair bit of energy to maintain our internal body temperature. The resting metabolic rate measures the amount of energy required per day to maintain essential life processes, at rest.

Of all the life processes requiring energy, evolution has ensured that movement takes priority. Our ancestors needed to run away from sabre-tooth tigers. So the energy we derive from food is allocated first to the demands of movement. The residual energy is known as energy availability. To stay healthy, energy availability per day needs to equate to resting metabolic rate. Energy availability can be expressed in terms of kilocalories per kilogramme of fat-free mass per day. Fat-free mass includes muscle, bone and other systems like the gastrointestinal system, circulatory system and nervous system. The brain is one of the greedier, energy-demanding organs.

Figure 10.2 illustrates the concept of energy availability. The person in the centre is happy and healthy, as total energy intake matches total energy demand. Energy intake is prioritised to cover movement (training load), and the residual energy availability matches the needs of fundamental physiological life processes. The same person can become unbalanced in different ways. On the right, a higher training load has increased energy demand, but energy intake has been held at the same level, by eating the same amount as before. The result is a reduction in energy availability, below the level required to maintain health. On the left, the same person might be intentionally restricting what they eat, possibly in the belief that this might improve performance, while keeping the training load steady. Once again, energy availability is diminished. The net result in either case, whether unintentional or intentional, leaves energy intake out of step with energy demand from exercise, leading to low energy availability.

Does low energy availability really matter? The answer is a resounding yes, as there are consequences for hormone networks.

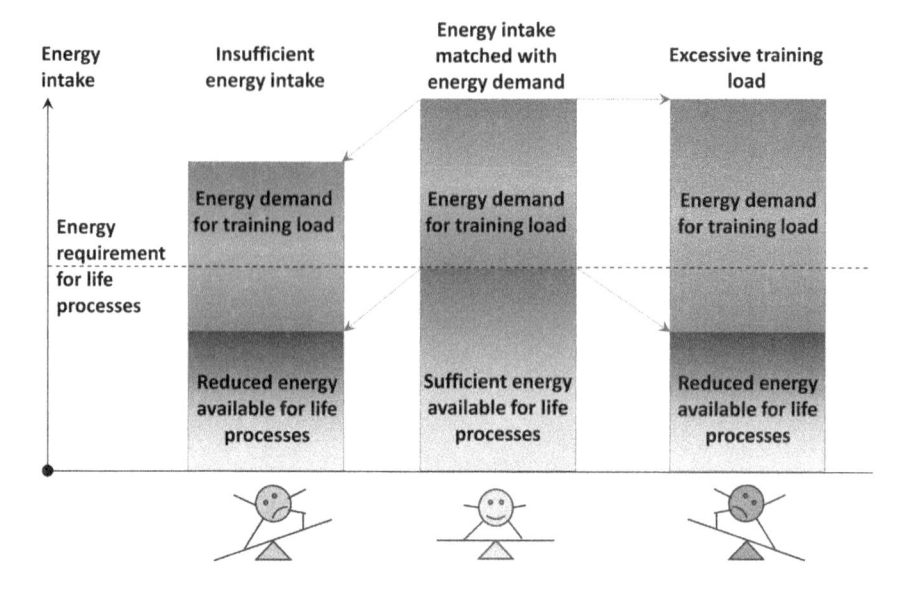

**Figure 10.2:** Matching energy intake with energy demand.*

## Low energy availability and the female athlete triad

During the 1980s a study of female collegiate runners found that even though there was no significant difference in dietary intake, athletes with a higher weekly mileage had a higher incidence of menstrual disruption and poorer bone health, in terms of lower bone mineral density[1]. Runners, who were not matching their energy intake with a higher-energy demand, were in low energy availability. They were on the right in the figure above, compared with their counterparts with adequate energy availability in the central column. This combination of insufficient energy intake, menstrual disruption and poor bone health became known as the female athlete triad[2].

Despite the unfortunate acronym, the description of the female athlete triad is crucial as it demonstrates the adverse health consequence of being in low energy availability. It is normal physiology for all women of reproductive age to have menstrual cycles characterised by regular menstrual periods, regardless of their level of exercise. Menstrual periods are a barometer of healthy hormone networks. Low energy availability, causing either irregular periods or cessation of menstruation (amenorrhoea), has a negative effect on bone health, with an increased risk of fracture. Amenorrhoea is an external sign that internal female hormones are not fluctuating in a healthy manner, characterised by low levels of ovarian hormones, in particular low oestradiol. Bone health deteriorates because it is dependent on oestradiol status (see Act 1, "Scene 7: Bare Bones").

Further refinement of the female athlete triad recognised that the female athlete triad should be considered as a clinical spectrum[3]. At one end we find healthy female athletes with eating patterns in step with demand, regular menstruation (eumenorrhoea) and good bone health. At the other end of the spectrum, athletes may have a clinically diagnosed eating disorder, amenorrhoea and osteoporosis. In between, there are athletes with varying degrees of disordered eating behaviours, menstrual dysfunction and bone health issues.

In a study of 67 female exercisers, although half the group had normal, ovulatory cycles, a range of menstrual disturbances were found in the remainder. These included a lack of periods (amenorrhea), infrequent periods (oligomenorrhea) and more subtle issues of ovulation, such as luteal phase defects and anovulation, which might not be picked up unless hormones were measured[4]. This does not mean that it is "normal" for periods to be disrupted if you exercise nor that exercise is "bad" for female hormone health. Rather it indicates that hormones need to be treated with respect. Balancing exercise, nutrition and recovery means that hormone networks respond to support both health and exercise performance. In fact, menstrual periods can be a personal, sensitive training metric, especially if combined with hormone testing (see Act 1, "Scene 6: Hormone Supermodels").

## Low energy availability and relative energy deficiency in sport (RED-S)

Although the female athlete triad is well established and researched, it became apparent that low energy availability was not an issue restricted to female athletes displaying menstrual dysfunction and poor bone health.

In 2014, the *British Journal of Sports Medicine* published the International Olympic Committee consensus statement on relative energy deficiency in sport (RED-S)[5], with a subsequent update published in 2018[6]. This described the broader concept of who and what low energy availability can impact. RED-S is a syndrome, a collection, of clinical health and exercise performance consequences of low energy availability occurring in both men and women.

## Hormone network disruption

Fully functioning, dynamic hormone networks are crucial to health and exercise performance in men and women. Low energy availability causes endocrine dysfunction, and this mechanism underpins the array of health and performance consequences of RED-S[7]. This downregulation mechanism was shown in a landmark study of women, where sequentially decreasing energy availability (specifically carbohydrate availability) was correlated with falling levels of many hormones across several networks, including leptin, thyroid axis hormones and the reproductive hormone network. The exception being an upregulation of the adrenal axis and production of the "stress" hormone cortisol[8]. This effect of low energy availability on hormone networks has also been shown to occur in men[9]. Figure 10.3 summarises some parts of the complex network of effects of misalignment between external behaviours and internal endocrine system.

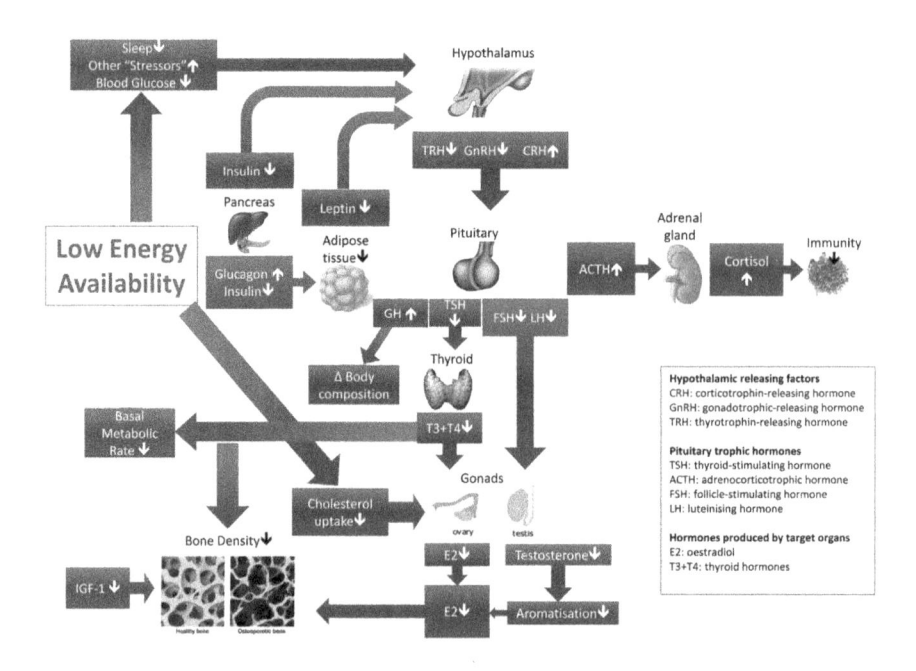

**Figure 10.3:** Effects of misalignment on hormone networks.*

Starting at the low energy availability box. This causes internal metabolic stress. Low blood glucose levels impact the control centre for blood glucose regulation found in the pancreas. This results in lower levels of the anabolic hormone insulin, alongside increased levels of the antagonistic hormone glucagon, which breaks down glucagon (carbohydrate) stores in the liver and skeletal muscle to maintain blood glucose levels. The adipose tissue found in fat stores is also broken down to provide energy. This, in turn, results in lower levels of the hormone leptin. In addition to these internal metabolic stress signals, other external psychological stressors such as poor sleep all funnel into the hypothalamus.

The hypothalamus is the neuro-endocrine gatekeeper, integrating external and internal inputs to determine which messages, about hormone production and release, to forward on to the pituitary. It is interesting to note that the hypothalamus cannot distinguish between external and internal stress, nevertheless if the net input is that of "high stress", as occurs in low energy availability, this results in downregulation of many endocrine networks including the reproductive and thyroid axes, in order to "save energy". The adrenal axis is the exception, being upregulated in low energy availability, with an increased, steady production of the stress hormone cortisol, which loses its usual diurnal variation[10]. The effect of this upregulated pattern of cortisol production is to bolster blood glucose. However, the downsides include the potential negative effect on immunity and indirect negative effects on other hormone networks, such as the reproductive axis and the thyroid axis in the conversion of thyroxine (T4) to triiodothyronine (T3).

## *Thyroid axis*

Downregulation of the thyroid axis, in the face of low energy availability, is an effective way for the body to conserve energy. The hormones secreted by the thyroid gland, T4 and T3, regulate metabolic rate: the rate at which energy is used. When the hypothalamus recognises the distress signal of low energy availability, it lowers the level of thyrotrophin-releasing hormone (TRH), causing the pituitary to decrease the production of thyroid-stimulating hormone (TSH). As the thyroid gland receives a lower TSH signal, it reduces the secretion of T4 and T3. It is known that T3 levels are correlated with decreasing carbohydrate availability[8,11], thereby providing an indirect indicator of energy availability in the clinical setting.

Downregulation of the thyroid axis has been shown to reduce metabolic rate, to "save energy", in men and women[12]. The reduction of metabolic rate explains why those in low energy availability may maintain a steady body weight, rather than actively losing weight.

A full house of low levels of all the thyroid hormones is very unusual, sometimes known as "sick euthyroid". Usually, feedback loops between the control and response hormones ensure homeostasis. So endocrine markers can be helpful objective indicators in identifying low energy availability, especially in someone not overtly underweight. Nevertheless, this unusual pattern of thyroid hormones can lead to confusion, especially if TSH is mid-range, while T4 and T3 are low range. This might tempt an eager prescriber to suggest thyroxine replacement. However, this is not advisable, as it externally overrides the safety feature of metabolic rate downregulation. Addressing low energy availability as the underlying cause of hypothalamic endocrine downregulation is the priority, as discussed in the section on realignment.

### *Reproductive hormone axis*

Amenorrhoea (lack of periods) is an important clinical sign of RED-S in women. What is the underlying endocrine mechanism? Stress signals caused by low energy availability, specifically low carbohydrate availability in females[8], feed into the hypothalamus. This includes low levels of leptin, due to adipose tissue breakdown. Interestingly, an early researcher in this field proposed the "minimum fat threshold" for women to have periods[13] and leptin appears to be the missing mechanistic hormone link[14]. Together with low leptin, other stressor signals, including high cortisol and low T3, are summated by the hypothalamus, which makes the executive decision to suspend the reproductive hormone axis, to preserve energy and divert what is available to essential life processes. From an evolutionary perspective, reproduction must wait.

A study investigated how this shutdown occurs in women whose energy availability was incrementally decreased. Levels below 30 kcal/kg of lean body mass per day caused scrambled gonadotrophin-releasing hormone (GnRH) pulsatility and subsequently the analogue code of LH secretion from the pituitary became disrupted[8] The LH signal to the ovaries is encoded in terms of frequency and magnitude. The ovaries do not recognise this scrambled signal, causing oestradiol levels to drop. Ovulation does not occur and periods stop.

This type of amenorrhoea (lack of periods) is called functional hypothalamic amenorrhoea (FHA). This is because the cause of amenorrhoea is the hypothalamus (as opposed to the ovaries), evidenced by consistently low range levels of LH. The word "functional" is put in front to indicate that an imbalance of behaviours is the cause of this shutdown. The good news is that as this is a temporary suspension of this axis, FHA is a reversible situation. That is not to say that changing behaviours is easy, especially in the case of intentional low energy availability. We discuss practical steps to address FHA in the section on realignment.

Men in low energy availability can experience a similar downregulation of the reproductive axis from the hypothalamic level. Disrupted LH secretion results in low testosterone. The rather cumbersome terminology for this situation is hypogonadotrophic hypogonadism or exercise-hypogonadal male condition (EHMC), which translates to functional hypothalamic low testosterone. This is the exact male equivalent of FHA in women.

There is some evidence to suggest that the energy availability threshold that triggers downregulation of the endocrine reproductive axis is lower in men compared with women[15]. It is nevertheless unlikely, for both men and women, that an absolute energy availability threshold is applicable to all individuals. In practice there are subtle differences in the presentation of low energy availability (how big a deficit and over what time period) and in the regulation of endocrine networks between individuals. In other words, there is not a specific threshold of energy availability below which all hormone networks switch off and above which all aspects of the endocrine system work perfectly.

For example, the magnitude of the daily energy deficit was found to influence the frequency, rather than the extent, of menstrual disruption in female athletes[16]. So, it is not an on/off effect of a threshold energy availability on menstrual function. In female students, whether at school or university, the end of summer term can be a time when periods might become irregular coinciding with exam stress, on top of training and limited time to eat and relax. However, if the student has ongoing low energy availability, rather than restricted to the summer term, she may report menstrual disruption at other times of the year.

Subclinical anovulatory cycles are where a woman experiences regular menstruation without ovulation. There is evidence that this subtle menstrual cycle disruption is associated with health issues[17]. Furthermore, psychological factors impacting hormone networks, particularly the reproductive hormone axis, cannot be overlooked. Different psychological factors come into play depending on the unintentional or intentional nature of low energy availability.

## *Growth hormone axis*

Growth hormone (GH) production is actually increased in an attempt to bolster blood glucose levels, with fat breakdown. Paradoxically the level of insulin-like growth factor 1 (IGF-1), which is made from GH in the liver, is reduced. This is partly because the binding transport proteins for IGF-1 are increased, resulting in lower bioactive levels of IGF-1. As IGF-1 is key player in bone and muscle turnover, lower levels of the active form of this hormone conserve energy.

### *Appetite regulation hormones*

Ghrelin is the "hungry hormone", secreted by the stomach. It influences the hypothalamus and pituitary control centre. In low energy availability, raised levels of ghrelin disrupt GnRH secretion and therefore LH pulsatility. This is independent of the same inhibitory effect on the reproductive hormone axis as low levels of leptin described above. To add yet further layers of complexity, there are some other hormones that play a role in appetite regulation (adiponectin from adipose tissue and peptide YY from the intestine) and eating behaviour (oxytocin from the posterior pituitary)[18]. Suffice to say that low energy availability disrupts all these interrelated endocrine feedback control loops in an attempt to conserve energy.

What is particularly interesting is the potential impact of psychological factors on these disrupted hormone networks. For example, if low energy availability causes an increase in the hungry hormone ghrelin, why do these individuals not eat more? Is there a physiological or a psychological suppression of the effects of ghrelin on appetite? Whichever mechanism is the case, this can be problematic for a person seeking to recover from low energy availability in recognising hunger cues and recalibrating hormones.

## Impact of RED-S endocrine disruption on health

All aspects of health: menstrual function in women, testosterone levels in men, bone health, metabolic rate, growth and development, psychological, cardiovascular, gastrointestinal and immunological and haematological systems are adversely affected by the underlying endocrine disruption of RED-S[19]. These occur over different time scales.

### *Make no bones about it*

Bone is not a static tissue; it is continually recycled. Bone turnover is one of the first systems impacted by the hormone effects of RED-S. Although weight-bearing exercise provides a bone-building, osteogenic effect, any benefit is negated, if not backed up with sufficient energy intake to support healthy hormone networks. Studies show that failure to refuel with carbohydrate and protein, shortly after stopping exercise, has a negative effect on bone turnover[20]. In other words, bone formation is decreased and bone breakdown, called resorption, is favoured. This situation can be detected by a decrease in the bone formation hormone, osteocalcin. Furthermore, a recent study in male athletes published in the *Journal of Bone and Mineral Research* demonstrated that specifically low carbohydrate availability, more than overall low energy availability, had an adverse effect on bone turnover. If this under-fuelling pattern around exercise is repeated and magnified with overall low carbohydrate availability, over days and weeks, progressive endocrine disruption and subsequent deterioration in bone health occur.

As energy deficits accumulate, more elements of the endocrine system are affected, see Figure 10.4.

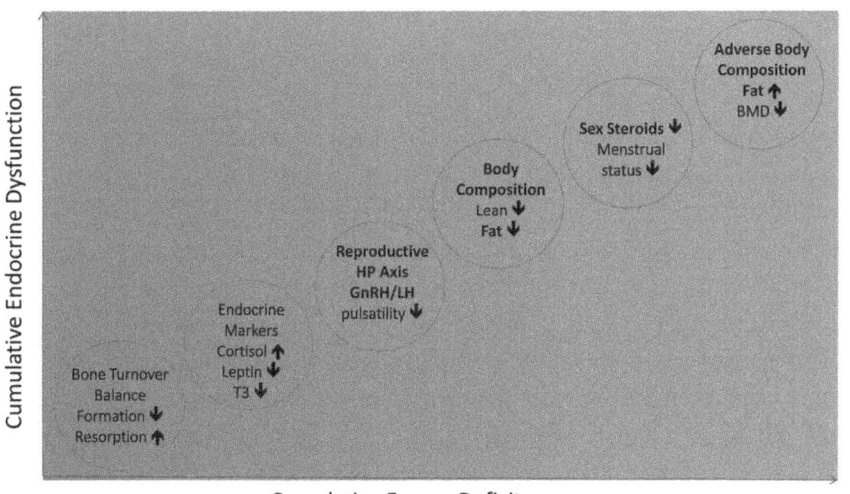

**Figure 10.4:** Cumulative energy deficit and endocrine dysfunction.*

## *Metabolic rate*

Metabolic compensation occurs next in the sequence of hormone dysregulation, with decreased thyroid hormones (specifically T3) and leptin, while cortisol starts to lose some of its diurnal variation and the reproductive hormone axis downregulate. IGF-1 levels also drop. These endocrine changes have further adverse effects on bone health, which is very dependent on IGF-1 and T3, alongside oestradiol (in men and women), over longer time scales. In a study of women with progressive energy availability reduction over five days, the bone formation hormone, osteocalcin, declined first, then reductions in the other hormones controlling bone turnover (T3 and IGF-1) were closely paralleled by a further reduction in bone formation and an increase in bone resorption markers[21]. To reiterate, after just five days of low energy availability, hormones and bone health were adversely affected.

Further prolongation of low energy availability and consequent disruption of endocrine networks, in particular the reproductive hormone axis, results in the clinical outcomes, such as bone stress fractures. In a study of adult male and female runners, there were far more bone stress fractures in those athletes with downregulated hormones, due to low energy availability (males with low range testosterone and females with amenorrhoea), compared with runners with adequate energy availability and normal endocrine function[22].

## Growth and development

The consequences of disrupted endocrine networks from low energy availability in younger exercisers have detrimental effects on growth and development[5]. Delayed and/or arrested puberty has an effect on the accrual of bone mineral density and peak bone mass[23]. The trabecular bone of the lumbar spine is most sensitive and therefore susceptible to any endocrine disruption, compared with the cortical bone of the hip. Not only is the mineralisation of bone affected, in the absence of the expected increase in hormones at puberty, the structure of bone, specifically the bone microarchitecture, can be adversely impacted[24]. Although stress fractures may not occur during teenage years, young athletes and dancers can find themselves in a vulnerable position as they move from junior to senior ranks, when training loads increase. If peak bone mass and bone microarchitecture have been compromised, then the early 20s can be when stress fracture incidence peaks[25].

## Cardiovascular system

Endocrine disruption caused by low energy availability can result in adverse effects on the cardiovascular system. In females, consequent FHA and low oestradiol levels are associated with less favourable lipid profile, reduced endothelial reactivity (inner lining of arteries) and blood pressure control[26].

## Neurological system

As hormones have important interactions with neurotransmitters found in the brain, disruption can be associated with low mood and impaired cognition.

## Gastrointestinal system

As mentioned earlier, hormones play an important part in appetite regulation. There are also "in-house" gastrointestinal hormones at play in absorption and assimilation. Ultimately, low energy availability disrupts digestion, and associated symptoms may be incorrectly attributed to eating certain food types. This can lead to a vicious circle of food restriction and increased symptoms. Counterintuitively, large amounts of fibrous food can contribute to constipation as voluminous food displaces more energy-dense foods, contributing to slowed gut transit time.

## Haematological and immune systems

The hormone erythropoietin controls the production of red blood cells in bone marrow. Reduced food intake limits both the availability of haematinics required to make red blood cells and the production of blood cells. This can impact the immune system and as mentioned above raised cortisol levels reduces immune response

# Time scales of endocrine disruption in RED-S

Energy deficits can accumulate in different ways. Even if an athlete takes on board sufficient energy over a day, an uneven distribution of fuelling over the day can have an adverse effect on endocrine function. Within-day deficits in men and women have been shown to increase cortisol and decrease testosterone or oestradiol respectively[27,28]. Inadequate fuelling around exercise can adversely impact endocrine networks. In our study of male cyclists, athletes doing three or more fasted training sessions per week had lower levels of testosterone, bone health and race performance[29]. Equally, failing to fuel with protein and carbohydrate, shortly after training, has a negative effect on recovery in terms of metabolism and immune function[30]. Ultimately, although the endocrine system has some resilience to transient, intermittent energy deficits, if athletes and exercisers fail to fuel systematically around training sessions the cumulative effect results in progressive endocrine dysfunction, as illustrated in Figure 10.4.

Ultimately, cumulative energy deficiency causes cortisol secretion patterns to lack the expected diurnal variation, with levels remaining consistently at the upper end of the range. Disturbed sleeping patterns can perpetuate this disruption. Cortisol is catabolic, favouring the breakdown of muscle and bone. Sustained high cortisol levels favour the deposition of the high energy reserve store, fat, as a survival tactic. In this way, ironically and rather sadly, some athletes aiming to change body composition in favour of muscle, by restricting energy intake, can end up with less a favourable body composition in the long run. This was found in a study of athletes, where the largest cumulative daily energy deficits were found to be linked with higher body fat[31].

## How you think impacts your hormones!

Psychological factors can be implicated in both cause and effect of RED-S. Individuals, who are very driven to achieve athletic prowess, may also apply this psychology to rigid eating and training behaviours, which increase the risk of endocrine disruption. The interconnection between psychological factors and both physical and physiological indicators of low energy availability was demonstrated in our study of male and female dancers. Female dancers with anxiety around controlling food and body weight, tended to (a) be anxious about missing training (psychological factor), (b) have lower minimum body mass index (a physical factor) and (c) have irregular menstrual cycles (a physiological factor). Statistically significant relationships were seen in each case, with hormones providing the underlying explanatory mechanism[32]. Further evidence for the impact of psychological factors on hormones comes from several other studies of exercising women where intentional, cognitive dietary restraint was linked to menstrual disruption[33] and the drive for thinness was linked with low T3, raised ghrelin and menstrual dysfunction[34] and further studies where cognitive restraint resulted in a range of menstrual issues, raised cortisol and poor bone health[35,36].

A similar situation was found in studies of male athletes, where indicators of exercise dependence and disordered eating were associated with endocrine markers of RED-S, in terms of low testosterone to cortisol ratio and high cortisol to insulin ratios[37]. In our study of male endurance athletes, cognitive restraint, that is, intentional low energy availability was linked with indicators of energy conservation[38]. In other words, how you think about food intake, body weight and exercise have an impact on your hormones.

## Performance consequences of RED-S

Even though there is undisputable evidence that RED-S has adverse effects on health, ultimately athletes and dancers of all levels are often more interested in the here and now of athletic prowess. However, there is mounting evidence that RED-S adversely impacts performance. For example, in young female swimmers, athletes with low energy availability with downregulated hormones (ovarian, T3 and IGF-1) did not improve their 400 m swim time compared with their energy sufficient teammates whose hormones were in range[39]. Impaired neuromuscular performance was found in female athletes with FHA, low T3 and high cortisol, due to low energy availability. These athletes had reduced reaction time and impaired muscle performance in terms of endurance and power production, compared with their eumenorrheic counterparts with healthy hormones[40]. These studies show that hormone dysfunction found in RED-S impairs athletic performance in females. The same applies to male athletes.

In our study, male cyclists clinically assessed as being in chronic low energy availability from clinical history (e.g. inadequate fuelling around training) and hormones levels (lower range testosterone) showed adverse effects on bone health and race performance. Not only did the male athletes, with low energy availability, lose bone mineral density at the same rate as an astronaut in space, but moreover they failed to win as many cycling race points, over the season, as their energy sufficient counterparts. The cyclists with RED-S underperformed relative to their predicted "potential" in terms of their functional threshold power[41].

This is the key message for athletes. Although, initially, the adverse effects of low energy availability might be apparent and performance might even improve temporarily, this is "fool's gold". Maintaining low energy availability over a longer timescale is not compatible with sustained performance. In a similar way to NFO and OTS, performance stagnates and ultimately declines in long term. An athlete with RED-S is never able to reach full potential, see Figure 10.5. I often show this figure to athletes and dancers to illustrate that RED-S limits performance. Increasing training load, in a periodised fashion, supported by sufficient energy intake improves performance. A levelling off is found as NFO is reached. Conversely in an athlete with RED-S, increasing training load does not improve performance, as hormones are downregulated.

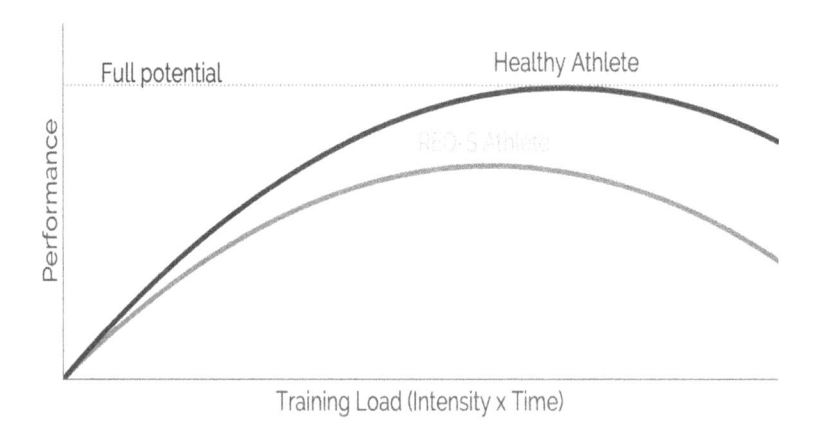

**Figure 10.5:** Implications of RED-S on sports performance.*

## Using hormones to identify those at risk of RED-S

As RED-S puts athletes at risk of career threatening injuries and/or adverse health outcomes, early identification and prevention are vital. Especially in view of the possibility that these adverse outcomes may not be reversible. In our study of retired pre-menopausal female dancers, those who had experienced indicators of RED-S during their career, in terms of low body weight, delayed menarche and secondary amenorrhoea, had lower than expected bone mineral density of the lumbar spine for their age[42].

Although low energy availability is the aetiology of RED-S, measuring energy availability in practical terms is challenging. Even if a value is calculated, this reflects a limited time frame, and it is difficult to interpret the meaning of the value for an individual[43]. A far more practical and relevant approach is to assess hormones. Hormone measurements provide direct access to how an individual is reacting physiologically to a given energy availability status. Repeating these hormone measurements adds a time dimension to the physiological outcomes of low energy availability. Measurements of many of the key hormones are readily available: thyroid function (TSH, T4 and T3), 9 am cortisol, LH, FSH, prolactin, oestradiol/testosterone. Although these hormones may be within range, recognising a pattern in those hormones at the lower or upper end of the normal range is key to interpretation. In the case of female exercisers, the early warning sign of subclinical ovulatory issues can be detected using mathematical modelling of hormones of a menstrual cycle (see Act 1, "Scene 6: Hormone Supermodels").

I work with many dancers. Unlike athletes competing in sports, dancers don't really have an "off season"; performances run continuously through the year. Having introduced a menstrual tracking facility to existing training and wellbeing monitoring, I thought this would pick up early warning signs of low energy availability in terms of menstrual disruption. I was surprised that by modelling female hormones I found that several dancers reporting regular menstrual cycles were in fact experiencing subclinical anovulatory cycles. In other words, their female hormones were not showing the full repertoire of hormonal fluctuations need for optimal health. This occurred especially around heavy rehearsal schedules. Having identified this situation, I was able to give personal recommendations and suggestions to dancers in terms of recovery and nutrition strategies to maintain healthy hormones for optimal dance performance. This illustrates the need to pay close attention to individual hormone patterns[44].

A detailed clinical history is vital, particularly as psychological factors play a role in RED-S. To this end, there are questionnaires that can be used as screening tools. The low energy availability female-questionnaire (LEAF-Q) was the first validated questionnaire for female athletes[45]. Activity-specific questionnaires are being developed, for example, a sport-specific energy availability questionnaire combined with an interview (SEAQ-I) has been used with male cyclists[29]. For male and female dancers, our dance energy availability questionnaire (DEAQ)[32] is being adopted by dance schools internationally. It is currently being adapted for other sport disciplines. Those identified from screening questionnaires as being at risk can have further tests to quantify hormone levels.

## The tip of the iceberg

Isn't RED-S just a concern for female elite athletes with eating disorders? Absolutely not! If anything, I would argue that non-elite, amateur and recreational exercisers are more likely to develop both unintentional and intentional RED-S, because they may not have easy access to reliable information from healthcare professionals with expertise in RED-S. The RED-S syndrome can occur in all levels of exerciser, whether male or female and at any age.

As described above, RED-S in a young, developing child or adolescent is of particular concern for long-term health in adulthood. Equally, in older, age-group athletes, RED-S could be mistaken for perimenopause in women. A careful review of hormones can distinguish a downregulated hypothalamic-pituitary axis in RED-S from reduced ovarian responsiveness in perimenopause. On the matter of eating behaviours, there is a spectrum from optimal nutrition to disordered eating to an eating disorder. Certain clinical criteria are used to make a diagnosis of an eating disorder. Although disordered eating may not meet these diagnostic criteria, an individual may be suffering the consequences of RED-S. Disordered eating includes regularly intentionally skipping meals or excluding/restricting certain food types: orthorexia[46]. Carbohydrates are often perceived in a bad light, despite their crucial importance for health, in terms of female hormone reproductive axis and performance in high-intensity exercise, as discussed earlier.

## RED-S: what to look out for?

From a practical point of view, what should athletes, dancers, teammates, coaches, parents and healthcare professionals look out for as warning signs of low energy availability? To raise awareness and provide reliable information, I lead the team that created the British Association of Sport and Exercise Medicine website www.health4performance.co.uk

Here is a summary of the key things to look out for as indicators of the risk of RED-S.

- Difficult relationship with food and/or exercise
  - Eating patterns: disordered eating to eating disorder
  - Exercise dependence
- Changes in behaviour, mood, sleep patterns
- Body weight: possibly an initial loss, although BMI may be in the normal range
- Arrest/delay in growth and development in younger individuals
- Menstrual function disruption (ranging from amenorrhoea, oligomenorrhoea to subclinical ovulatory disturbances)
- Reduced libido
- Increased, recurrent and/or slow to recover injuries (soft tissue and bone) and illness
- Gastrointestinal issues (may present with symptoms similar to irritable bowel syndrome)
- Fatigue and inability to recover
- Exercise performance (stagnation to deterioration)

## Different facets of the same hormone issues?

It is important to bear in mind that the hypothalamus is astute to all types of input. This neuro-endocrine gatekeeper does not distinguish between internal or external sources of stress nor whether these stressors are physical or psychological. Although I have described the imbalances in the key behaviours for hormone health as separate entities, there is no clear cut-off between overtraining and under-fuelling, in terms of aetiology and biological mechanism[47]. If you are a driven, determined person, this attitude is likely to apply in you to exercise and food. Exercise dependence is closely linked to disordered eating patterns[48].

## Overtraining and RED-S overlap

Evidence for overlap between overtraining and RED-S comes from a study of male athletes who undertook a four-week intensive training block. Reduced improvement in performance was observed in those athletes who demonstrated indicators of RED-S (decreased T3 and increased cortisol). The conclusion is that tracking hormones provides a sensitive clinical tool to identify athletes at risk of low energy availability during training blocks[49].

Similarly, in female athletes undertaking a four-week training block, those that did not increase energy intake developed non-functional overreaching (NFOR) and indicators of low energy availability in terms of suppression of ovulation. As RED-S includes both health and performance effects this would suggest that low energy availability (whether intentional or unintentional) is the underlying cause of NFOR and OTS[50].

## Diagnosis of exclusion

Clinical history and screening questionnaires are important tools in identifying those at risk of RED-S, but ultimately RED-S is a diagnosis of exclusion. In other words, there can be other "organic" medical causes. This is why measuring hormones is important in the process of making a diagnosis and risk stratification. The RED-S clinical assessment tool (RED-S CAT) collates clinical features to stratify athletes according to a traffic light system[51].

# Realignment

> *"Before you heal someone, ask him if he's willing to give up the things that make him sick."*
>
> Hippocrates

As discussed above, psychological factors are important aetiological factors in the origin and maintenance of RED-S. The challenge of changing behaviours in terms of training and nutrition cannot be underestimated. Often it is not actually about food. Rather the anxiety around controlling eating, body weight/shape and exercise behaviours is about self-esteem[32]. This is why cognitive behavioural therapy (CBT) has proven value FHA[52].

# Eat more to regulate body weight!

Paradoxically it is important to eat more to enable the body to regulate body weight in the situation of RED-S. Once the energy deficit has been cleared, thyroid function reboots, and metabolic rate increases. Just like clearing an overdraft, energy intake needs to be increased above baseline requirement to cover the overdraft and the accumulated interest. This was demonstrated in a study of exercising women with menstrual irregularity, where increasing baseline intake over 12 months restored menstrual function and increased T3[53]. Thereafter, the intake needs to be maintained at a level to meet to the demands of a higher, healthy metabolic rate.

Athletes may be anxious about gaining a lot of weight, but in reality, the aim is to restore weight to a level where endocrine networks can function normally. Initial weight gain often takes the form of water, which is required to accumulate glycogen, the storage form of carbohydrate, in the liver and skeletal muscles. Ultimately weight on the scales is a measurement of earth's gravity and does not reflect body composition. The weight loss associated with RED-S may have resulted in increased body fat[31] and increased body dimensions because fat takes up more volume than muscles. This means that restoration of weight may reflect a change in body composition with an increase in denser muscle and a decrease in fat.

As described above energy availability, particularly carbohydrate, is essential for hormone network function. Recovering from RED-S requires consistency of intake over the day, to prevent any within-day deficits is also crucial[27, 28].

Specifically, fuelling around training is important. Follow the maxim of "fuelling for the work required" on a forward-looking schedule to meet demand and prevent energy deficits[54]. Fasted training in the morning puts a particular strain on endocrine networks. This was shown in a study of male cyclists, where those performing three or more fasted rides per week were left with lower T3 and testosterone[29]. Apart from being important for hormone health, fuelling in a pre-emptive manner is important to establish and engrain beneficial nutrition strategies. Following "mechanical eating" patterns can also be helpful from physiological or psychological point of view, where hunger cues of raised ghrelin levels cannot be relied upon, until hormones have recalibrated.

## I want to train!

You can't eat yourself out of RED-S. It is important to address other sources of stress and energy output. Energy expenditure outside of formal training can be overlooked: walking, running or cycling to work or intense study. Some jobs involve more energy expenditure than desk-based work. Training itself may well need temporary modification: a reduction in intensity in favour of a focus on strength work helps both body composition and bone health. Even if an athlete has not suffered a bone stress injury, some disruption of bone health is inevitable in the low energy availability state. Strength work that includes multidirectional loading of the skeleton, such as changing direction jumping and hopping, in conjunction with adequate nutrition has been shown to be beneficial for bone health[41].

## Restoring hormone health

Rebooting hormone networks is not necessarily a smooth course. As the endocrine system recalibrates, there can be mistiming, which can be confused with de novo medical conditions. For example, women restoring energy availability can experience a transient lag between the increase in LH and testosterone, prior to the ovaries producing sufficient oestradiol for ovulatory cycles. This can result in a diagnosis of polycystic ovary syndrome (PCOS), when in fact it is a temporary situation; this is discussed in further detail in Act 2 Scene 4.

Once menstrual cycles have been restored, initially these may have an insufficient luteal phase, and it is advisable to delay an increase in training load until at least three menstrual cycles have occurred and ideally confirmed that full female hormone fluctuations and ovulation is occurring (see Act 2 "Scene 6:

Hormone Supermodels"). Combining close hormone monitoring and access to on-demand virtual clinical discussion has proved to be very successful and well received among professional dancers that I work with[55,56,57].

In a similar way, the thyroid axis may show some lag between TSH increasing and T4 responding. Careful monitoring helps avoid the inappropriate prescription of thyroxine[58].

Another misconception is that the combined oral contraception pill (COCP) is suitable for women suffering from FHA due to RED-S. The Endocrine Society guidelines advise against using the COCP in FHA, as it suppresses internal female hormones[59]. The withdrawal bleeds experienced on the COCP are not the same as periods that result from natural internal female hormones. Therefore, this external source of artificial hormones acts as a masking agent.

Furthermore, there is no evidence that the COCP is protective of bone health. In contrast, hormone replacement therapy (HRT) is bone protective and recommended where the bone mineral density Z-score (age matched) of lumbar spine is below −1 and/or two or more stress fractures have occurred[60]. Ideally, HRT should be applied in the form of transdermal oestradiol and cyclic micronized progesterone, in conjunction with support for the exerciser to make behavioural changes with nutrition and training load.

Having seen many female exercisers with FHA due to RED-S being erroneously advised to take COCP, I am pleased to report that following a letter to National Institute of Clinical Excellence (NICE), the Clinical Knowledge Summaries (CKS) were swiftly updated in February 2022 to align with Endocrine Society guidelines[61].

## Hormone story

*Vanessa* *was a 28-year-old exerciser, who had been restricting her carbohydrate intake in the belief that she would become lighter and therefore run faster. Initially her times were improved, but then her periods stopped and she started to run slower. Vanessa started to eat some more carbohydrate and although she restored some weight, her periods did not come back. She had been told that having no periods meant that she should take the COCP to "restore her hormones and protect her bone health". Unfortunately, she went on to sustain several bone stress fractures. When I saw Vanessa, she stopped taking the COCP (and used barrier methods of contraception) and had a DXA scan. Unsurprisingly her bone health was compromised and her own periods did not restore.*

*Blood tests taken after cessation of the COCP showed FHA and a downregulated thyroid axis. After talking through the results and the situation, Vanessa agreed to increase further her carbohydrate intake. However, this was a challenge psychologically and would take time to overcome. So as an interim measure she took HRT for 3 months.*

*Happily, she worked hard to re-establish eating patterns that would support healthy hormones. So shortly after stopping HRT her periods recommenced. We checked that full fluctuation of her female hormones had restored through modelling of her hormone results. Vanessa is gradually increasing her training load, being careful to match increased energy demand with increased energy intake.*

*We discussed that often we default to rigid, familiar behaviours in times of stress. So, the process of overcoming intentional RED-S increases resilience. Although life may throw up challenges, being aware that returning to old familiar, unhelpful behaviours is just a coping mechanism and not the long-term solution, can be a constructive way to think about intentional RED-S.*

Unlicensed bisphosphanates should not be used for treating poor bone health in RED-S, as this family of medicines suspends bone turnover. Oestradiol in both (men and women) is the lead player in favouring bone formation. In men testosterone is converted to oestradiol.

For male exercisers, testosterone therapy is not advised as this hormone is on the World Antidoping Agency (WADA) banned list and a therapeutic use exemption (TUE) cannot be obtained for treating a functional condition. Furthermore, taking external testosterone suppresses internal production of testosterone, so it is not helpful in restoring hormone function, just as the COCP is not helpful for women with FHA. As with females with RED-S, the mainstay of management is a multi-disciplinary team approach to support change of behaviours around training, nutrition and recovery[62].

## Hormone story

**Samuel** *was a 32-year-old high-level competitive road cyclist. He thought reducing weight would bring success on the road. So, he increased training and reduced carbohydrate intake. After an initial loss in body weight and improvement in power output per kg of body weight, things started to go awry. Despite further reduction of what he ate, he did not lose any further weight and his performance stagnated. Furthermore, he felt fatigued, reported poor sleep and reduced libido. He had been* *offered external testosterone, but he knew that this was on WADA banned list. When we met, blood tests confirmed RED-S: low range hormones across the board. His DXA also showed low bone mineral density (BMD) for his age, especially at lumbar spine.*

*We discussed strategies to reboot his hormones by increasing his carbohydrate intake in a consistent way, together with temporarily reducing his training intensity and doing some strength work. Although he was very fearful this would result in an uncontrolled increase in body weight, we discussed that initially an increase in weight would actually be water to store glycogen (storage form of carbohydrate) and also to bear in mind that muscle is denser than fat. With reduced cortisol levels and increased strength work and testosterone, this would favour change in body composition to muscle. So, although body weight would increase body shape should improve. Furthermore, once hormones re-equilibrate and metabolic rate increases, then the hormone networks stabilise body weight. I am pleased to report that Samuel's hormone networks rebooted and his physical and mental health improved. He also rediscovered his enjoyment of riding his bike.*

## Strategies to prevent and address adverse effects on hormone networks from low energy availability

### Exercise

- Training should be periodised and polarised, in the short and long term.
- Intensity of exercise may need to be reduced temporarily in suspected low energy availability
- Place emphasis on strength work
- Recovery between exercise sessions needs to be sufficient for hormone networks to maintain health and support positive adaptations

### Sleep

- Sleep is an essential part of any training schedule and essential for hormone function.
- Reviewing sleep hygiene strategies is important

## *Nutrition*

- Fuelling consistently throughout the day is crucial to support healthy hormones.
- Eat meals at regular times and avoid long gaps
- Every meal should include a portion of protein and slow-release complex carbohydrates (cereals, rice, pasta, bread, potatoes) appropriate for body size, age and activity levels
- Fuel for the work required on a forward-looking schedule around exercise
    - Before exercise: take on carbohydrate. Do not exercise in a fasted state
    - During exercise: top up with carbohydrates, in a drink form or banana or cereal bar
    - After exercise: within 20 minutes, refuel with protein and complex carbohydrates

## *Further information*

- See the British Association Sport and Exercise Medicine website https://health4performance.basem.co.uk/

# Entr'acte

*"All the world's a stage,*
*And all the men and women merely players;*
*They have their exits and their entrances;*
*And one man in his time plays many parts,*
*His acts being seven ages."*
*Shakespeare, As You Like It*

**Subtitle:** We have explored the clandestine work of hormones to support our health and the ways our behaviour choices can influence hormone networks. Now we move on to examine how this interaction plays out over the lifespan. This will be staged through the seven ages of man (and woman!) according to Shakespeare's "As You Like it".

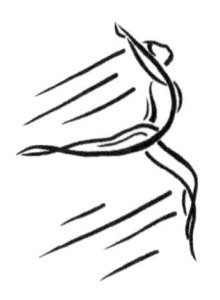

# Act 2

# Scene 1
## Infancy

*"At first the infant,*
*Mewling and puking in the nurse's arms."*
*Shakespeare*

**Subtitle:** Even before birth, hormone networks play a vital role in determining the future health of the developing foetus, over the entire lifespan: from infancy to adulthood. The mother's hormones communicate features of the external environment to the foetus through the placenta, to prepare the foetal endocrine system for the anticipated external world after birth. A mismatch between the realities of the external world and the pre-tuned hormone network, especially during early infancy, can increase the risk of health issues moving into childhood and adulthood.

## Hormone stories

**Polly** was a 29-year-old woman, hoping to become pregnant. She wanted to be as healthy as possible, as she was aware that being overweight and "unfit" may not be beneficial for her or the future health of her baby. Polly had seen a plethora of "diets" on social media, claiming to miraculously transform someone from being overweight to svelte in just a few weeks. The quick fix seemed too attractive not to try.

## Setting the hormone scene in utero

Hormones play a key part in our future health, even before we are born. Metabolic and cardiovascular health are to a large extent determined by the tuning of hormone networks during the critical period of intrauterine development[1]. During the nine-month period of gestation, the fertilised egg does not simply grow in an isolated internal incubator. The development of the foetus is affected by the mother's hormones, which, in turn, depend on her interactions with the external environment.

It is well documented that adverse lifestyle behaviours, including lack of exercise, overeating, smoking and drinking alcohol, negatively impact health. This applies from conception to the end of the lifespan.

During early infancy, the endocrine system that has been tuned to the predicted external environment in utero meets the challenge of the real world. Any mismatch can be a problem for health in infancy and over the lifespan.

The genotype describes the collection of genes that an embryo inherits, half from the mother and half from the father. The phenotype describes the observable traits and characteristics of an individual: the consequence of the interactions of the genotype with its environment. The mechanism by which these interactions trigger gene expression is called epigenetics. But have you ever wondered what determines which genes are expressed and when? The answer is the hormone networks. And these hormone networks start working while the foetus is still in the mother's womb.

Babies who are born prematurely or who are small for their gestational age have an increased risk of endocrine dysfunction, causing diseases including type 2 diabetes mellitus and cardiovascular disease in adulthood. This is especially true when these new-borns have a rapid increase in weight in early infancy. These infants are also more likely to experience a mistiming of adrenarche (adrenal gland hormone secretion) and the awakening of sex hormone production that heralds the onset of puberty[2]. How does intrauterine life have such a profound effect on long-term health after birth in infancy and beyond?

## Determinants of health in infancy and beyond

The developing foetus is affected by the mother in many ways. The most obvious is through genetic inheritance: half of the foetus' DNA comes from the mother. The foetus is also influenced by the mother's genotype and phenotype, indirectly, through intrauterine programming via epigenetic effects.

Intrauterine programming is the term used to describe the interactions between the external environment, via the intrauterine microenvironment, and the expression of genes in the foetus. Variations in the uterine environment can alter gene expression and produce a different infant phenotype from exactly the same set of genes. This developmental plasticity in utero has profound effects on future health throughout life, potentially even more potent than lifestyle choices and health once born[3].

An epigenetic effect[4] is the way in which external factors influence genetic expression, without changing the sequence of the base pairs in DNA. However, these effects are not limited to the lifespan of the individual; they are heritable. In other words, epigenetic effects can be passed on to future generations, even if the original environmental stimulus is no longer present[5].

How do epigenetic effects work? Methylation is a natural process that silences genes and is thought to be one of the main molecular mechanisms to bring about epigenetic effects on gene expression. A methyl group is added to the promotor region of a gene, where the promotor region can be thought of as a capital letter marking the beginning of a sentence in the genetic code. After fertilisation of the egg, there is a wave of demethylation. This takes the brakes off gene expression so that the cells are "pluripotent" and have the freedom to become any type of cell. Sequential waves of methylation ensure a structured time sequence, thereby avoiding a chaotic free for all. Flexibility in the process of methylation enables interaction between the intrauterine environment and the expression of genes in foetus. This determines the phenotype of the infant.

Developmental Origins of Health and Disease (DOHaD) describes the ways that the future life-long health of a newborn can be affected by environmental factors starting from preconception and gestation (pregnancy)[4]. This is based on pioneering work by Dr David Barker, who demonstrated that external conditions, especially poor nutritional status of the pregnant mother, during foetal development had an adverse effect on future cardiovascular health in adulthood[6]. The foetal origins hypothesis (Barker hypothesis) is based on latency (effects of intrauterine environment present in later life), persistency (these effects are long term) and gene programming (genetic expression is determined by intrauterine conditions)[7]. Evidence comes from the effects on adult endocrine and metabolic health of those conceived during times of poor nutrition and/or stressful situations; for example, during the Dutch Hunger Winter of Second World War[8], the siege of Leningrad[9] and more recent events such as climate environmental-related events. Furthermore, even after these adverse situations had been resolved, the epigenetic tags and consequences on gene expression and endocrine function were passed on to future generations. These profound effects of intrauterine conditions on future health are mediated by hormones.

## Hormones at work in utero

> *"The fetuses' adaptations to undernutrition are associated with changes in the concentrations of fetal and placental hormones. Persisting changes in the levels of hormone secretion, and in the sensitivity of tissues to them, may link fetal undernutrition with abnormal structure, function, and disease in adult life."*
>
> The Lancet 1993

This quote from a prominent medical publication highlights the role of hormones in mediating and directing internal responses to external factors. Hormones orchestrate foetal adaptation to maternal nutritional status and direct the gene expression of hormone production that is maintained throughout adult life[10].

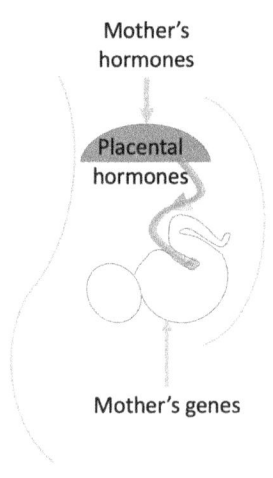

**Figure 11.1:** Epigenetic tuning of foetal endocrine system

The placenta, shown in Figure 11.1, acts as the go-between for the maternal environment and the foetus. Just one cell thickness at the placenta separates the blood of the mother from the circulation of the developing foetus. This presents no barrier to hormone communications and the placenta itself also produces an array of hormones. The foetus is awash with maternal and placental hormones in utero. This repertoire of hormones influences the development and settings of the foetal endocrine system, in preparation for the anticipated outside world.

*Scene 1: Infancy*

# Endocrine effects of undernutrition

Maternal undernutrition drives developmental plasticity towards the foetus developing an energy-saving "thrifty phenotype"[11]. Endocrine networks adjust in anticipation of the baby being born into an environment where food is in short supply. How exactly does this happen? The placenta increases the production of insulin-like growth factor-1 (IGF-1) to try to compensate for restricted nutrition available for the foetus. Placental hormones induce increased insulin production and insulin sensitivity to facilitate catch-up growth once the baby is born. However, if, in fact, the baby has plenty of food available, this catch-up can be very rapid and an overshot may occur. In this case, the infant lays down a lot of visceral fat, increasing the production of the hormone leptin, by adipose tissue. Insulin sensitivity switches to insulin resistance and an increase in markers of cardiovascular risk is observed in the first three months of life. Ironically this adverse endocrine profile for health in infancy is due to epigenetic changes in utero favouring a thrifty metabolism, in (mistaken) anticipation of continued low nutritional availability once born[12]. See Figure 11.2.

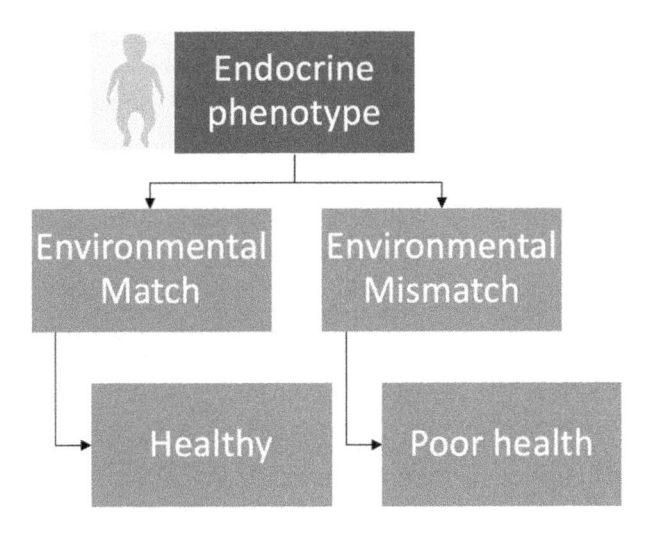

**Figure 11.2:** Outcome of tuning the foetal endocrine system

## Endocrine effects of nutrition surplus

Just as undernutrition can have adverse effects on foetal endocrine function, so can surplus maternal nutrition. Diabetes mellitus is the most common medical complication of pregnancy with risks for both foetal and maternal health[13]. For this reason, mothers who have pre-existing diabetes mellitus or have risk factors for developing gestational diabetes are carefully monitored in medical antenatal clinics during pregnancy. Why does pregnancy present a challenge to blood glucose control that can have a knock-on effect on foetal and subsequent infant health? Increased levels of placental and maternal hormones such as growth hormone, progesterone and cortisol increase blood glucose levels that spill over to the foetus. High levels of blood glucose (hyperglycaemia) cause the baby to grow very large (macrosomia), which is linked with delivery complications. Poor blood glucose control early in pregnancy increases the risk of malformations in the embryo. Hyperglycaemia later in pregnancy increases the risk of stillbirth. High blood glucose levels also put the mother's health at risk. Pre-eclampsia is a hormone-mediated syndrome of increased blood pressure and deterioration of renal function, which can be serious for both mother and baby.

Obesity is a further maternal risk factor. Having a body mass index (BMI) over 35 kg/m$^2$ increases the likelihood of thromboembolic disease (blood clotting). If not already diabetic, mothers who are overweight are at higher risk of developing diabetes during pregnancy (gestational diabetes), which in turn doubles the risk of subsequent type 2 diabetes mellitus post-partum. All pregnant women are screened for gestational diabetes with an oral glucose tolerance test (OGTT) around 24–28 weeks into pregnancy: blood tests are performed two hours after consuming a sugary drink. However, earlier screening with an OGTT is recommended for women who are at risk of gestational diabetes, including being overweight. Surplus nutrition and inactivity are risk factors for developing type 2 diabetes mellitus, which is magnified by the effects of an increase in the anabolic hormones associated with pregnancy.

The reason it is so important to be alert to impaired glucose control in pregnancy is that not only does it increase the risk of foetal and maternal health, but it also has repercussions for infant health after birth. Increased foetal production of insulin, in response to intrauterine hyperglycaemia, has an anabolic effect on insulin-sensitive tissues resulting in increased abdominal fat, heart and liver size, as well as an increase in foetal pancreatic cells to pump out high levels of insulin to bring blood glucose down into a healthy range. After birth, the baby continues to produce high levels of insulin, which can cause insulin resistance.

Cells lose their responsiveness to insulin. This is the underlying cause of type 2 diabetes.

Ironically, this is the same sequence of endocrine system maladaptation that occurs when the foetus is undernourished. Therefore, the same adverse consequences on health tend to occur in infancy and adulthood, if in utero nutritional conditions are not optimal.

On a positive note, if intrauterine nutrition is optimal, the foetal endocrine system is set fair for health in infancy and beyond.

Although many of the early studies focused on the influence of maternal nutritional status on the long-term health of the developing foetus, it is now recognised that a broad range of intrauterine environments play a role in determining the future health of the infant throughout its life.

## Other maternal endocrine conditions

Due to the close hormonal communication between mother and foetus, other maternal hormone conditions can affect the development of the foetal endocrine system settings.

The foetus is dependent on maternal thyroxine until its own production starts, 12 weeks into gestation. Thyroxine is important for neurological development, including intellectual and cognitive development. Therefore, when mothers known to be hypothyroid and already on thyroxine become pregnant, they are advised to increase their dose by about 30% to cover the extra demand and they are monitored during pregnancy. When the baby is born the heel prick test screens for a range of metabolic conditions, including thyroid function, as any hormone issues need to be detected as soon as possible to prevent adverse health effects on the infant.

For mothers with known Graves' disease, an autoimmune condition causing an overactive thyroid, symptoms tend to be exacerbated in the initial third of pregnancy (first trimester). Autoimmune conditions tend to become worse in pregnancy, because the immune system is dialled down, to "accept" the growing foetus. This, of course, can impact the baby. If a mother with Graves' disease has high levels of thyroid-stimulating autoantibodies, they can cross the placenta and induce hyperthyroidism in the baby. On the other hand, a baby may become hypothyroid, if high doses of antithyroid drugs are needed to keep maternal thyroid function in range, as these medications can cross the placenta.

Temporary, physiological gestational hyperthyroidism (as opposed to Graves' disease which is a permanent state of hyperthyroidism) can cause severe vomiting and weight loss in early pregnancy (hyperemesis gravidarum). It is not unusual to feel a bit nauseous during the first 12 weeks of pregnancy, although "morning sickness" is often not restricted to the morning. The reason is the early-pregnancy hormone beta-human chorionic gonadotrophin (β-hCG) is produced by the mother's cells surrounding the fertilised egg, which go on to become the placenta. Home pregnancy tests measure the level of β-hCG. This hormone is very similar in structure and action to luteinising hormone (LH), produced by the pituitary. So, the β-hCG instructs the corpus luteum (the remnant of the ovulated egg in the ovary) to continue producing progesterone. This maintains the lining of the endometrium in order to accommodate the fertilised egg. This process continues until the placenta is able to produce a local source of progesterone. Although β-hCG plays this very important role, the downside is that this hormone can cause nausea in early pregnancy. The explanation is that β-hCG is not only very similar to LH; it is also similar to another hormone: thyroid-stimulating hormone (TSH). This results in a temporarily overactive thyroid that causes nausea and suppresses the pituitary's production of TSH. The degree of thyroid stimulation from β-hCG corresponds to the severity of vomiting[14].

## Stressful intrauterine life

Floating around carefree in the warm, amniotic fluid of the uterus might seem stress-free for the developing foetus. However, the foetus becomes exposed to stress if nourishment and/or oxygen are restricted. Cortisol is a hormone produced by the adrenal glands, nestling above the kidneys, whose production increases in response to external or internal stressors. The foetus responds to adversity in intrauterine life by an upregulation of the hypothalamic-pituitary-adrenal (HPA) axis and increased production of cortisol. The placenta acts as the hormone go-between for a mother under "stress" and her foetus. Increased placental production of adrenal activating hormones contributes to the increased activity of the foetal HPA axis. The net result of the foetal response to stressors in utero is a reprogramming of the HPA axis that persists after birth. Raised adult levels of cortisol are associated with insulin resistance, hypertension and risk of developing metabolic syndrome.

## Hormones rule after birth

After birth, the effects of the intrauterine hormone milieu continue to impact the development of hormones secretion and tissue sensitivity to these instigators of gene expression[10]. In-utero alterations in hormonal networks in response to restricted nutrition continue into childhood. Adrenarche is when the adrenal glands start increasing hormone production in line with adult levels. It is considered premature when this occurs before eight years of age in girls and before nine years in boys. Premature adrenarche is associated with insulin resistance and metabolic syndrome (suboptimal blood glucose control and lipid profile, with hypertension). Abdominal fat increases the adverse effect of premature adrenarche on increasing the risk of cardiovascular disease and type 2 diabetes mellitus. In girls, this endocrine profile is also associated with the development of polycystic ovary syndrome (PCOS) where there is a mistiming of the female hormone axis resulting in overproduction of testosterone, irregular periods and the observation of multiple follicles in the ovaries on ultrasound[2].

Reprogramming of the hypothalamic-pituitary-gonadal axis is also reported in those born small for gestational age. Although the onset of puberty occurs in the expected range, it tends to be earlier and at a faster rate[15]. Girls may have an early age of menarche and end up being smaller than their peers[16].

The development of endocrine network function, in utero, that does not match external conditions after birth can have an adverse impact beyond infancy: in the timing of the maturation of other endocrine systems such as the adrenal and reproductive axes. The net result is potentially compromised adult health.

## Mismatch of in utero tuned hormone networks and post-natal environment

Darwinian evolution by natural selection describes how a species and its environment become well matched. The mechanism is through heritable changes in DNA being passed down to future offspring, with the survival of those best adapted to the environment. Developmental plasticity is a short-term solution to preparing offspring in utero to meet the challenge of a changing environment, exploring the range of phenotypic outcomes available in the existing DNA sequence. The phenotype that most closely matches the predicted external environment is induced in utero through the action of hormones. The endocrine profile of a thrifty phenotype is potentially advantageous for a baby born into an environment where the prediction of food scarcity is a reality. However, it would be a disadvantage in an environment where food turned out to be abundant. Maladapted infants may suffer long-term health effects, such as increased risk of adult cardiovascular disease, in particular. This is especially relevant for women, where the leading cause of death after menopause is from cardiovascular disease[17].

Mothers who bore children during the time of food rationing during and just after the Second World War (1945–1950) may have passed on thrifty phenotypes to the benefit of their offspring, but their grandchildren (born 1970–1975) who grew up with adequate food were susceptible to becoming overweight. Potentially their great-grandchildren (born 1995–2000), who grew up with plentiful cheap, fast food and low activity levels, were even more likely to become overweight and obese compared with previous generations.

The degree of mismatch between the endocrine phenotype and the subsequent external environment determines the degree and range of negative health outcomes[18]. Originally the thrifty endocrine phenotype may have been a survival advantage for the "mewling, puking" infant in Shakespeare's time. However, in a modern environment shifted more towards high energy intake and low energy expenditure in infancy and beyond; this type of prenatal endocrine adaptation can be contributing to the increase in metabolic and cardiovascular disease over the lifespan and generations[19].

## Hormone stories: what happened next?

*Polly was a 29-year-old woman looking for a way to lose weight quickly, to benefit the future health of the baby she hoped to conceive. She had read on social media that doing high intensity exercise in the morning and eating a single very low-calorie meal in the late afternoon would guarantee the attainment of her goal quickly. Initially her weight declined but then it plateaued. She was starting to feel dizzy and suffered from headaches. She noticed that her menstrual cycle was becoming shorter. She realised that she needed medically-based advice.*

*Although being a healthy weight is certainly important, better approaches produce sustainable effects. Polly spaced out three meals over the day, ensuring small portion sizes. She maintained regular exercise, but at a more moderate intensity and never in a fasted state. Polly was able to attain a healthy weight that she could maintain and her cycles resumed their regularity. This provided a more stable internal environment for her future baby to match its developing endocrine system with the environment.*

## Strategies to support hormone health in infancy

### Considerations

- Before pregnancy, preconception, it is advisable for the mother to aim for a healthy weight and eating patterns
- Where possible, pregnant mothers should match nutrition to demand, avoiding both undereating and overeating, to regulate pregnancy weight gain

*Scene 1: Infancy*

- Any pre-existing maternal endocrine conditions, such as diabetes mellitus or thyroid dysfunction, need monitoring in a medical antenatal clinic
- After birth, monitoring infant growth relative to charts of height and weight for age is helpful. Where catch-up growth is hoped for, it should not be too rapid

# Scene 2
## Childhood

> *"And then the whining school-boy with his satchel*
> *And shining morning face, creeping like a snail,*
> *Unwillingly to school."*
>
> Shakespeare

**Subtitle:** During infancy, a child's hormone networks that were primed during pregnancy adapt to the reality of the external environment. Childhood is the time when the hormone networks enter the phase of growth and development, in preparation for the transition towards adulthood. The habits and behaviours adopted by young people can influence these processes.

## Hormone stories

*Charlie* was a 12-year-old schoolboy who was upset at being the smallest in his class. Some of his peers had recently become much taller. As a fast runner, he had enjoyed playing as a winger in rugby, but suddenly the opposition had become a lot bigger than him. He faced the risk of injury each time he was tackled. He was losing confidence both on the pitch and in the classroom.

*Jane* was an 11-year-old schoolgirl. She was one of the taller girls in her class and a keen gymnast. She was also top of the class academically. Jane enjoyed being good at both sport and schoolwork. She wanted things to stay like this. She saw some of her friends changing shape towards a woman and some had started their period. Jane thought that a change in her shape would mean she wouldn't be so good at gymnastics. She decided to take control of the situation and reduce eating carbohydrates. Jane felt satisfied seeing her weight drop. However, her mother, teachers and school friends were concerned that she was not eating enough and becoming withdrawn.

*Scene 2: Childhood*

# Hormone networks in children

## Growth spurt

The main endocrine event that occurs during later childhood is a surge in growth hormone (GH) production, supported by the thyroid hormone thyroxine, which causes the childhood growth spurt. This sets the stage for progression into puberty when the production of the sex steroid hormones ramps up.

The main internal biological clock, the hypothalamus, times the initiation and progress of hormone network changes occurring in childhood. It directs the pituitary gland to increase its production of GH. GH is converted peripherally into insulin-like growth factor 1 (IGF-1), which acts on the various tissues in the body. This process depends on the synchronised timing of the sensitivity and response of tissues to childhood hormonal changes. The tissue response rates to these hormone changes can vary, as described below.

## Physical and psychological effects

GH promotes the growth of all the tissues in the body. It does this through the anabolic "body-building" action of IGF-1. GH also has an impact on body composition, favouring lean body mass (muscle and bone) over fat[1]. This is why the percentage of fat in older children starts to reduce towards adult levels. The thyroid hormone thyroxine also plays an important part in the changes occurring during childhood, backing up the actions of GH in terms of physical growth and continuing to support brain neural development.

The onset of the childhood growth spurt starts earlier in girls than boys, as shown in Figure 12.1. At around the age of 11 or 12, girls are taller and faster than boys. This is reflected in qualification times for swimming competitions, which are faster for girls than boys at that age. However, despite a later start in GH surge, boys soon catch up and overtake the girls. Ultimately when adults, men are on average 13 cm taller than women[2].

## Height versus Age

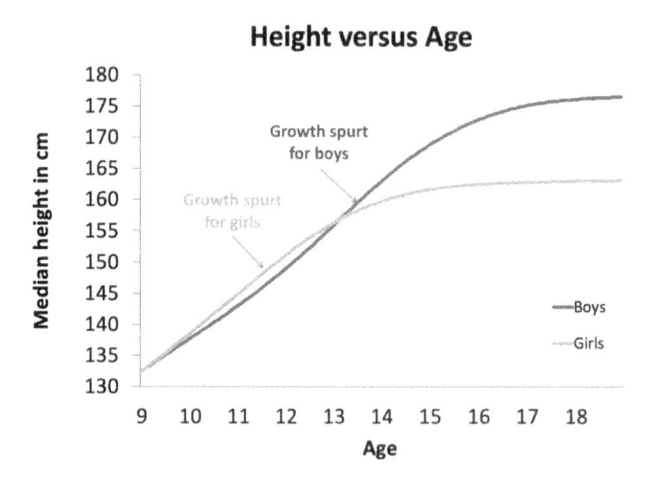

**Figure 12.1:** Growth spurt

The profile of the changes in height with age is reflected in standard childhood growth charts. These include percentile lines indicating the spread of heights across children of the same age. Although the growth spurt of an individual child does not progress in a smooth manner, with weeks of alternating growth and stasis, there is a tendency to remain close to the same percentile line over time. A child who is tall before the growth spurt can expect to become a taller adult.

The growth spurt causes a change in body proportions, which does not occur in a synchronous way. The initial rapid growth in the long bones of the limbs can make youngsters look awkward and gangly, until the growth of the axial skeleton (the spine) catches up. The adult arm span closely matches height, as first described by the Roman writer Vetruvius and recorded for posterity in Leonardo da Vinci's drawing of the "Vetruvian man". Individual variation in the "ape index" gives some adults slightly longer reach, which can be an advantage in activities such as climbing and boxing.

Similarly, following the growth spurt the proportions of the upper and lower segments of the body settle to be roughly equal, with the dividing line being set at the pelvic rim. As with the ape index, individual variation can be advantageous to certain types of sports. Some top swimmers have relatively longer upper body segments and shorter legs. To quantify the change in body proportions during this time of flux, anthropometric measurements in children include measurement of standing height and sitting height. Subtraction provides a calculation of leg length.

This dyssynchronous growth pattern in children during the growth spurt influences proprioception: awareness of where your body is in space. Picking up a glass requires accurate computation of how long your arm is and how far away the glass is. If your arm is now longer than before, a period of familiarisation is required to recalculate movements accurately. This can result in a broken glass. Temporary growth-induced "clumsiness" can have psychological effects. Precision movements required in certain activities maybe be impacted, so a previously skilled athlete can temporarily become very average. Those experiencing an earlier growth spurt compared with their peers may enjoy early success in some sports, like swimming. However, subsequently these children may have to contend with being caught up and overtaken by those experiencing a later growth spurt.

The effect of the hormone-driven growth spurt on the musculoskeletal system can present some physical issues for children. This is because the growth of bone and soft tissues occurs at different rates. Rapid increase in the length of the long bones of the limbs means that the soft tissues of the tendons, ligaments and muscles are stretched. Tendons are made of robust connective tissue called collagen that anchors the tapered end of a muscle onto the bone. Tendons are generally found across joints, allowing skeletal muscle groups to create movement. For example, when the thigh muscle group, the quadriceps, contracts, the force is transmitted via the patella (kneecap) tendon embedded in the upper part of the tibia (shin bone). This results in knee extension, a straightening of the leg. If rapid growth in the length of the femur (thigh bone) and tibia has not been matched by an increase in the lengths of muscles and tendons, the force exerted at the muscle attachment point to the bone is increased. Repetitive, high forces can result in traction on the bone that causes bone damage and even detachment of some bone.

In growing children, the area of bone close to the joint where tendons attach is called an apophysis. This is an area of bone undergoing growth, which is close to, but not securely attached to, the "mother" bone. The growth spurt predisposes children to traction apophysitis. At the knee, this is called Osgood-Schlatter disease (although not really a "disease", but rather a result of expected hormone physiology). A youngster typically complains of pain, tenderness and swelling just below the knee cap. A similar situation can occur at the heel, where the Achilles tendon inserts into the calcaneus (heel bone). This is called Sever's disease. Due to the susceptibility to these types of injuries, this is one of the reasons why it is advised that children should not undertake the same type and volume of exercise training as adults[3].

From a physical and psychological point of view, childhood is a window of opportunity to develop good movement patterns by working on improving neuromuscular skills: the fine tuning of neurological control of movement[4]. This has maximal beneficial effect when the neurological system is in a state of flux, called neuroplasticity, at the same time as physical change. This is why it is harder to learn a new skill, like ballet for example, at a later age, as this requires refined, precision movement. Children have a golden window of opportunity to develop efficiency of movement and reduce injury in the short and long term.

## *Variations on a theme*

A child's genetic height potential can be estimated using a simple formula. Take the average height of the mother and father, then add 7 cm (3 inches) for a boy or deduct 7 cm for a girl. Since there is a wide variation around this central estimate, it is also useful to project forward a child's height percentile on a standard growth chart.

Environmental and behavioural factors play a part in the attainment of adult height, acting via hormone networks and gene expression. The importance of nutrition for fully functioning hormone networks during childhood is reflected in the increase in average height over the past several hundred years in the UK. The adult clothes from centuries ago would fit some children of today. In England, from 1972 to 1994 children's heights increased by 1cm [2].

The timing of the growth spurt is partially genetically determined. Constitutional delay is the term used to describe children whose biological age, in terms of growth and development, is behind chronological age. This can run in families. However, it is always important to exclude underlying medical conditions that might be causing delay, for example, systemic illness, such as malabsorption found in coeliac disease. Coeliac disease is where the gut does not absorb sufficient nutrients and energy to support growth. Although there are no underlying issues with hormone networks, this shows how external factors such as nutrition can downregulate the expected hormone timing in children. In the case of coeliac disease, modification in diet enables hormone networks to reboot and regain expected timing.

Hormone-specific issues can impair childhood growth and cause short stature (height more than 2 standard deviations below the mean for age and sex). Top of the list are issues with underproduction of GH and thyroid hormones. GH production is tricky to assess as the main stimulus to release is sleep, when it is produced in pulses. A GH stimulation test can be performed to assess the system. A lack of GH response to stimulation indicates an issue in production, which could either be genetic or due to medical conditions impinging on hypothalamic-pituitary function. Rarely, the stimulation test can show an increased GH production response, in which case the problem in the system lies at the level of tissue responses to GH.

Thyroid function is easier to assess as this hormone network acts over longer time scales. A static test of the pituitary control hormone, thyroid-stimulating hormone (TSH) and the thyroid-response hormones, thyroxine (T4) and tri-iodothyronine (T3), is usually sufficient. A child born with a congenital underactive thyroid (hypothyroidism) would be picked up at neonatal screening. If hypothyroidism develops during childhood this is usually autoimmune in nature, where the body makes antibodies to the thyroid gland, rendering it less effective in producing the hormones T4 and T3.

Where underproduction of either of these hormones, GH or thyroxine, is identified, treatment with the appropriate external hormone can help the child move up the growth chart.

On the other hand, some children with very rapid growth attain a tall stature (more than 2 standard deviations above the mean for age and sex). As with delayed growth, this may simply be a variation in biological timing. Hormonal causes would include the overproduction of the usual suspects: GH and thyroid hormones. In cases of suspected overproduction of GH, a suppression test is performed. Failure to suppress the production of GH indicates the rare situation of "uncontrolled" GH production. Occasionally low-dose sex steroids might be used to advance puberty and limit further height gain.

## Interaction of hormone networks and external behaviours

Throughout this book the emphasis has been on how our lifestyle behaviours act via our internal hormone networks to influence gene expression. This interaction holds true in children[5].

### *Sleep rules supreme*

For children, sleep duration is associated with telomere length[6]. The telomere region of a chromosome is located at the end, like a cap. This telomere region is effectively the control switch for DNA expression, allowing hormones to initiate or suppress gene expression. Shortened telomeres can disrupt gene expression, with potential health consequences. In adults, it is well documented that poor sleep causes shortening of telomeres. A large study of children showed the same effect. This is of particular concern as effects of inadequate sleep on DNA in children are carried through to adulthood and have potential long-term adverse health effects.

What about the effects of sleep on hormone networks? Circadian misalignment, with suboptimal sleep patterns, is known to impact hormone network function in adults, with subsequent adverse consequences on health. The same situation pertains to children[7]. However, sleep is an even more crucial requirement for children, not just to maintain health but to support growth and the healthy transition from adolescence to adulthood. An adequate quantity of good quality sleep is needed to support the development of cognitive, emotional and social health. One of the main stimuli for GH release is sleep. GH production wakes up while the child sleeps, with regular pulses of GH released every three hours or so.

Conversely, insufficient or poor-quality childhood sleep can cause issues with metabolism and a tendency towards insulin resistance, which in turn can lead to a cascade of metabolic health issues[8].

Sleep patterns influence health through the interaction of hormones and gene expression. This interaction is even more important for children than adults, given that consequences can be carried through into adult health.

## *Activity and exercise*

Recent years have witnessed a surge in childhood obesity. Genetics plays a part in obesity, but, as ever, hormones determine gene expression. A reduction in the physical activity of children impacts hormones. Rather than the schoolboy walking to school in Shakespeare's time, albeit reluctantly, nowadays children are frequently ferried around in motorised transport. Overall activity levels have fallen, and many leisure activities tend to be sedentary. Specifically, research shows that screen time is linked to adiposity in children[9]. There were no televisions or computers in Shakespeare's day.

In a large study of children aged 6–8 years, the balance of exercise and sedentary time was found to be an important determinant of reading and arithmetic skills[10]. Physical activity was measured via motion sensors and fitness was measured with a bike test. Hormones were the mediators of this effect of physical activity on academic achievement in children. In boys higher body fat and the hormone, leptin, produced by this adipose tissue, were linked to a lower level of reading fluency and comprehension. This was reflected in reduced neuromuscular performance which was assessed through tests of agility (ability to change direction quickly), speed and balance. For girls in this study, reading fluency was found to be liked with indicators of suboptimal cardiometabolic health. Higher levels of a particular liver enzyme were found in less active girls. This is surprising and somewhat concerning as this profile is found in adults with metabolic syndrome and is linked with poor cardiovascular and metabolic health. Evidence of the adverse consequences of a sedentary lifestyle in children as young as six years of age is clearly a concern[11].

These findings in children are also very striking because of the potential for long-term effects on health. During childhood, lifestyle factors acting via hormone networks are determining not only the physical and academic potential of a child in real-time. The actions of hormones in childhood are setting the pattern for health and potential in adulthood.

On the other hand, at the other end of the spectrum, early sport specialisation, not seen in Shakespeare's day, can be equally problematic, with an increased risk of injury, concussion and psychological burnout[3]. Children pursuing training programmes better suited to adults face an increased likelihood of adverse outcomes of exercise. Children do not have the established adult hormone networks to be able to cope with, or benefit from, excessive levels of exercise training. During childhood, low levels of sex steroid hormones (testosterone and oestradiol) are found in both girls and boys. In terms of metabolism, substrate (food fuel) utilisation is similar at rest and during exercise[12]. This means that both boys and girls are less able to cope with high-intensity anaerobic exercise, where carbohydrate is the sole substrate. This explains why the type of exercise for children should be more focused on the aerobic system. For example, in competitive swimming, sprint distances are not introduced until around the age of 13. The lower levels of GH and sex steroid hormones found in childhood are similar to the situation at the other end of the lifespan. In old age when hormone networks start winding down, the profile returns to that of a child before the growth spurt. This is part of the reason that masters athletes start to lose "top-end" performance, in terms of sprint ability.

Exercise training for children should focus on enjoyment and general neuromuscular skill acquisition, rather than specialisation. This approach promotes the positive effects of activity on developing endocrine networks.

## *Nutrition*

The positive effects of adequate nutrition, in terms of quantity and quality, can be seen historically, as adult height has increased in step with improvements in diet. Protein is particularly important both as a stimulus for GH release and to provide the building blocks for the growth of tissues during the childhood growth spurt. Conversely, excessive nutrition, especially when in presence of low activity levels, has contributed to the increase in childhood obesity[13]. The quality of diet is also a major factor. Studies show that ultra-processed "convenience food" diets cause excess calorie intake and weight gain[14]. Compared with the food rationing that occurred during the Second World War, we now have unlimited access to ubiquitous cheap processed food from a very young age. The fact that this has occurred in a relatively short space of time, alongside a decrease in activity levels, is a major health problem. This situation can disrupt developing hormone networks and increase the risk of metabolic and cardiovascular diseases in adulthood.

Having sufficient levels of vitamin D is especially important during childhood. In spite of the name, vitamin D is actually a steroid hormone, whose main source is the action of sunlight on the skin. It is not possible to obtain sufficient vitamin D from diet alone. Vitamin D is crucial for bone health. Since bones are growing rapidly during the childhood growth spurt, vitamin D is in demand to support the action of GH. Lack of vitamin D during childhood results in the deformation of bone known as rickets. As sunlight is in short supply in higher latitudes, including the UK, vitamin D supplementation is necessary[15].

## Hormone stories: what happened next?

***Charlie*** *was the schoolboy who was upset and losing confidence because he was the smallest in his class. Charlie had his birthday in late August, close to the end of the academic year group. So some of his classmates with September birthdays were nearly a whole chronological year older than him, meaning they had already started their growth spurts and entered the early stages of puberty. On further discussion, it transpired that family members tended to be "slow developers". Charlie's predicted mid-parental height indicated that he was most likely to attain an average height. Reassuringly he had been consistently tracking his personal growth percentile. In other words, Charlie was experiencing constitutional delay. After explaining the situation Charlie and his parents were reassured. His personal biological timing of hormone production for growth spurt and puberty was running a little slower than his chronological age. A situation made more prominent by being relatively young for* his class. Charlie was also a fast swimmer, so he decided that for time being he would focus more on water polo, which he described as being like rugby in water. A year later Charlie and his parents got in touch to say that Charlie was now making ground on his peers, in terms of height, and he was becoming a very successful water polo player.

**Jane** was a 11-year-old schoolgirl, a keen gymnast and strong academically. Jane wanted things to stay the same. She thought she could achieve this by reducing what she ate. Although she had started her childhood growth spurt, being one of the tallest in her class, progression into puberty and the start of periods did not follow, due to insufficient energy. She was in a state of low energy availability, resulting in down-regulation of developing hormone networks, which were attempting to "save" energy. To restore hormone function and progression through puberty, Jane required support to overcome psychological barriers to eating sufficiently to meet the internal energy requirements of this most active time for hormone networks.

## Strategies to support hormone networks in childhood

### Sleep

- Good sleep patterns are crucial for both DNA and hormone health in childhood, with important repercussions on adult health
- The hours of sleep are when GH is released to support the growth spurt

### Exercise

- Exercise at an appropriate level for children supports healthy hormone networks and subsequent physical and cognitive development
- Childhood is a window of opportunity to focus on developing the neuromuscular skill aspect of exercise
- Conversely, children performing adult-level exercise training are at increased risk of injury and burnout

### Nutrition

- Nutrition is particularly important during childhood for hormone health
- Diet needs to provide sufficient energy, include all food types and be of good quality to support the demands of a changing hormone function
- Good nutrition supports the child's physical and cognitive development

# Scene 3
## Teenager

*"And then the lover,*
*Sighing like furnace, with a woeful ballad,*
*Made to his mistress' eyebrow"*
*Shakespeare*

**Subtitle:** The teenage years are when puberty occurs. This is marked by the awakening and establishment of the reproductive hormone axis. A rapid increase in the production of the sex steroid hormones, oestrogen and testosterone, propagates seismic physical and mental changes. Lifestyle choices can influence this transition to adulthood.

## Hormone stories

*At 17 years of age, **Jake** was training to be a dancer at a vocational school. Although he loved dancing, he was finding it tough living away from home and missed his mother's home-cooked food. He knew that a career as a professional dancer was very competitive and looked at himself critically in the dance studio mirrors. He convinced himself that he did not look slim enough and that he would be a better dancer if he lost weight. However, rather than improving, he felt tired, slept badly and lacked the energy to jump high.*

***Jenny** was a keen 18-year-old athlete, participating in many school sports, as well as training and competing in sports teams outside of school. Jenny was also very successful in her academic work at school and looking to gain a place at university.*

*Scene 3: Teenager*

*Everything seemed to be going very well for Jenny; however, her periods had not started. Jenny experienced a sharp pain in her foot during a running session, which turned out to be a fracture.*

## Awakening of sex steroid production

The teenage years are when sex steroid hormone production starts ramping up, stoking the emotional furnace. The sex steroids are oestrogen and testosterone. Both hormones are produced in males and females, but in different proportions. Puberty is a time during adolescence when these hormone network developments cause physical and physiological changes. By the completion of puberty, sexual maturity is reached[1].

In the two years before puberty, the production of adrenal androgens increases in both boys and girls. In this process, called adrenarche, the steroid hormones dehydroepiandrosterone sulphate (DHEAS) and androstenedione contribute to pubic hair growth. However, adrenarche is a precursor to that main hormone event of puberty: the awakening of sex steroid production by the gonads: ovaries in females and testes in males.

*Hormones, Health and Human Potential*

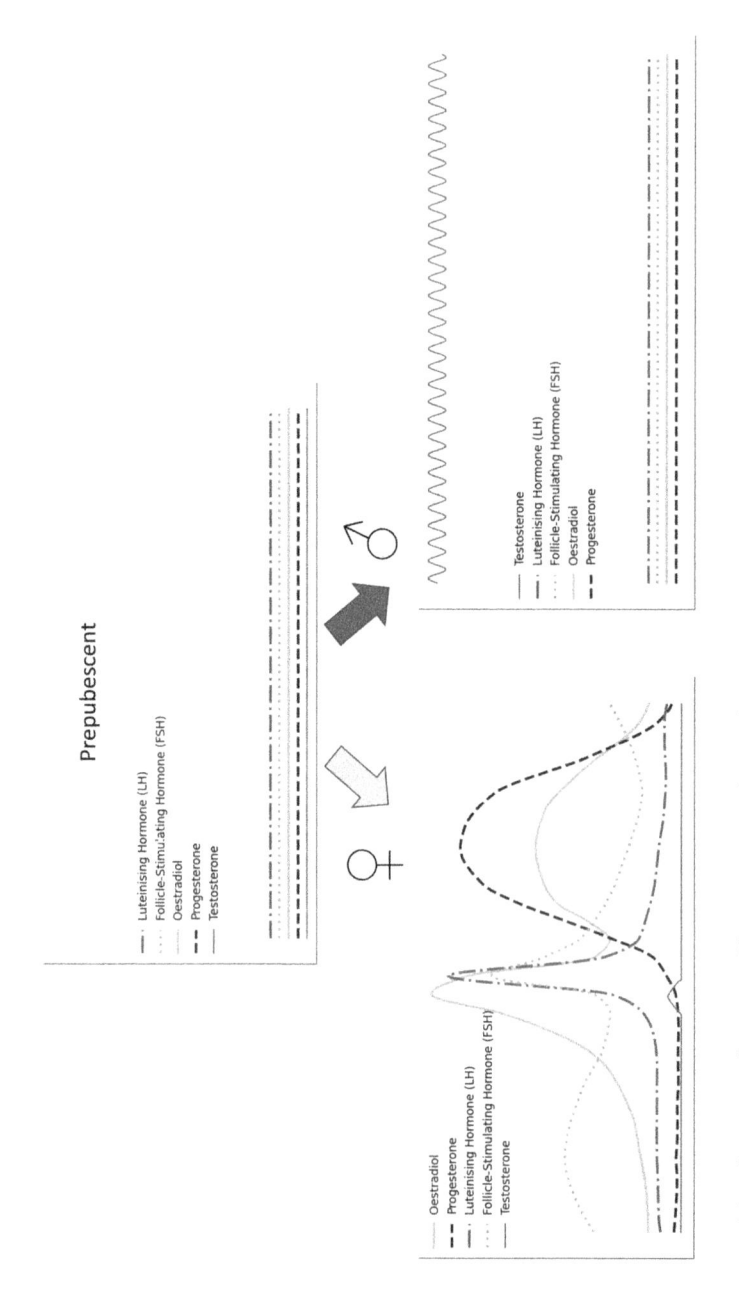

**Figure 13.1:** Transformation of sex steroid hormone networks at puberty

## Scene 3: Teenager

The top part of Figure 13.1 shows the sex steroid hormone network in a quiescent state prior to puberty. In both boys and girls there are low levels of the pituitary control hormones, follicle-stimulating hormone (FSH) and luteinising hormone (LH), alongside low levels of the sex steroid hormones, oestradiol (the most active form of oestrogen), progesterone and testosterone. However, by the end of puberty a transformation has occurred, with adult patterns of sex steroid production. Women experience significant cyclical variations every 28 days or so, while men have small diurnal variations in testosterone. What has brought about this awakening?

The conductor of the endocrine orchestra is the hypothalamic-pituitary control centre located in the brain. The setting in motion of sex steroid production starts here. The hypothalamus produces bursts of gonadotrophin-releasing hormone (GnRH) in a characteristic pattern. This occurs during sleep, and these GnRH signals travel the short distance to the pituitary via an exclusive blood supply. Physical changes begin to occur once communication is established between the hypothalamus and pituitary. When the pituitary receives the GnRH messages, it responds in turn with the pulsatile release of LH. The pulsatile release of LH causes the gonads to start sex steroid production. In boys, the action of LH on the testes increases testosterone production. In girls, LH acts on the ovaries to increase oestradiol production.

What controls the timing of the activation of the GnRH pulse generator? The hypothalamus is described as the neuroendocrine gatekeeper. It picks up cues from both hormone and neural sources. The hypothalamus is ideally located in the brain to process signals from both outside and within the body, as they are transmitted through chemical and electrical channels. However, the hypothalamus needs to be in a receptive state to be able to decode and act upon these neuroendocrine messages. So, the timing of the initiation of puberty depends on the development and plasticity (ability to change) of the hypothalamus[2].

This process of hypothalamic development, to set it on course to initiate puberty, starts in utero. The brain "gonadostat" theory describes how, at puberty, the GnRH pulse generator is finally released from the shackles that have held it in check. Initially, in early pregnancy the foetal gonadostat is insensitive to the negative feedback of sex steroid hormones. Towards the later stages of pregnancy, when the gonadostat has matured it increases in sensitivity, and high maternal circulating levels of oestradiol and testosterone cause suppression of foetal production of FSH and LH. This sensitivity of the gonadostat increases during childhood, reportedly becoming ten times more sensitive to negative feedback than in adults. This results in suppression of the GnRH generator. In other words, the gonadostat is under inhibitory control. At puberty, a decrease in sensitivity to circulating sex steroid hormones weakens the inhibitory signals, allowing the release of GnRH[3].

## Hormone-driven changes in puberty

### Physical changes

The average age for the onset of puberty is around 11 years in girls and 12 years in boys, though this can vary up to two years. The first physical signs of sex steroid hormones initiating puberty are breast development in girls and an increase in testicular size in boys. For each sex, puberty progresses in a set pattern of five physical phases known as the Tanner stages of puberty. These external physical changes reflect what is happening internally as the hormone networks progress through the gears to establish adult levels and patterns of hormone production.

### Oestrogen at work

Oestrogen has a variety of effects on bone as puberty progresses. The pubertal growth spurt occurs for girls at Tanner stages 2–3 and 3–4 in boys. This growth spurt is due to increases in oestrogen levels in both sexes. In girls, oestrogen is produced by the ovaries. In boys, testosterone is converted to oestrogen by the process of aromatisation. Increasing levels of oestrogen promote the secretion of the eponymous growth hormone (GH).

Although the initial increase in oestrogen underpins the pubertal growth spurt, as levels rise further, this sex steroid hormone plays a different role in growth. Oestrogen arrests growth in both boys and girls, by causing the epiphyses, the growth plates located at the ends of the long bones, to close. The progression of epiphyseal growth plate fusion can be measured on X-ray, to calculate bone age. This measure of biological age during puberty may differ from chronological age. The difference between bone age and chronological age can be used to estimate growth potential and help predict final adult height. The start of puberty bone age in girls is around 10.5–11 years and for boys 11–11.5 years of age. Skeletal maturity, with near-complete epiphyseal closure and limited further growth potential, occurs at a bone age of 15 years in girls and 17 years in boys[1].

The increase in oestrogen production during puberty has yet another role in bone health, which becomes particularly important once skeletal maturity is reached: the mineralisation of bone. Bone mineral density increases very rapidly during puberty, driven by increasing levels of oestrogen in both sexes. This results in the attainment of peak bone mass. This is shown in Figure 13.2. The rapid accrual of bone mineral density is essential to maintain bone strength following the increase in size and protect against the risk of fracture. Temporary physiological weakening of bone can occur, while mineralisation catches up with bone growth. Imbalances in lifestyle behaviours, particularly exercise and nutrition, can also delay bone mineralisation by holding back hormone changes, particularly the increase in sex steroid production.

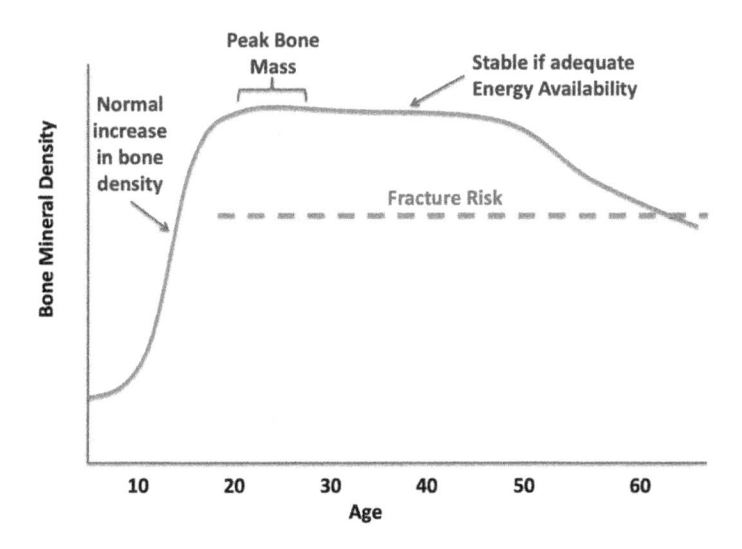

**Figure 13.2:** Attainment of peak bone mass: change in bone mineral density with age

## What about testosterone?

As with oestrogen, an initial increase of testosterone in both sexes plays an important role in puberty. Testosterone impacts body composition, favouring lean mass (muscle) formation over fat deposition, allowing the development of musculature. Nevertheless, as puberty progresses, so does the divergence in the relative amounts of sex steroid hormones in boys versus girls. As we explore below, it is essential for girls to have a certain amount of fat to support hormone health and the onset of the cyclical production of oestrogen and progesterone during menstrual cycles. In boys, increasing levels of testosterone over puberty boost muscle bulk. This has an indirect positive mechanical effect on bone mineral density (BMD), as larger muscles exert more force on bone. Higher testosterone levels in boys, established during puberty, can also have an effect on the geometry and size of bones.

## The period of the period

In girls, menarche (the start of menstrual periods) occurs at Tanner stage 4, near the completion of puberty. The average age for menarche is at 12.8 years, with some variation on either side of this age. A slightly later onset of menarche can run in families, where genetic elements cause a constitutional delay in puberty. Environmental and behavioural factors can also play a part in the timing of menarche. Interestingly, over the last century, the age of menarche has decreased: in 1900 the average age of menarche was 17 years. The decrease is thought to be due to improved environmental conditions, especially nutrition.

Puberty can occur early in girls who are overweight. Conversely, strenuous exercise and low body weight can delay puberty and the age of menarche, as found in dancers and gymnasts. Early work in this area found that the number of years of training before menarche delayed the onset[4]. There was a higher incidence of lack of periods (amenorrhea) and irregular cycles (oligomenorrhoea) in this group, compared with girls who started training after menarche.

The reason appears to be related to hormones, specifically leptin which is a hormone produced from adipose tissue (an adipokine). Leptin comes from the Greek word meaning "thin". Exercise training favours reduction in fat and increase in lean mass (muscle). However, low levels of fat lead to low levels of leptin. This impedes the ability of the hypothalamus to complete the hormone changes associated with puberty. In particular, low leptin reduces LH secretion from the pituitary. This is important because the increased pulsatile release of LH initiates and establishes menstrual cycle fluctuations of female hormones. In a study I conducted, female dancers in vocational training had lower levels of leptin and a later start of periods than their non-dance counterparts[5]. Low leptin and LH secretion have been found in young amenorrhoeic athletes[6]. Does this matter? Yes[7]. As oestrogen is essential for bone health, a delay in the onset of menarche can have adverse effects that are discussed in more detail below.

Regardless of how much exercise a girl is doing, if periods have not been established by the age of 16 years, at the very latest she is said to be experiencing primary amenorrhoea. This warrants investigation to exclude any underlying medical condition requiring appropriate intervention[7]

## Psychological changes

Neuroplasticity encompasses the ability of the nervous system, including the brain, to change in structure, function and connections in response to stimuli from outside and inside the body. Hormones are the mediators of neuroplasticity.

Sex steroid hormones influence brain structure from early in life. The big increase in sex steroids at puberty produces effects on brain organization and structure[8]. The surge in pubertal sex steroid hormones also affects brain function. For example, experience-dependent plasticity enhances during adolescence, corresponding to the teenager seeking to develop independence[9]. In terms of higher-order cognitive function, there seems to be an initial enhanced plasticity of cortical circuits in early puberty, followed by a decline as sex steroids settle into adult patterns. The ability to learn new skills quickly is enhanced, but then subsequently suppressed, with language skills being a good example[10]. Maybe there is some truth in the adage that "you can't teach an old dog new tricks". The fact that puberty is now occurring at an earlier age than in Shakespeare's time may impact learning potential[11].

## When pubertal hormone changes don't go according to plan

**Precocious puberty** is when puberty starts earlier than expected: under eight years in girls or under nine in boys. The reason could be a mistiming in the production of gonadotrophins from the hypothalamus or unexpected peripheral production of sex hormones, independent of central gonadotrophin control. It is important to identify the cause of precocious puberty and treat it accordingly. One of the considerations is that early puberty, apart from creating psychological challenges, may compromise final adult height as early sex steroid production causes early closure of bone growth plates.

**Delayed puberty** is where there is a failure to progress into puberty by the age of 14 in girls and 15 years in boys. Sometimes puberty may have started, but then progression to the next stage is delayed by more than two years. Among the causes of delayed puberty, the most common is constitutional delay. This is a consistent slower timing of growth and development without a medical cause. Occasionally external sex steroids can be given to initiate puberty, when delay is causing concern and psychological distress. This may be a small dose of testosterone for a boy over 13 years of age or a small dose of oestradiol in a girl over 12 years. Although this helps with bone mineralisation, the downside is that treatment with external sex steroids can cause growth plate fusion, so careful discussion is required.

Other causes of delayed puberty include chronic systemic disease, for example, conditions causing malabsorption. Imbalances in behaviours relating to exercise and nutrition can delay puberty.

There are some medical conditions impacting hormone production that impact puberty. These can be divided into conditions resulting in a lack of gonadotrophin production characterised by low levels of gonadotrophins or problems with the production of sex steroid hormones from the gonads (ovaries or testes), where gonadotrophins are high. Once the underlying cause has been identified, management can be tailored accordingly.

## Sleep rules supreme (again)

It is when a teenager is asleep that the master endocrine controller, the hypothalamus, initiates the start and progression of puberty. The optimal amount of sleep for sex steroid production to switch on and establish itself is around eight hours. Sleep is essential both directly and indirectly for neural plasticity during puberty. Sleep supports the awakening of sex steroids for the development of neural plasticity. Neural networks are pruned and refined during sleep[12].

Sleep is also important for the hormones involved in the metabolic health of teenagers. Having too much or too little sleep interferes with this biological timekeeping of hormone release. Too little sleep, especially at the start of puberty, is associated with fat gain. This is because insufficient sleep disrupts appetite hormones, increasing the tendency to eat more, which has the effect of reducing insulin sensitivity. High blood glucose levels cause an increase in insulin production to move glucose out of the bloodstream into the cells. However, sustained, high insulin levels result in a drop-off in the cellular response to the presence of the hormone. This "fatigue" in response is similar to when you become unaware of persistent background noise. The transition from reduced insulin sensitivity to insulin resistance occurs in type 2 diabetes. Exercise improves insulin sensitivity directly: by increasing cellular demand for glucose, cells are obliged to be responsive to insulin, in order to absorb glucose from the blood. Exercise improves insulin sensitivity indirectly via improved sleep after exertion[13].

*Scene 3: Teenager*

## Nutrition

Adolescence is a time of high energy demand to drive and complete the physical and physiological changes of puberty. In addition, the teenage years are a busy time with the energy demands of exercise, academic and social events. Whether unintentional or intentional, insufficient energy intake to meet the sum of these demands can result in low energy availability. The body reacts to low energy availability with a compensatory downregulation of hormone networks, in an attempt to "save" energy. In particular, low carbohydrate availability, rather than the "stress" of exercise per se, results in low levels of leptin (produced by adipose tissue) and subsequent reduction of LH pulsatility[14].

When this occurs during the teenage years, it can cause a delay or arrest in the sex steroid production hormones of puberty. This puberty hormone dysregulation has a knock-on impact on the accrual of peak bone mass. This was found in our study of youngsters at vocational dance training school mentioned earlier. Compared with girls of similar age at an academic school, with lower levels of exercise, but similar food intake, the ballet students with higher energy demand from exercise had lower levels of leptin, delayed menarche and higher report of disrupted menstrual cycles. In other words, the ballet students had lower levels of oestrogen compared with their contemporaries with sufficient energy availability.

This low oestrogen state during adolescence was directly related to lower bone mineral density, especially in the lumbar spine, which is rich in the trabecular bone type that is particularly dependent on oestrogen. This is not to say that exercise is a bad thing for teenagers. The good news was that the best bone mineral density was found in dance students in the musical theatre stream. These students appeared to have an optimal balance between exercise and nutrition, favouring hormone health in terms of regular periods and consequently the best bone mineral density compared with either the ballet students or the academic students[15].

Figure 13.3 shows the hormone effects on peak bone mass accrual. The upper curve traces what happens to bone mineral density when there is sufficient energy availability to support sufficient oestrogen production for the rapid increase in bone mineral density to reach peak bone mass. Measurements of the musical theatre group of dancers in the study were consistent with this profile. Conversely, the bone mineral accrual of the ballet dancers was more like the lower curve. They could potentially have the bone mineral density of a 60-year-old woman, while they are still in their 30s. This shows the effect of low energy availability, which reduces the expected oestrogen production during puberty and consequently limits the rate of bone mineralisation.

Does this matter? By missing the window of opportunity to attain peak bone mass, these teenagers were at risk of developing stress fractures, particularly when they increased their exercise training load after transitioning to the more senior ranks of sport or dance[16]. Furthermore, oestrogen not only affects bone mineralisation, it also plays a role in optimising the microarchitecture that allows bone to withstand force[17]. From a biological bone age health point of view, the timing of increased sex steroid production during puberty is essential for bone health not only during adolescence but also for future adult life. A 10% decrease in peak bone mass is predicted to bring forward by 13 years the development of osteoporosis ("brittle bone disease")[18]. In our study of retired, premenopausal dancers, those who had experienced delay in menarche had a lower bone mineral density than those of the same age in the general population[19]. This illustrates how the timing of hormone changes occurring during the teenage years is crucial to health moving into adulthood and for the rest of the lifespan.

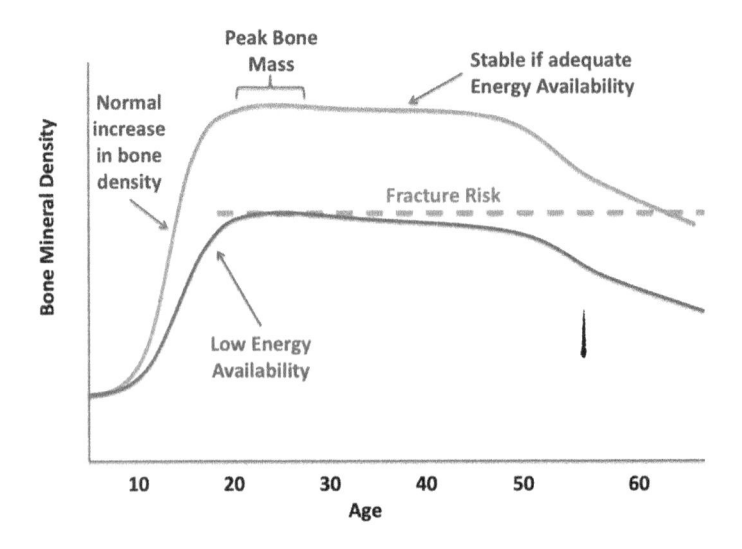

**Figure 13.3:** Importance of adequate diet during adolescence for bone health

## Exercise and activity

As described above, excessive exercise relative to energy intake can have negative effects on the development of hormone networks during the teenage years. Equally, inactivity can also have negative effects on developing physiology and metabolism[20]. The adverse consequences of obesity are well documented. Ideally aiming to include activities that encompass the various components of fitness (cardiovascular, muscle strength and endurance, motor skills and flexibility) supports the timing and effects of developing hormone networks.

It is human nature to prefer doing things that we are good at. Working with teenagers, boys tend to want to do strength work, whereas the girls prefer flexibility exercises. It is important to cover all aspects of fitness, so that everyone can enjoy the class and, in the long term, avoid injury[21]. Although the hormone changes associated with puberty allow teenagers to perform higher intensity exercise than children, the timing of puberty can vary. Physiological capacity is more related to biological age than chronological age. Exercise that hones neuromuscular skills and proprioception is universally beneficial[22]. The brain produces complex and adaptable movements. This is achieved through a learning process, combining sensory feedback with prior knowledge of movement outcomes[23]. On the surface it seems strange when playing tennis that "following through" with a stroke, even once the ball has left the racket, helps ensure a good shot. It turns out that learning and perfecting the full movement pattern from start to finish results in a better quality of movement delivery.

## Hormone stories: what happened next?

*Jake was a 17-year-old dancer who felt tired and lacked energy after trying to lose weight. Although initially he said that he was eating less because he didn't like the school food, it transpired that he was avoiding carbohydrates because he wanted to lose weight. As a result of low energy availability his hormones had downregulated. This was why he was feeling fatigued and experiencing poor sleep. When we discussed the situation, he realised that under-fuelling had deprived him of what he valued the most: the ability to perform.*

*Back home during the holidays, he started eating as he had done previously. Jake regained energy and better sleep. When he returned to dance school, he was able to jump high again. Jake realised that you need energy to fuel hormones and you need healthy hormones for dance performance. Jake also felt a lot happier and more confident about his future as a resilient dancer.*

***Jenny*** was an 18-year-old athlete, without periods, who fractured her foot, while juggling the sporting and academic demands of school with extra-curricular commitments. Since her periods had not started by 16, she was experiencing primary amenorrhea. This required investigation to rule out medical causes. Although the investigations did not show any medical conditions, blood tests revealed low, prepubescent levels of FSH, LH and oestradiol.

*Although Jenny had not intentionally restricted what she was eating, she was not matching the high energy demands of her activity-filled life. With so much energy being burned up on the running track, there was not enough energy left over for the female reproductive axis to fire up for the initiation of periods. She was experiencing arrested puberty. The consequence was that bone mineral density had not increased as expected during puberty. However, Jenny was training at the level of a sexually mature female. So, bone strength was not sufficient to withstand this type of loading, resulting in fracture.*

*After explaining the situation to Jenny, she agreed to scale back her exercise training. She was finding it stressful to maintain all these sports commitments on top of academic work. A few months later her periods started.*

## Summary of the strategies to support hormone networks during adolescence

### *Sleep*

- Good quality and quantity of sleep are vital for the establishment of hormone network timing, particularly the production of sex steroids, which ramp up during puberty to reach adult levels and patterns of secretion
- Avoiding screens, including mobile phones, near bedtime is particularly relevant for teenagers.

### *Exercise*

- Variety of exercise types that cover all components of fitness, with particular attention to refinement of neuromuscular muscular skills
- Avoid early specialisation where possible, rather focus on enjoyment and skill acquisition
- Be aware of individual physiological and physical development in transitioning to adult-level exercise training

## Nutrition

- Energy demands are high for adolescents with busy schedule of work, exercise and socialising
- Good quality and timing of food are important to establish and maintain the sex steroid hormone networks

## Other considerations

- For young exercisers, a good starting point is the British Association of Sport and Exercise Medicine website https://health4performance.basem.co.uk/ which has information for athletes, parents, coaches and healthcare professionals
- For female exercisers, parents and coaches, online courses, endorsed by the British Association of Sport and Exercise Medicine, provide the latest professional-level training and medical performance strategies on how young exercisers can reach their full potential. Practical, actionable strategies around exercise training, nutrition and recovery ensure that these behaviours are supporting the development and establishment of healthy internal hormone networks. There are separate streams for athletes[24,25] and dancers[26,27].

# Scene 4
## Young Man (and Young Woman!)

> *"Then a soldier,*
> *Full of strange oaths, and bearded like the pard,*
> *Jealous in honour, sudden and quick in quarrel,*
> *Seeking the bubble reputation*
> *Even in the cannon's mouth"*
>
> *Shakespeare*

**Subtitle:** The period from adulthood through to middle age should be the time when hormone networks are established and working smoothly to support health and attainment of full individual potential. Nevertheless, balancing lifestyle behaviours can be challenging. We explore the potential pitfalls and how to avoid hormone disruption, with a particular focus on female hormones.

## Hormone stories

***David*** *is a 30-year-old working full time, with frequent long hours. He also has a young family. He gets up early to exercise before work and tries to fit in some more exercise after work, as he feels his job is mainly sedentary. David reports feeling tired, with poor sleep and loss of libido. What do you think might be going on for David?*

***Susie*** *is a 29-year-old woman. She works full time as a PE teacher and is a keen amateur athlete, training with her running club every day. Susie wants to start a family soon; however, since coming off the combined oral contraceptive pill a year ago, her own periods have not returned. What do you think might be going on for Susie?*

## Hormones at their peak

Shakespeare describes a man in his prime when hormone networks would be expected to be working at their optimal level. This is an important stage of life for men and women to be supporting and harnessing their hormones effectively. Sex steroid hormones reach their peak for health. In the case of female hormones, this provides women with the potential to bear children.

## Balancing act for lifestyle factors

Since Shakespeare's time, there has been a shift towards more sedentary lifestyles. Communication and technology have reduced the need to physically move and allowed work to continue beyond daylight hours. The uncoupling of the balance between physical activity, sleep and eating patterns leads to a discordance between our behaviours and internal biological clocks. This circadian misalignment results in hormone network dysfunction (described in Act 1 "Scene 9: A Balancing Act"). It manifests itself in the adverse outcomes described in metabolic syndrome[1]: abdominal obesity, insulin resistance and ultimately type 2 diabetes mellitus. Other consequences include raised blood pressure, adverse lipid profile, inflammatory state and non-alcoholic fatty liver disease, which are all recognised risk factors for cardiovascular and cerebrovascular disease (heart attack and stroke).

Hormone networks can also be disrupted by excessive exercise relative to food intake and rest. This clinical syndrome is known as relative energy deficiency in sport (RED-S), described in detail in Act 1 "Scene 10: In the Red". Although, as the name suggests, RED-S was originally described in sports athletes, it is now recognised as a situation that can occur in any man or woman, whether they describe themselves as an athlete or not. For some, the desire to become "healthier" can tip over into an unhealthy obsession that disturbs hormone networks. Although this functional hormone disruption can occur at any age, young adults can be vulnerable, as they navigate work, family and social commitments.

## Female hormone challenges

The intricate variations in menstrual cycle hormones form part of the most complex of all the hormone networks. Although these cycles have typically settled and work reliably in young adulthood, they are, nevertheless, particularly susceptible to lifestyle imbalances. This can present challenges for some women, balancing a busy schedule of work, family, leisure time and social demands.

I decided to examine the non-medical and non-scientific sources of advice available for women about the potential challenges of fluctuating female hormones and how to address them. This was certainly not a reassuring experience. The Internet and social media are full of conflicting and sometimes puzzling explanations and advice. A tiresome, but irritatingly persistent myth is repeated, suggesting that most women feel a certain way during certain phases of the menstrual cycle. The implication is that anyone not feeling that way must be abnormal. But the fact is that there is a high degree of variation in the way that individual women experience different cycles.

A wide range of recommendations was proposed for what to do to feel a particular way during a certain phase of the cycle. Many of these included expensive courses of supplements or special foods. It is not hard to imagine women becoming despondent when a certain "magic" recommendation did not leave them feeling amazing, as the sales message had suggested they "should". Why are there so many conflicting views and advice?

The simple answer is that women are not clones. Each of us has very subtle, yet important, differences in the levels and timing of our female hormones during a menstrual cycle and even from cycle to cycle. Moreover, each of us responds slightly differently to the same level of a hormone. There cannot be any generic course of action that is applicable to all women, a point recognised in scientific published studies[2,3]. Even in studies of female athletes, whether power or endurance sport, where there is a big emphasis on how to improve performance, the level of individual variation means that no "winning formula" has been found[4,5]. Although the "null" outcomes of studies are important, they do not grab the headlines, are often downplayed and do not receive much airtime. The key message is that hormone levels and timing are highly individual.

To measure accurate hormone levels and timing for an individual woman would require daily blood samples, which would be hard to implement in practice. Fortunately, as described in Act 1, "Scene 6: Hormone Supermodels" artificial intelligence techniques can be very helpful. Knowledge of precise levels and timing of hormones during the menstrual cycle for an individual woman can be linked to how she is feeling: her personal response to these hormone levels and timings. Otherwise, we cannot be certain that applying the theoretical knowledge of hormone effects during the menstrual cycle is either correct or helpful. Even in high-performance sport, where marginal gains are crucial, applying the best theory "blind" is not effective[6].

Women should not resign themselves to a fate decided by their hormones. In fact, the secret to feeling at your best, both physically and mentally, throughout the menstrual cycle is to appreciate that your behaviours and lifestyle choices can have a feedback effect on your hormones and how you feel. What are the facts?

Gentle exercise during menstruation can help with cramps and discomfort. Keeping well hydrated and ensuring adequate iron intake are also important. Severe pain occurring every period requires medical input to exclude conditions such as endometriosis, described below.

During the later follicular phase of the cycle, in the build-up to ovulation, oestradiol, being the dominant hormone, supports the use of glycogen, which is the storage form of carbohydrate found in skeletal muscles. As carbohydrate is used for higher intensity exercise, some women find this can be a good time to perform this type of exercise[7]. On the other hand, it is not unusual for other women to report that exercise actually feels harder: higher perceived exertion. Knowing about this natural individual variation can help you to be psychologically prepared and to avoid being frustrated when others are overtaking you on bike or running sprints, saying how great they feel in this phase of the cycle!

During the luteal phase of the cycle, hormones have a more direct impact on the way women feel. Although there are particular cases, known as anovulatory cycles, when ovulation does not occur, for the majority of healthy women ovulation takes place around the midpoint of the menstrual cycle. Following ovulation, progesterone levels increase significantly, relative to oestradiol, resulting in a rise in resting metabolic rate. This means you need a bit more food to meet energy requirements, particularly carbohydrate, because progesterone impairs the body's ability to use the stored form of carbohydrate, glycogen. So, if you have ovulated and progesterone levels are high, you need to be especially aware of maintaining a consistent intake of complex carbohydrate[7]. For some this might be a good time for longer, endurance-type exercise, provided that increased body temperature is not problematic. It can be helpful to factor in more recovery time, to allow for slightly compromised ability to store glycogen. Unfortunately, a slightly raised body temperature can make sleep more difficult in the luteal phase. Keeping cool and sleeping in a well-ventilated room helps.

The way you feel during your menstrual cycle is a personal thing. To tune into your menstrual cycle hormones, a very good starting point is to note down how you feel over your cycle. Look out for cyclical patterns and try out straightforward strategies of eating, exercise and sleep patterns that work for you. This does not have to be complicated or expensive. In fact, this approach is recommended by the Royal College of Obstetrics and Gynaecologists as a way to identify phases of the cycle that are problematic for you and try some evidence-based suggestions. This is particularly helpful for premenstrual syndrome.

## Heightened sensitivity to female hormones

### Premenstrual syndrome (PMS)

Although fluctuations in female hormones over the menstrual cycle are normal physiology and important for health, sometimes they come with challenges. PMS is a situation where a woman experiences difficulties during the two weeks before menstruation, in a repeating fashion over several cycles. Psychological symptoms include depression, anxiety, irritability and mood swings, alongside possible physical symptoms, such as feeling bloated and breast tenderness. PMS is particularly prevalent in women between 35 and 45 years of age, with 40% of women experiencing symptoms[8].

Though there are various theories around the exact mechanisms, the fact is that PMS is driven by the fluctuations in female hormones. Symptoms resolve when menstruation arrives and female hormone levels are low across the board. Since PMS is a diagnosis based on cyclical symptoms linked with the timing of menstrual cycle hormones, the Royal College of Obstetrics and Gynaecologists advises keeping a diary with a daily record of symptoms over at least two cycles.

As premenstrual symptoms occur during the luteal phase of the cycle, both oestradiol and progesterone have been implicated. For example, progesterone may affect a particular neurotransmitter in the brain called γ-aminobutyric acid (GABA). Oestradiol is known to influence another neurotransmitter called serotonin. There is particular interest in the possibility that there may be a genetic predisposition to the sensitivity of oestrogen receptors in the brain. This might explain why some women might be more prone to oestrogen-dependent conditions such as PMS, perimenopause and even post-natal depression. On the other hand, the oestradiol/progesterone ratio might be the key, as there are variants of PMS seen in anovulatory cycles (low progesterone in luteal phase) and also due to the type of progestogen used in certain combined oral contraceptive pills (with higher levels of progesterone).

What are the options for women experiencing PMS? The first port of call is a review of lifestyle factors such as exercise, nutrition and stress management.

Evidence-based complementary therapies include vitamin B6, vitamin D and Vitex agnus castus. Otherwise, as this is a condition driven by female hormones, rather sadly, the best option may be to suppress the natural cycle with continuous combined oral contraceptive pill use (making sure this contains the most "modern" type of progestogen). Giving progestogen alone is not effective and not recommended[8]. There are also other more "heavy-duty" pharmacological ways of suppressing female hormones described in the Royal of Obstetrics and Gynaecology guidelines.

## *Endometriosis*

Endometriosis is a condition dependent on fluctuations in the ovarian hormone, oestradiol. In women who have endometriosis, endometrial tissue, which is sensitive to oestradiol, is found outside the uterine cavity. This is most commonly within the pelvis, such as the ovaries, and/or "misplaced" endometrial tissue outside of the reproductive tract, such as the bowel and bladder. It causes high levels of pain, especially in a cyclical fashion: during menstruation, originating from both the reproductive tract (uterus and ovaries) and pain from the bowel during defaecation and bladder during urination. Other times when pain may be felt is deep pelvic pain associated with intercourse.

One of the reasons it can be challenging to make the diagnosis of endometriosis is that it is difficult to differentiate from other chronic pelvic pain conditions. This includes the psychological effect of living with chronic pain. There is also currently a lack of a non-invasive biomarker test. NICE guidelines[9] advise it is important that doctors discuss the possible diagnosis and offer a three-month trial with pain relief and the possibility of hormonal contraception to suppress ovarian hormones if fertility is not a priority. For women who continue to suffer from symptoms, onward referral for specialist hospital care is recommended. There are non-hormonal options with neuromodulator medications, psychological and physiotherapy interventions. Sometimes surgery is an option, although this may not be curative.

Although female hormones are essential for health, sometimes, especially during this phase of life when hormones are in full action, individuals with elevated sensitivity to these hormones can encounter challenges. The most important point is to seek medical advice if symptoms are impacting your quality of life.

## Mistiming of female hormones

A "mistiming" of female hormone interactions is seen in PCOS (polycystic ovary syndrome), the most common endocrine condition in women of reproductive age. In PCOS, there is a relatively high level of oestrogen associated with lower levels of progesterone, as a mistiming in the endocrine networks results frequently in anovulatory cycles, when the ovaries fail to release an egg.

## When is PCOS not PCOS?

PCOS is something of a misnomer. Rather than ovarian "cysts", we are talking about multiple follicles. Follicles are the hopeful "eggs" that vie with each other to be the chosen follicle that is ovulated during a menstrual cycle. Really PCOS should be called "polyfollicular ovary syndrome". Aside from semantics, the issue of focusing on the physical appearance of the ovaries in PCOS is that the endocrine and metabolic implications can be overlooked. Given that PCOS is the most common endocrine disorder among women of reproductive age, reported as occurring in 10% of women in this age group, focusing on the metabolic consequences of PCOS is advisable for female health[10].

Considering the diagnostic criteria for PCOS, you might have thought it should be relatively straightforward to diagnose this condition. According to the Rotterdam criteria[11], two out of the following three clinical aspects are required to make a diagnosis, *after the exclusion of other medical causes.*

1. Irregular menstrual cycles (oligomenorrhoea or amenorrhoea)
2. Clinical or biochemical evidence of high levels of androgens (raised testosterone on a blood test or excess hair growth/acne on skin)
3. Multiple follicles in the ovaries on pelvic ultrasound scan, known as PCO (polycystic ovaries)

Problems can arise when the criteria are applied without excluding other potential causes of these clinical aspects. It is not unusual for a woman to experience some irregular menstrual cycles, but it would be incorrect to diagnose her with PCOS without considering other causes. In a similar way, having multiple follicles is not diagnostic of PCOS. In a study of young women, 68% were reported to have multiple follicles on pelvic ultrasound scan: PCO (or "polyfollicular" ovaries)[12], suggesting that the third criterion is rather common. Is this important? The resounding answer is absolutely yes! PCOS is a combined endocrine and metabolic dysfunction. From the endocrine point of view, oestrogen is mid-range/high and progesterone is low due to anovulatory cycles. From a metabolic point of view, insulin sensitivity is low with an increased risk of metabolic syndrome. Conversely, as we explore later, a woman whose clinical findings include PCO and/or moderately raised testosterone might be recovering from low-energy availability with low oestrogen and high insulin sensitivity. In other words, the manifestation of PCO can arise independently of the full spectrum of PCOS. This is where a detailed clinical history is crucial. Each situation has distinct potential adverse consequences, requiring distinct management paths.

Turning the spotlight on PCOS, which has an increased risk of metabolic syndrome, there appears to be a contribution from both genetic and environmental factors. The result is an overproduction of testosterone by the ovaries and increased insulin resistance. What is less clear is what comes first. It could be that the ovaries produce high levels of ovarian testosterone. While testosterone is important in the initial development of follicles in the ovary, excessive levels arrest follicle development by decreasing the responsiveness of follicles to LH. This situation amplifies the effect of anti-mullerian hormone (AMH) in arresting follicle development. AMH is released by the granulosa cells of the ovary. Usually, high levels of AMH indicate good ovarian reserve; however, in the case of PCOS because of the mistiming of hormone communications, the combination of high AMH and oestradiol results in erratic ovulation and frequent fertility issues.

On the other hand, insulin resistance could be the primary event, as high levels of insulin disrupt the lines of communication between the pituitary and ovaries. This mistiming of hormone network interactions is often seen with relatively high concentrations of LH and prolactin[13].

Another complicating factor is that not all women with PCOS present as the personification of the first description of PCOS or Stein-Leventhal syndrome as it was initially described in 1935: as women who were overweight and somewhat hairy. Rather it is now recognised that there is a spectrum of phenotypes for PCOS. In other words, you can be slim and yet still have the metabolic signature of PCOS with insulin resistance[14].

What is known for sure is that whatever the physical appearance of a woman with PCOS, the syndrome can cause internal endocrine and metabolic health issues in terms of the risk of developing metabolic syndrome and fertility problems. Although the focus is often on the fertility aspect of PCOS in younger women, lack of ovulation is a contributing factor to metabolic dysregulation. Unique to other causes of anovulation, unopposed oestrogen, in the absence of progesterone, can contribute to fat deposition and weight gain[13]. This is a prime example of where considering menstrual cycles only from reproductive perspective can, quite literally, have adverse health implications for a woman.

Improving insulin sensitivity is helpful for women with PCOS, for example through lifestyle measures of increasing activity levels[15] and modifying diet, sometimes alongside an oral medication used in type 2 diabetes. Dealing with the consequences of raised testosterone and oestrogen depends on whether the woman wishes to become pregnant or not. To assist conception, medication directed towards more co-ordinated communication between hypothalamus-pituitary and the ovaries has been shown to be effective. If pregnancy is not the priority, the combined oral contraceptive pill (COCP) is effective at reducing ovarian production of both testosterone and oestrogen. Unopposed levels of oestrogen, in addition to contributing to metabolic dysregulation, can also cause endometrial hyperplasia: thickening of the lining of the uterus[16].

*Faux Amis? PCOS and PCO*

So where has the confusion arisen between a diagnosis of PCOS and the presentation of irregular cycles and/or the clinical sign of PCO, when there are potentially very different things going on in terms of endocrine and metabolic function? Imagine the situation of a woman whose menstrual cycles have been disrupted, due to low-energy availability. In other words, she has been experiencing relative energy deficiency in sport (RED-S), which is characterised by functional hypothalamic amenorrhoea (FHA) with low levels of oestrogen (in fact all hormones downregulate apart from the stress-response hormone cortisol). Insulin sensitivity is typically high. This female exerciser now starts to restore energy availability by eating more and calming exercise training load. As her hypothalamic-pituitary axis starts to "wake up", LH pulsatility restarts. However, just like a teenager approaching menarche, this can be a stuttering start. So initially there can be some discoordination between pituitary and ovary communications, putting the menstrual cycle hormone choreography somewhat out of step.

This situation results in transient confusion among the ovarian follicles and ultrasound appearance may be that of multiple follicles (PCO): seen in both teenagers and those restoring energy availability. Blood testing might even reveal transient raised LH and testosterone levels as normal hormone service resumes. But PCOS cannot be diagnosed until these other causes have been excluded.

## Scene 4: Young Man (and Young Woman!)

Those with PCO recovering from RED-S have low oestrogen and high insulin sensitivity. To fully restore menstrual hormone choreography and ovarian morphology, these women need to fuel consistently, with a particular focus on complex carbohydrate intake and moderate exercise. In contrast, women with PCOS need to moderate carbohydrate intake and increase activity levels to mitigate adverse metabolic effects. Therefore, it is crucial to distinguish between situations with similar ovarian morphologies, but entirely different endocrine and metabolic pictures. In personalising advice for the individual, it is important to determine when PCOS is PCOS and not simply the observation of PCO.

*Let me introduce you to two women, both 28 years of age, called Katherine and Katie. Both were of similar BMI (body mass index) around 21 and both reported irregular periods for the last six months or so, with cycle lengths more than 35 days. Both women also had slightly raised testosterone, and pelvic ultrasound was reported as showing multiple follicles in the ovaries. Do both Katherine and Katie have PCOS? Although so similar, they are also so different.*

***Katherine*** *explained that her mother and sister both had PCOS, and she had always had trouble controlling her weight. Her ultrasound showed that in addition to multiple follicles she also had quite a thick endometrium (lining of the uterus) and blood tests also had a slightly high range of LH and prolactin.*

***Katie*** *on the other hand explained that she had experienced no periods for the last eight years, due to relative energy deficiency in sport (RED-S) causing functional hypothalamic amenorrhoea (FHA). Over the last six months she had been working on restoring her body weight to the level where she used to have periods, by training less intensely and eating more consistently. Katie's ultrasound showed thin endometrium and blood test showed that LH and T3 had improved from being very low in range to more mid-range.*

*Although their symptoms were similar in many respects, there were big differences between Katherine and Katie in their clinical histories and details of their clinical tests. Katherine had PCOS, whereas Katie was recovering from RED-S.*

*As Katherine was not seeking to become pregnant and was bothered by hair growth, she opted to take combined oral contraceptive pill (COCP) to lower testosterone levels and prevent further thickening of the endometrium. She started doing more exercise to help with metabolic component of PCOS.*

*Katie needed to keep going with low key exercise and consistent intake of carbohydrate to support "rebooting" of her female hormones. A few months later her periods became more regular with hormones fluctuating as expected.*

# Hormonal contraception

While it is every man and woman's individual choice what form of contraception to use, there are some important considerations for each individual when making an informed decision. Especially in the case of hormonal contraception which wasn't around in Shakespeare's day. To set the scene, before putting the spotlight on hormonal contraception, some of the other possibilities for contraception are briefly mentioned by way of prelude[17].

Ovulation thermometers provide women with an indication that ovulation may have occurred. Ovulation results in increasing levels of progesterone, which raises metabolic rate and body temperature. So a slight increase in body temperature indicates the time of ovulation. Avoiding sexual intercourse during the most fertile time in the cycle as either side of ovulation offers a "natural" family planning method that can be effective if you have reasonably regular cycle and time of ovulation. However, as there is individual variability in menstrual cycle hormone choreography, it is not possible to be absolutely certain about the exact timing of ovulation and fertility for every cycle.

Barrier methods of contraception, such as condoms, can be very effective. Condoms have the added advantage of being the only method of contraception described here that reduces the risk of contracting sexually transmitted diseases. A barrier method specific for women is the copper coil. Some women can experience heavy periods for a few cycles when a coil is initially inserted, though this generally settles if the coil is positioned correctly.

The next option is hormonal contraception. Although male hormone contraception involving lowering of testosterone has been trialled, this was not well received by men due to side effects on mood[18]. So hormonal methods are directed towards women.

## *Progestogen-only contraception*

Progestogen is the type of progesterone contained in hormonal contraception. Progestogens are externally produced (exogenous) "sisters" of the internally produced (endogenous) progesterone. In other words, progestogens are very similar in molecular structure but not identical to endogenous progesterone. There are various ways of taking the progestogen-only contraception: pill, implant, injection and coil impregnated with progestogen (not to be confused with a copper coil which does not contain any hormone). Some of the oral types of progestogen-only contraceptives do not suppress the physiological variation of internal menstrual cycle hormone fluctuations and therefore do not prevent ovulation. Others, such as the long-acting depot injection and the newer generation of oral forms of this type of hormonal progestogen do suppress ovulation.

Even in the case of progestogen-only contraception products that do not suppress ovulation, menstrual bleeds often do not occur. The unvarying levels of progestogen maintain the thickness of the endometrium and create an environment in the female reproductive tract that is adverse to fertilisation and implantation of the embryo, thereby preventing pregnancy. While the suppression of menstrual bleeds can be convenient, it also makes it difficult to be sure that the physiological variation in female hormones is impacted by a change in lifestyle such as exercise levels or modification of diet, as there is no obvious clinical sign from menstrual periods. Assessing hormones from a blood test will not necessarily be helpful either. Without orientation from the date of the start of a menstrual period, it is very challenging to interpret blood test results. If the result shows a high LH level, is this because by chance it was taken around ovulation or does it indicate that ovaries might have reduced responsiveness?

The other important consideration when deciding on this form of hormonal contraception is the exact type and the age of the woman. Long-acting progestogen injectable contraceptives render the woman in a hypothalamic amenorrhoeic state. This results in suppression of ovulation and cessation of the production of ovarian oestradiol, which is the key hormone for bone health. Having low oestrogen adversely affects bone mineral density in adult premenopausal women and adolescents, which has led to a US Food and Drug Administration warning for this type of contraception[19]. In a large study, previous use of this type of contraception in women in their younger years was found to be linked to an increased risk of fracture up to 30 years of age[20]. During teenage years and young adult life, oestradiol is key in the accrual of peak bone mass. Lack of this bone health hormone during this crucial time impacts this process and can have long-term effects. Bones don't forget. Ultimately it comes down to weighing up the risk of bone loss against the benefit of an effective hormonal contraception for the individual woman, considering her age.

### *Combined Oral Contraceptive Pill (COCP)*

The COCP[21] contains an exogenous type of oestradiol (usually ethinylestradiol) and a progestogen. They come in various combinations. The mechanism of action of the COCP is to suppress the production of all internal female hormones. Starting at the control centre of the hypothalamus and pituitary, the external hormones enforce a reduction of the control hormones FSH and LH. This means that the ovaries receive no messages to produce ovarian hormones of oestradiol or progesterone, thereby suppressing ovulation. The net result renders the woman in a state of hypothalamic amenorrhoea, as shown in Figure 14.1.

The suppression of all female hormones makes the COCP very effective as contraception. Indeed, this medication can be very helpful in certain conditions, which are driven by the internal fluctuations of female hormones, for example, endometriosis, premenstrual syndrome and polycystic ovary syndrome (PCOS). On the other hand, there are situations where the benefits of suppression of internal female hormones need to be weighed up against potential adverse effects. There are also some situations where the COCP is not recommended.

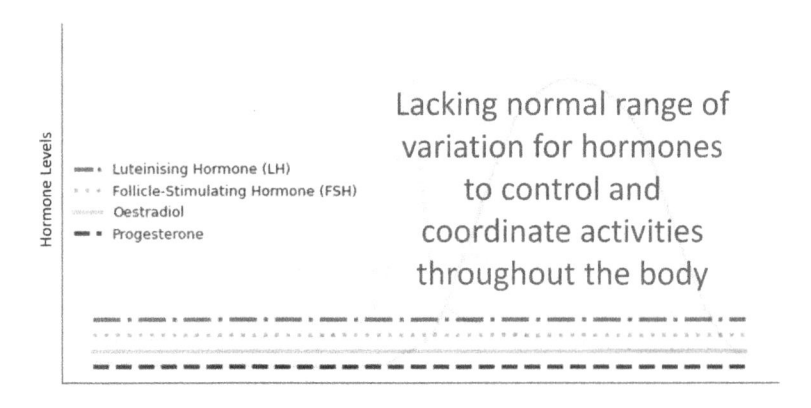

**Figure 14.1:** Endogenous hormones suppressed by certain hormonal contraception or due to functional hypothalamic amenorrhoea (FHA).*

Although the COCP contains "sister" molecules of oestradiol and progesterone, they are not identical to the body's naturally occurring hormones. These subtle differences mean that although some tissues in the body are fooled by the disguised hormones, others are not. The exogenous hormones in the COCP persuade the hypothalamus and pituitary to take a break, as shown by low levels of LH and FSH. There are various types and ways of taking a COCP. Taking the COCP cyclically, for example for 21 days with 7-day break, produces a withdrawal bleed. The endometrium (lining of the uterus) follows the instruction of the exogenous hormones to thicken and then shed. The reason this is called a

## Scene 4: Young Man (and Young Woman!)

withdrawal bleed and not a menstrual period is that the instructions are issued by the external hormones in the COCP and not those of internally produced hormones, which have been shut down.

The distinction between a withdrawal bleed and a menstrual period is very important. Bone is a key tissue in the body that is not fooled by these external hormones. There is now increasing evidence that the COCP can compromise bone health in young women[22]. In some ways this is unsurprising on two counts: female hormones are crucial for bone health, and the adolescent years are when bone mass accrues rapidly to attain peak bone mass in early 20s. So hormonal contraception, whose mechanism of action is to suppress hormone networks, specifically that for endogenous oestradiol production, can potentially impact bone health.

The other situation where the distinction between a withdrawal bleed and a menstrual period is crucial is for women experiencing functional hypothalamic amenorrhoea (FHA). The functional part of the term means that there is no medical cause, rather amenorrhoea (lack of periods) is due to stress and/or behaviours, which include reduced food intake and/or high levels of exercise. In FHA the hypothalamic-pituitary control centre shuts down to conserve energy. This results in low levels of FSH and LH. As no control hormones arrive at the ovaries, the production of oestradiol drops off and no periods occur. Therefore, FHA creates exactly the same hormone signature as the COCP, shown in Figure 14.1: flat line FSH, LH, oestradiol and progesterone. So, putting a woman with FHA on the COCP simply reinforces the downregulation of the female hormone network. For this reason, the Endocrine Society guidelines advise against this practice[23].

Unfortunately, some women with FHA continue to be offered the COCP. This may be because it gives a psychological boost by inducing a regular withdrawal bleed. However, as pointed out in the guidelines, the COCP effectively acts as a masking agent. Having seen several women with FHA being erroneously advised to take COCP, I am pleased to report that following a letter to the National Institute of Clinical Excellence, the Clinical Knowledge Summaries (CKS) were swiftly updated in February 2022 to align with Endocrine Society guidelines[24]. Furthermore, recent evidence indicates that rather than having a neutral effect, the practice of prescribing hormonal contraceptives for young women to "regulate" disrupted menstrual function can have adverse effects on bone heath[25].

Of course, if you have regular menstrual periods, then as discussed initially, hormonal contraception can be a good choice as an effective method of contraception. Forms of contraceptives that suppress ovulation can be a good choice if you are experiencing particular problematic symptoms from conditions dependent on female hormones as described above (e.g. PCOS, endometriosis). For exercising women with regular periods, the COCP is not reported to affect performance[26]. On the other hand, a recent study showed that COCP usage was associated with an increase in an inflammatory marker[27]. While some inflammatory response is part of the expected physiological response to exercise, it is not known if more is necessarily better or worse. So as ever, it comes down to making an informed decision taking account of your personal lifestyle choices and preference.

Although medical understanding has advanced since Shakespeare's day, so that hormonal contraception is a possibility, informed choice of the method of contraception should take account of all the facts at hand. This is especially the case when it comes to hormonal contraception for women, each woman is well advised to base her choice on her age, menstrual status and personal preference.

## What about men?

Returning to Shakespeare's description of a testosterone-fuelled soldier, for many men of this age, hormones attain their peak function. The fundamental physiology of sex steroid production is the same in men and women. The pituitary produces FSH and LH which act on the gonads (testes or ovaries) to produce predominately testosterone in man or oestradiol and progesterone in women.

Although men do have a diurnal variation in testosterone, the timing of the male hormone network is far less complex than its female counterpart. Nevertheless, men share the susceptibility of women to imbalances in lifestyle behaviours. On the one hand, a sedentary lifestyle with excess food intake relative to requirements can increase the risk of metabolic syndrome and lower levels of testosterone. On the other, excessive exercise, relative to energy intake, can lead to downregulation of hormone networks described in Act 1, "Scene 10: In the Red". So arguably, modern lifestyles promote extremes in both the tails of the distribution.

## Fertility: men and women

While those seeking to avoid pregnancy may consider contraception, fertility becomes the primary concern of those wishing to start a family. Many things need to fall into place for a woman to become pregnant. Not least, a healthy sperm is required to fertilise an egg. Each gamete (egg or sperm) brings half the complement of DNA, so the combination results in the full set of double-stranded DNA. When a couple is unable to conceive, one of the early tests is semen analysis, to check that the sperm are ready for action and male hormones are active.

*Tim* was a 30-year-old, working full time with a heavy training load. He wanted to compete in an Ironman before starting a family. He would often train early before work, as well as in the evenings. He found it very challenging to take on enough fuel to match the calories he was burning. Unintentionally he found that he lost weight and felt very fatigued. He also reported decreased libido, which was not helping in starting a family. His blood tests showed low male hormones across the board in the presence of a normal level of prolactin. His thyroid function showed low-range levels. This picture indicated that low-energy availability was impairing his fertility. Easing back on training improved his well-being and hormone levels. He was able to compete in the Ironman, and he and his partner were happy to report back that she was pregnant.

For women, confirming that menstruation is happening is the starting point. If not, then the priority is to identify any medical conditions causing the lack of periods (amenorrhoea). This process of elimination, based on clinical history and blood tests, is shown in Figure 14.2. The process takes into consideration the type of amenorrhoea: primary amenorrhoea means no start of periods by her 16th birthday; secondary amenorrhoea means no periods for six consecutive months in a woman with previously regular periods; and oligomenorrhoea means fewer than nine periods per calendar year. The diagram shows how hormone levels can be used to identify or exclude a range of causes. Only once medical conditions have been ruled out can the diagnosis of functional hypothalamic (FHA) be made.

*Jane* was a 30-year-old woman looking to become pregnant. However, her periods had stopped (amenorrhoea) for the past year. The first important tests to consider were the levels of FSH and LH, which although in range, were at the low end. This indicated that the "control centre" of the hypothalamus/pituitary was on a "go slow". In other words, hypothalamic amenorrhoea is opposed to an ovarian issue. High levels of prolactin can be a cause of hypothalamic amenorrhoea, but Jane's prolactin was not raised. Furthermore, her thyroid function tests were normal, albeit low in the range. Jane had functional hypothalamic amenorrhoea. It turned out that over the past few years, Jane had started a new demanding job with long hours, so she *had been doing her exercise training early before work, fasted and often did not eat anything till lunchtime. She had also been reducing carbohydrate intake.*

*While waiting for referral to a fertility unit for further tests (hysterosalpingogram: HSG checks for patency of Fallopian tubes), Jane made changes to her lifestyle: eating breakfast and carbohydrates again. She also took a break from running and decided to do Pilates and yoga. I advised her that this could well restore her periods. A few months later her periods returned. She went on to conceive "naturally" without treatment for ovulation induction.*

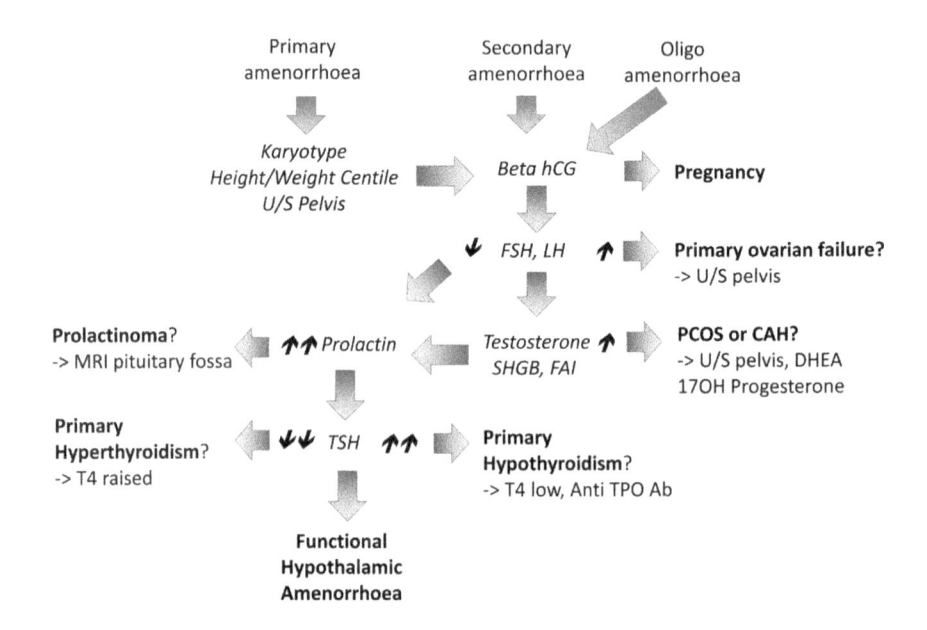

**Figure 14.2:** Functional hypothalamic amenorrhoea: a diagnosis of exclusion.* Figure key: U/S= ultrasound. CAH = congenital adrenal hyperplasia. SHBG = sex hormone binding globulin. FAI = free androgen index. MRI = magnetic resonance imaging. Anti TPO Ab = anti-thyroid peroxidase antibodies

Of course, not all women with amenorrhoea have FHA; there may well be other causes of fertility issues which are grouped by the World Health Organisation as follows:

- WHO group I: Hypothalamic-pituitary-gonadal axis failure
- WHO group II: Hypothalamic-pituitary-gonadal axis dysfunction. WHO group II is the most common cause of ovulatory disorders, and the most frequent reason is PCOS

- WHO group III: Ovarian insufficiency
- WHO group IV: Hyperprolactinemia

For women with a hypothalamic-pituitary-gonadal axis dysfunction, ovulation induction, with oral medication, dramatically lowers oestradiol levels "shocking" the hypothalamus-pituitary to produce LH and FSH for ovulation. Injections to stimulate ovulation can also be used. In the case of hyperprolactinemia, if caused by excess production from a macroprolactinoma in the pituitary, this requires medication to reduce prolactin levels and re-establish menstruation and ovulation.

In all cases, the support and advice must be personalised for the individual.

## All change for female hormones: pregnancy

One of the most dramatic times of physiological hormone change is during pregnancy. This starts relatively quietly: a pregnancy test is based on detecting β-hCG, which is a subunit of the hormone human chorionic gonadotrophin (hCG). This hormone is secreted from the cells surrounding the fertilised egg, which goes on to form the placenta once the embryo implants in the endometrium of the uterus. The α subunit of hCG is very similar to LH, so it acts on the ovary to persuade the corpus luteum to keep producing progesterone until the placenta is ready to take over this hormone production duty. Progesterone is important to keep the endometrium "welcoming" and maintain the pregnancy; it is pro gestation. It has been suggested that hCG plays a role in maternal immunoregulation, allowing the mother to "accept" the growth of the embryo. Mothers with pre-existing autoimmune conditions can experience a flare-up during pregnancy, when the immune system is somewhat downregulated. This hormone may also be the cause of "morning sickness", up to around 12 weeks into pregnancy. It is worth remembering that feeling slightly nauseous in the early weeks of pregnancy, although not great, can be a positive sign. After 12 weeks, hCG levels fall and the corpus luteum regresses as the placenta takes over hormones-producing duties producing high, stable levels of oestradiol and progesterone.

From conception, if the pregnancy progresses, the mother experiences nine months of physiological amenorrhoea. In other words, no menstrual periods. This is because initially high levels of progesterone from the corpus luteum, then high sustained levels of oestradiol and progesterone from the placenta, suppress the cyclical pituitary production of LH and FSH. The hormone pregnancy "signature" is that of high prolactin, low FSH and LH with high oestradiol and progesterone.

As indicated in Figure 14.2, high prolactin can also be due to a macroprolactinoma, which can also cause amenorrhoea by suppressing LH and FSH. However, the distinguishing feature is the level of oestradiol and progesterone. After birth, breastfeeding is associated with continued high levels of prolactin, which is why there may be a delay in periods restarting. However, unlike during pregnancy, oestradiol and progesterone are low.

Pregnancy is divided into three stages or trimesters. Counting starts from the first day of the last menstrual period (LMP).

- First Trimester (0 to 13 Weeks): this is the time from when the fertilised egg nestles into the endometrium to when the placenta takes over from the corpus luteum in terms of hormone production of oestradiol and progesterone. Amazingly, by the end of this trimester the major organs of the foetus have already formed. From now on it is down to the serious business of growth.
- Second Trimester (14 to 26 Weeks): during this trimester, growth and maturation of the foetus occur. The mother feels her baby moving.
- Third Trimester (27 to 40 Weeks): more growth and maturation, culminating in birth. Usually, timing is pretty much like clockwork. Occasionally if a baby is enjoying the friendly home too long or a medical situation arises that puts either mother or baby at risk, the birth can be induced. This involves the injection of a hormone to get contractions underway.

Relaxin is a hormone that is specific to pregnancy. This appropriately named hormone influences ligaments to increase their laxity. This allows the pelvic ligaments to give during childbirth. On the other hand, this is not a good time to try to increase flexibility, as injury risk can be increased. Maintenance stretching is best. This is especially relevant for dancers, where flexibility is sought. It is important for dancers to avoid getting carried away with the possibility of increased stretching, bearing in mind that relaxin circulates after birth in the post-natal period[28].

Staying active and taking exercise during pregnancy is very beneficial for the health of both mother and baby. Taking up to 150 minutes of exercise per week is advocated by European and American guidelines to help optimise weight gain during pregnancy and mitigate the risk of gestational diabetes and raised blood pressure[10]. On the other hand, this is not the time to take up a new type of intense exercise. For example, Pilates teachers are trained around suitable exercise for women who are pregnant and in post-natal stage[29]. On a personal note, I continued to take regular ballet classes and I was swimming when my initial contractions started. Using perceived exertion as a guide is helpful: exercise to a level where it remains easy to have a conversation. Ensuring maintenance of hydration and fuelling is also particularly important when exercising during pregnancy[30].

## Hormone stories: what happened next?

***David*** *was a 30-year-old working full time, frequently long hours. He also had a young family. In order to fit in exercise, he was getting up early to train before work. He tried to fit in some more exercise after work as he felt his office job was mainly sedentary. David reported feeling tired, with poor sleep and loss of libido.*

*When we discussed David's motivation for doing up to four hours of exercise every day, it transpired this was not for performance. Rather he described feeling obliged to stick rigidly to this exercise schedule, even if he was feeling very tired. He often avoided social and even family events, as this would disrupt and curtail his exercise routine.*

*David's blood tests showed low-range hormones in thyroid function and male hormones, including testosterone. LH was in low range with prolactin in range. Cortisol was slightly raised. These results indicated downregulation of the hypothalamic-pituitary axis due to low energy availability caused by high energy expenditure from exercise, not matched by adequate energy intake. This was in keeping with his clinical history of exercise dependence.*

*After we discussed the situation, he agreed to reduce his exercise sessions to a maximum of once a day and to have at least one rest day per week. A few weeks later he reported feeling less fatigued. After six weeks his repeat blood test showed a big improvement, and he reported feeling much happier.*

***Susie*** *was a 29-year-old woman whose periods had not resumed after she stopped taking the combined oral contraceptive pill a year ago. Susie had a very active job as a PE teacher and was doing a lot of training daily.*

*When we discussed Susie's exercise in detail it transpired that in addition to having an active job and training with her running club every day, she was also running to and from work every day but did not count this as training. In the morning she skipped breakfast and sometimes could not eat anything till mid-morning as she had* to organise before-school football club training. She did not eat anything after school before running home and then went straight to her club training.

Susie's blood test results showed lower range hormones across the board: thyroid function and female hormones. We recognised that she did not have enough energy on board to cover all her demands. Low-energy availability had downregulated her hormones to "save energy". This was why her periods had stopped. Susie started eating breakfast and driving to/from school. She took a full rest day from exercise each week. After a couple of months, I received a message saying that her period had returned. I encouraged her to keep everything steady. She was happy to do so as she was not feeling so tired. The next message I received was that initially Susie had been concerned that she did not get the third period, only to discover, to her delight, that she was pregnant.

## Strategies to support your hormones as a young adult

During this time in your life, your hormone networks have the potential to be at their optimal. So, making choices to work with your hormones is very important and beneficial in achieving your personal goals. What are the keys areas to consider?

### *Exercise*

- Mix it up and focus on the type of exercise that you like. For example, if you don't like running or lifting weights at the gym, then explore other options.
- Try to do exercise that involves the various components of fitness: include exercise that promotes cardiovascular fitness like swimming, running, cycling or dancing, together with exercise that is good for muscular strength like resistance exercise and climbing
- If you are exercise training, at any level from recreational to elite, then it is particularly important to treat your hormone networks with respect as these drive the adaptive processes you seek from training
- Periodised, polarised training: don't do the same training every day, all year round. Mix up higher and lower intensities
- For women be flexible where possible and try and synchronise the type of exercise with times in your cycle when you feel ready to train and rest when you need more recovery. Bear in mind that every woman is different, so a personalised approach is essential

- Timing of exercise: If you need to exercise before work, then try to eat something small, or at least liquid-like diluted fruit juice, before you go start
- Recovery is an important part of any exercise schedule

## *Nutrition*

- Match your nutrition with your activity levels and body composition.
- Surplus intake can lead to metabolic syndrome
- Conversely, insufficient fuelling risks low-energy availability and hormone network disruption
- Sex steroid hormones are particularly sensitive to the timing and composition of energy intake. Consistent fuelling over the day and either side of training is important.
- For women, be aware that you are more dependent on carbohydrates as fuel during the luteal phase of your menstrual cycle. You can pre-empt hunger urges by being particularly mindful of consistent intake during this phase of the cycle.

## *Sleep*

- As ever, sleep is crucial for hormone health, ensuring circadian alignment of internal biological clocks and the timing of external behaviours
- Both quality and quantity of sleep patterns help maintain this alignment
- During this phase of life, a particular challenge can be balancing work, exercise and social commitments. Aim to go to bed and get up at consistent times
- Avoid frequent late exercise, alcohol, caffeine or nicotine

## Female specific: menstrual cycle

- Menstruation is the barometer of internal health hormones, if the regularity and/or nature of periods persistently changes, medical advice should be sought
- Oestradiol is dominant in the later follicular phase. Many, though not all women feel at their best around this time.
- Progesterone prevails in the luteal phase of the cycle, after ovulation. An increase in metabolic rate can disturb sleep and cause hunger urges.

Ensure a consistent intake of complex carbohydrate during the day, factoring in more recovery between bouts of exercise and sleeping in a well-ventilated room.
- Painful periods: gentle exercise can help, alongside keeping well hydrated. If pain limits usual daily activities on a regular basis, then medical advice should be sought
- Premenstrual Syndrome (PMS) is where a woman experiences recurrent cyclic symptoms in the luteal phase of her cycle, two weeks before menstruation. Modifying behaviours can help alongside evidence-based complimentary therapies
- Polycystic ovary syndrome (PCOS) comprises two out of three clinical aspects of irregular periods, raised testosterone levels and multiple follicles on pelvic ultrasound. Lifestyle factors are important, due to the metabolic component of PCOS.
- Hormonal contraception options include combined preparations of synthetic oestradiol and progesterone which supress ovulation, or progestogen-only forms. Choice is based on personal preference although for women with PMS, combined hormonal contraception is a more suitable choice. Hormonal contraception should not be given to a woman with functional hypothalamic amenorrhoea (FHA).

# Scene 5
## Middle Age

> *"And then the justice,*
> *In a fair round belly, with good capon lin'd,*
> *With eyes severe, and beard of formal cut,*
> *Full of wise saws, and modern instances."*
>
> *Shakespeare*

**Subtitle:** Middle age sees the start of physiological age-related decline in some key hormones such as growth hormone and the sex steroids testosterone and oestradiol. Since this hormone transition can impact both health and exercise performance, adopting specific strategies around exercise type, nutrition and sleep can help mitigate these consequences. Women face the dramatic reduction in female hormones associated with menopause, which is addressed and discussed in detail.

## Hormone stories

*Gerald* was a 53-year-old man who had practised sport in his youth, but had slipped into a very sedentary life. He enjoyed good food and wine "maybe a bit too much". He had put on weight around the belly over the past few years, necessitating investing in a new wardrobe. He wondered, with some degree of trepidation, what a forthcoming company medical assessment might reveal.

*Tim* was a 51-year-old keen competitive, amateur cyclist. He had heard that being lighter would give him an advantage riding up hills in races. So, he decided to train more and eat less. Although this resulted in some weight loss, he also started to feel fatigued, and his race results did not improve as he had hoped. He felt he needed a change, so he started to do some running. Unfortunately, he suffered a stress fracture of his hip.

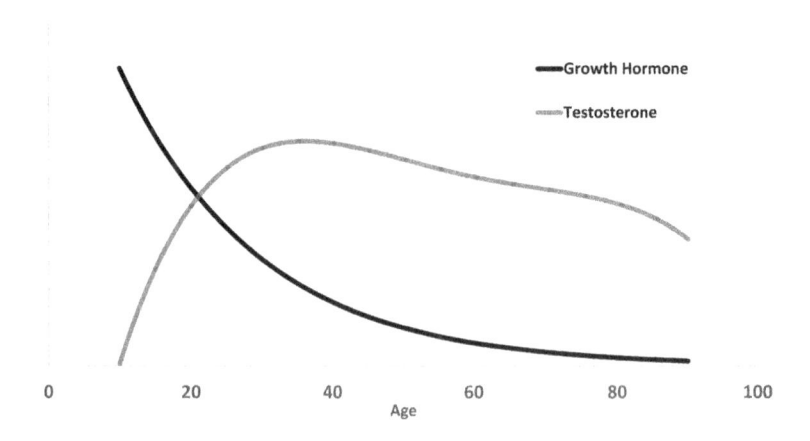

**Figure 15.2:** Decline of testosterone in men with age

Although middle-aged men may lament the physiological consequences of declining levels of testosterone, spare a thought for women of this age, who see the precipitous decline in oestrogen shown in Figure 15.3. This is due to the ovaries becoming less responsive, producing only very low levels of the ovarian hormones, oestrogen and progesterone. This change affects body composition, cardiovascular health, bones and many other aspects of health. We catch up with men shortly in: What about men?

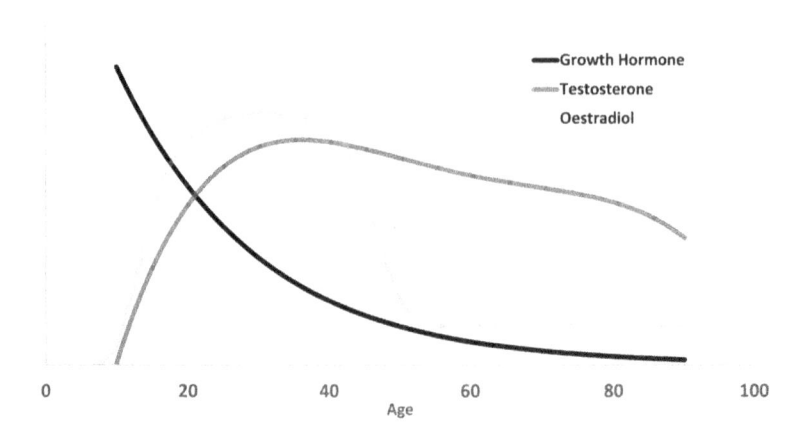

**Figure 15.3:** Decline of oestrogen in women with age

## Perimenopause: the bumpy road to menopause

Although the rapid decline in oestrogen shown in Figure 15.3 is a smooth curve, it can follow a very bumpy and circuitous route. From around the age of 40, the ovaries can start to falter in their production of ovarian hormones. This is called perimenopause, marking the transition towards menopause, when the ovaries eventually retire in their role of producing oestradiol (most active form of oestrogen) and progesterone. If the reduction in ovarian response and production of hormones occur before the age of 40, it is known as premature ovarian insufficiency (POI) and occurs in 1% of women. For 0.1%, this occurs under the age of 30.

Menopause is the final destination of the perimenopause journey, where the ovaries no longer respond to the control hormones from the pituitary gland, follicle-stimulating hormone (FSH) and luteinising hormone (LH). The production of the ovarian hormones, oestradiol and progesterone, drops back down to pre-pubertal levels and menstrual bleeds/periods cease. The average age of menopause is 51, with a typical range from 45 to 55 years of age. POI may lead to early menopause, occurring between 40 and 45, or premature menopause, occurring before 40 years of age.

Over the course of the perimenopause, the feedback between the ovaries and the pituitary breaks down and the female hormones become stuck at constant levels, as shown in Figure 15.4. However, this change very rarely occurs overnight, unless a woman has had a medical menopause from surgery to remove the ovaries, or from medication.

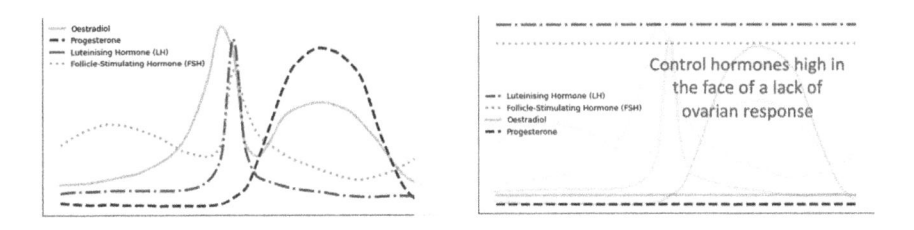

**Figure 15.4:** Menstrual cycle hormones before and after menopause

Although I reason there could be a theoretical progression of hormone stages from perimenopause to menopause, women experience this journey in different ways. Some hormone stages may last longer, while others may be skipped entirely.

Subclinical ovulatory issues: this is where a woman may experience no change in the length of her menstrual cycle. FSH and LH are in the normal range, but oestradiol and progesterone levels are lower than expected.

Clinical anovulation or insufficient luteal phase: this is where a woman might start to notice changes in the nature of her periods. For example, variable cycle length and variable flow of her periods from cycle to cycle. This is a reflection that the ovaries are not producing previous levels or/and timing of progesterone and oestradiol. Nevertheless, the FSH and LH could still be in range as the control centre of the hypothalamus-pituitary has not yet responded.

Decline in the responsiveness of the ovaries: eventually the hypothalamus-pituitary registers a decline in the responsiveness of the ovaries. So, the control centre ups the ante: FSH and LH start to rise. This explains why some women experience a temporary restoration of ovulatory cycles: the control centre compensates for the recalcitrance of the ovaries. For this reason, it is still possible to fall pregnant in the perimenopause.

Decompensation: ultimately the coda ends with "decompensation", when even the high levels of FSH and LH cannot cajole the ovaries into producing oestradiol and progesterone to previous levels. Periods become very erratic in timing and nature, until they stop completely. Menopause is defined as a woman not having had a period for 12 consecutive months[2]. So this is a retrospective diagnosis.

The erratic decline of ovarian hormones during the transition to menopause can cause some challenging symptoms outlined in the recently published Menopause Practice Standards by the British Menopause Society July 2022.

- Changes in the menstrual cycle. Cycles can become erratic in timing and nature. Sometimes long or short cycle lengths, with heavy or light bleeding, reflecting the flux in hormone patterns described above
- Issues with body temperature regulation. Yes, the dreaded hot flushes, when you feel like you are burning up for no apparent reason. Not only does this disturb sleep but can occur at an inopportune moment in a work or social setting
- New onset of headaches and random joint and muscle discomfort and/or pain, not related to injury. This may be due to low-grade inflammation which occurs with decreasing oestrogen levels
- Brain fog: is where short term memory and concentration issues can occur. This can contribute to loss of self-esteem and mood issues

- Changeable mood: from low mood to anxiety and anger
- Dry skin, itchy skin throughout the body. Yes, I mean everywhere. Vaginal dryness is not something easy to talk about, but sometimes this can be one of the worst symptoms with itchiness and burning. Once again, this is down to dropping oestrogen levels which impact the quality of skin (independent of ageing) and blood supply
- The lower urinary tract can also be impacted by declining oestrogen levels, leading to increased need to urinate
- Sexual difficulties: not only you don't feel like it, having a dry vagina makes having sex physically uncomfortable

While every woman experiences the physiological hormone transition into menopause differently, it is suggested that those who might be most susceptible to associated symptoms might have particular sensitivity to ovarian hormones. These might include women who have experienced pre-menstrual syndrome or postnatal issues following the sharp decline in oestrogen and progesterone secreted by the placenta during pregnancy.

## All change for "the change"

Although "the change" is an old-fashioned euphemism for menopause, it does indicate that there are significant vicissitudes at this point in a woman's life, from both physical and psychological points of view. These changes can be a direct consequence of hormone changes, potentially impacting her physical and mental well-being. About 25% of women report debilitating adverse effects on their personal and professional lives[3]. Other life changes and realisations come at this time in your life. Even if a woman has made an active decision not to have children, menopause closes the chapter on this possibility. It can also be a time of life where things are changing: grown-up children are leaving home, parents may become infirm and new work colleagues seem to look very young.

The menopause is a natural, expected physiological event. However, it does not mean that a woman should resign herself to, or accept, a reduced quality of life. After all, with increasing life expectancy, women may live at least a third of their lives in the menopausal state. A couple of hundred years ago, even if a woman survived childbirth, not many reached the age of menopause. Far more women than ever before experience the consequences of low female hormones that come with menopause, potentially for 30 years or more of their lives.

Fortunately advances in medical knowledge and practice mean that there are better resources to support women navigating this stage in their hormone odyssey. Many of these resources have been jointly designed by non-medically and medically qualified people for the benefit of all, such as the British Menopause Society, Women's Health Concern and the Royal College of Obstetrics and Gynaecology. Dissemination of this information is essential.

As a female doctor having experienced perimenopause symptoms and menopause, I fully appreciate this would have been an even more disconcerting and indeed an alarming experience, if I had not known that my hormones were changing in a normal and expected way. The task of challenging misconceptions and changing attitudes to "the change" remains a work in progress.

"Think menopause" is the message from the current NHS England and Improvement (NHSEI) initative which encourages heathcare professionals to consider perimenopause as a possibility in all women over 40 years of age.

## How do I know if this is perimenopause or something else?

The typical symptoms of perimenopause can also be caused by medical conditions and/or reversible external factors. A good starting point is to unravel and consider other underlying causes. This starts with a review of your work/life "stresses", exercise levels, nutrition and sleep patterns. For example, if you exercise or train without fuelling sufficiently to cover all your demands, as discussed in Act 1, Scene 9, relative energy deficiency in sport (RED-S) can occur in non-elite, age group athletes. Any combination of imbalances in your exercise, nutrition and sleep patterns can disrupt menstrual function and contribute to lower levels of ovarian hormones. However, the key difference and distinguishing feature between perimenopause and reversible causes can be found in your hormone networks.

While it is true that a single snapshot blood test cannot diagnose perimenopause, monitoring and potentially mathematically modelling female hormones as discussed in Act 1, Scene 6, can help distinguish between progressing perimenopause and external functional causes of low ovarian hormones, especially in the 40 to 45 age group. These are typical hormone patterns I see.

> Perimenopause: decreasing ovarian responsiveness is indicated by consistently *upper*-range pituitary control hormones, LH and FSH,

throughout the menstrual cycle with simultaneous low-range ovarian response hormones, oestradiol and progesterone, particularly in the mid-luteal phase. This pattern tends to become more pronounced over time. External causes of low ovarian hormones, in contrast, are indicated by consistently *lower* range pituitary control hormones, LH and FSH, throughout the menstrual cycle with simultaneous low-range ovarian response hormones, oestradiol and progesterone, particularly in the mid-luteal phase.

In the case of suspected external functional suppression of ovarian hormones, supporting evidence can be gathered from other hormones: for example, in masters athletes with RED-S, thyroid function tests (TSH, T4 and T3) would all be expected to be in the lower end of range, with prolactin in range and cortisol at the upper end of range. These would suggest downregulation of hormone networks at the "control" level of the hypothalamus. I find checking these additional hormone levels with a routine blood test can be a particularly useful approach if the woman is on hormonal contraception that prevents ovulation, by suppressing all female hormones.

Excluding other underlying medical causes of symptoms similar to perimenopause is also important. For example, with advancing age, women are more prone to developing autoimmune conditions, such as underactive thyroid and rheumatoid arthritis. Low levels of vitamin D and iron can also cause well-being issues that are readily reversible.

Once perimenopause has been indentified as the cause of symtoms, what are the options for women progressing through perimenopause to support quality of life and long-term health?

*"Treat women as individuals, not statistics."*

*Professor Janice Rymer, Vice President of the Royal College of Obstetrics and Gynaecology*

This inspirational statement comes from a leading female professor, who advocates that the focus should be on the quality of life and long-term health for menopausal women. After many years of misinformation and scaremongering surrounding hormone replacement therapy (HRT) Professor Rymer urges "we must all work together to avoid another damaging setback in women's health". This means producing and disseminating unbiased, high-quality information to empower women to make informed decisions[4].

It is tragic and bewildering that a replacement therapy that restores hormones to physiological levels and improves the quality of life for women has been misrepresented. The focus seems to be on the potential side effects of taking HRT, rather than the significant risks of not taking HRT in terms of reduced quality of life, increased health risks and risk of death (mortality). This contrasts with replacement therapies for other hormones, where the emphasis is on the benefits. For example, diabetics need insulin injections and those with a diagnosed underactive thyroid gland need thyroxine replacement. Although menopause is a natural physiological event, nevertheless treating every woman as an individual and peroanslising hormone health should be a priority to support quality of life.

For younger women there are no qualms about giving supra-physiological doses of hormones, in non-identical molecular forms, found in many combined oral contraceptive pills, to suppress internal hormone production (ironically suppressing natural oestradiol and progesterone to the low levels seen in menopause). These external forms of hormones are even given, in some cases, to women with functional hypothalamic amenorrhoea (FHA), against the advice of the Endocrine Society[5] and updated guidelines from the National Institute of Clinical Excellence (NICE)[6].

A pervasive perception suggests that female hormones are solely about fertility. Although there is no denying that this is the evolutionary purpose of ovulation, female hormones are crucial to all aspects of health. This applies whatever the age of a woman.

## HRT: a story of misinformation

HRT typically comprises physiological doses of oestradiol and progesterone, restoring their levels to those a woman had when she was of reproductive age. This is a very effective way of alleviating the symptoms associated with the decline in ovarian hormones that occurs during the menopause. In this way, a woman's quality of life is maintained and improved above what it might otherwise be. This enhanced quality of life covers the increasing time women can expect to live in the menopausal state, typically longer than their premenopausal reproductive years[4]. Furthermore, HRT improves the long-term health of women in terms of reduced overall mortality (death from all causes). Importantly, HRT mitigates the risk of bone and cardiovascular health issues that increase at menopause, when natural levels of ovarian hormones drop[2].

Yet in the early 2000s there was a dramatic decrease in the uptake of HRT. The underlying cause was a press release, suggesting an increased risk of breast cancer from using HRT that came out before the formal medical publication of the Women's Health Initiative Study. This would certainly be a concern, if it were true. However, once the medical details of the study emerged, it became clear that bias in the sample of participants played a big part in the results. The mean age was 63 years (more than 10 years post menopause) and participants were considerably overweight with a mean body mass index (BMI) of 28, where the overweight threshold, quoted by the NHS, is a BMI of 25. Since being overweight is a recognised risk factor for developing breast cancer, it is not possible to conclude definitively that HRT causes breast cancer[7]. In fact, being overweight and making less healthy lifestyle choices are far more important risk factors, in both clinical and statistical terms, for developing breast cancer.

For every 1,000 women aged 50–59 years, there are 23 cases of breast cancer reported. Being overweight increases the cases of breast cancer by 24 extra cases per 1,000 women[8]. Conversely, there are seven fewer cases for women taking regular moderate exercise of at least two and a half hours per week. HRT accounts for an extra four cases, which is about the same as taking the combined oral contraceptive pill, drinking more than two units of alcohol per week, or smoking. In other words, taking regular exercise, maintaining body weight in a healthy range, not smoking and limiting intake of alcohol are the important things you can do to reduce your risk of developing breast cancer. This is why considering these lifestyle choices is always the first port of call, especially when approaching menopause[2]. This reduces your risk of health issues per se and puts you in a good position when/if you decide to opt for HRT.

There are some women for whom HRT is not recommended: those with a personal or close family history of breast cancer, especially if breast cancer was oestrogen receptor positive. For these menopausal women, there are alternatives with supporting evidence of helping some women, discussed shortly.

## What is the best HRT choice?

Having addressed imbalances in your lifestyle behaviours and excluded other causes for your symptoms, if you do come to the conclusion that you are progressing towards menopause, and have no contra-indications, what are the options for HRT?

Please be aware that a range of pharmacological substances may be offered to menopausal women. In addition to medically licensed HRT, various other unregulated compounds purporting to be "bioidentical hormones" are offered in the marketplace. The British Menopause Society advises against resorting to unregulated compounds, because their efficacy and safety are unknown.

Licensed, regulated HRT, containing "body indentical" hormones, molecularly identical to those internally produced in the body, is available on the NHS[9]. This is the logical choice. Your body and more precisely the receptors for these hormones have no problem "recognising" these hormones as old friends. In practical terms that means HRT containing oestradiol and the particular form of progesterone called "micronised progesterone". Progesterone must always be taken alongside oestradiol, unless you have had a hysterectomy.

What is the best way to take HRT? Taking oestradiol transdermally, through the skin, has a big advantage over taking it orally in tablet form. Any tablet taken via the mouth needs to travel to and be processed by the liver. In contrast, oestradiol going straight into the bloodstream from the skin reduces the risk of clots (venous thromboembolism) in the lungs or brain. Opting for "mild" micronised progesterone reduces the risk of blood clots, breast cancer and has less androgenic side effects, compared with other progestational agents. This optimal form of HRT, transdermal oestradiol (gel or patch) with micronised progesterone in soft capsules is available, in England and Wales, on the NHS.

In terms of practicalities of taking HRT, I find the advantage of oestradiol gel is that it is unobtrusive, applied daily, so that it is easy to adjust the dose, under medical supervision, according to symptoms. The only practical thing to remember is not to take a shower or go swimming within an hour after applying, otherwise it washes off! It is advisable to take micronised progesterone in the evening, before bed, as it can cause some drowsiness. This is not such a bad thing if you are having issues with sleep. Microionised progesterone can be taken continuously (every evening) or a higher dose sequentially typically for 12 days every month. The sequential regime appears to have slight advantage in terms of even lower risk of breast cancer than continuous[2], although the potential, downside for some is that you can get a withdrawal bleed and you may have had enough of buying sanitary wear.

The other important consideration is that taking HRT before the age of 60 (or within 10 years of menopause) has a particularly good risk/benefit profile in terms of improving quality of life and reducing the risk of heart disease. The same principle applies to younger women who have experienced an earlier than expected menopause. There are some women who experience premature ovarian insufficiency (menopause before the age of 40 years), whether as a variation in physiology or due to surgery. If you have a hysterectomy (removal of the uterus) always double-check if that included removal of your ovaries (oophorectomy) as that produces a "surgical menopause". On the other hand, if your ovaries have been left in situ, yet you have no uterus, then you do not have the cue of irregular periods for perimenopause and you need to be extra attentive for perimenopausal symptoms. For younger women experiencing earlier menopause, prompt HRT is very important and possibly at a higher dose[10].

Ultimately, doing your own research on HRT sooner, rather than later, is valuable so that you are in the best possible position to make a personal, informed and timely decision.

## Topical HRT for vaginal dryness

This consequence of menopause can be one of the worst. Feeling uncomfortable, with discomfort having sex and passing urine is not pleasant. As oestrogen is very important for skin health, very low-dose, small oestrogen pessaries can be very helpful, alongside external lubricants. Although this can be a difficult topic of conversation, it is definitely worth discussing, if you are not directly asked about these symptoms by your doctor. There are solutions.

## What about testosterone?

It may come as a surprise, but at some times during the menstrual cycle, women can produce more testosterone than oestrogen, though this is still around ten times less than men. In women, the main sources of testosterone and its precursors are the ovaries and adrenal glands. Testosterone can affect tissues directly or indirectly by conversion through aromatisation to oestradiol. As the ovaries reduce the production of all sex steroid hormones during perimenopause and at menopause, female levels of testosterone levels are about half at the age of 40 compared with 20. So, adding testosterone replacement, alongside HRT is a possibility, for women with residual symptoms after being on HRT for several months. So-called hypoactive sexual desire disorder (HSDD) is currently the only indication for testosterone replacement in menopausal woman. Although in Australia there are female-specific testosterone replacement preparations, to date in the UK, the male version has to be prescribed, needless to say, in smaller doses than you would give to a man. As with all unregulated "bioidentical" hormones, the British Menopause Society advises against alternatives to regulated testosterone replacement, like dehydroepiandrosterone (DHEA)[11]. For women competing in sporting events under World Anti-Doping Authority (WADA) jurisdiction, it is important to note that all forms of testosterone replacement are banned.

## Alternatives to HRT

There are some women for whom HRT is not recommended, including those with a personal or close family history of breast cancer, especially if breast cancer was oestrogen receptor positive. For these menopausal women, there are herbal preparations, which have been reported to help women. These include St John's Wort and Black cohosh. Checking for the Traditional Herbal Registration (THR) and any potential interactions with prescribed medications is important. There are also alternatives such as acupuncture, aromatherapy and phyto-oestrogens (plant sources of oestrogen): isoflavones found in legumes, such as soy, have been reported to be helpful. Fortunately, low-dose vaginal oestradiol is fine, even if systemic HRT is contraindicated, or in addition to HRT, for vaginal dryness[2]. Of course, always check with your medical prescriber.

## What about men?

Although testosterone replacement therapy (TRT) might seem an attractive proposition for men, it is not a panacea and should only be prescribed as clinically indicated by medical professionals. In the first instance, there may be other causes for symptoms of fatigue that should be addressed such as low levels of vitamin D or a primary underactive thyroid. Thereafter it is important to identify and address any underlying causes for consistently low testosterone levels. This would include reviewing reversible lifestyle factors causing low testosterone, such as relative energy deficiency or energy surplus, due to unbalanced food intake relative to demand, exercise levels and sleep patterns. Taking testosterone, where not clinically indicated, can present health risks[12]. For athletes competing in events under WADA jurisdiction, testosterone is banned, where the underlying cause of low levels is functional. In other words, if low testosterone is the result of an imbalance between training load and nutrition, a therapeutic use exemption (TUE) cannot be obtained.

## Bone health

Oestrogen is the key hormone for bone health, in both men and women. In men testosterone is converted to oestrogen, which in turn supports bone health. The reason why osteoporosis ("brittle bone disease") is more prevalent in women is that with menopause comes the dramatic drop in oestrogen. In men, the more gradual decline in testosterone means a gradual concomitant decline in oestrogen. For both men and women, reducing levels of GH also have an impact on bone health.

To maintain bone health, in the face of declining hormone levels, it becomes important to ensure that exercise includes particular types of activities. Bone health is supported by exercise that loads the skeleton in a multidirectional way: in other words, movement involving changes in direction, such as dancing or ball sports. If these are not your thing, then there are alternatives. In a study of male cyclists, which included age group competitive riders, I devised some simple exercises that could be done at home for 15 minutes, 3 times a week. These included multidirectional hopping, resistance and body weight exercises. When combined with good nutritional strategies and sufficient vitamin D, these cyclists saw a clinically significant improvement in bone mineral density (BMD) over 6 months. Conversely, those male cyclists who did not adopt these fuelling strategies and did not do the "bone health" exercises not only showed lower levels of testosterone but also a significant loss of BMD, commensurate with an astronaut in space. Worse still, the race performance of these cyclists suffered in comparison with those who modified their behaviours in the recommended positive ways and subsequently enjoyed stronger race results[13].

Resistance exercise helps bone health, both directly and indirectly. Putting extra weight/load through the skeleton provides a direct mechanical osteogenic, bone-building stimulus. The resistance element indirectly supports bone health, by recruiting many muscle groups that pull on the bone to which these muscles attach. This strengthens both muscle and bone.

## Muscle health

Sarcopenia is the loss of muscle mass that occurs with advancing years. Skeletal muscle (muscle that attaches to bone) is essential for movement and provides storage and utilisation of the energy source called glycogen, derived from carbohydrate in our diet.

This means sarcopenia causes a decline in the important functions of muscles, in terms of reduced mechanical strength and less metabolically active tissue. Why does sarcopenia occur? Once again, it is down to declining levels of both sex steroid hormones and GH. A particular derivative of GH, called IGF-1, and specifically a form of IGF-1 that acts locally on skeletal muscles, supports muscle protein synthesis. The good news is that muscle remains responsive to mechanical stimulus: exercise. However, this exercise needs to be more than just going about daily life, which might be sufficient in younger years when hormone levels are higher[14]. To compensate for lower hormone levels, as you get older you need to do resistance-type exercise to mitigate the tendency to sarcopenia.

If, like me, you are not keen on the prospect of "pumping iron" in a gym or investing in a set of dumbbells: don't worry. There are other ways to do resistance work. For example, Pilates and the use of resistance bands provide resistance through all stages of muscle contraction: concentric (shortening of muscle with contraction) and eccentric (lengthening of muscle with contraction). This type of resistance exercise is known as a closed kinetic chain and is the most effective way to make your muscles work through all phases of contraction. This contrasts to an open kinetic chain with free weights, where you can be tempted to just focus on the concentric phase of muscle contraction, where you lift the weight and then let it fall under gravity to the ground. So, if you are using hand weights/filled water bottles at home make sure you take advantage of the full range of muscle contraction to get maximum benefit (and prevent damaging your floor).

## Nutritional considerations

Muscle and bone are both dynamic tissues. There is a continuous cycle of new tissue formation and breakdown: a recycling process. With declining hormones, the balance swings in favour of tissue breakdown. For muscle protein this means a decrease in synthesis. To mitigate this effect, ensuring a good protein intake is important: in the region of 1.2 g to 1.5 g of protein per kilogramme of body weight per day. For a person weighing 70 kg this would mean 84 g to 105 g of protein per day. As protein is a complex molecule to breakdown, splitting protein intake up into digestible 20 g to 25 g portions spread out over the day is recommended[15].

Another aspect of timing is also crucial: taking on board protein after exercise. As discussed above, resistance/strength type exercise provides an anabolic (muscle building) stimulus, so backing up this exercise stimulus with the building blocks for synthesising muscle is ideal. Combining with complex carbohydrate is also a good strategy to replenish glycogen stores ahead of your next exercise session. A banana milkshake is a convenient and tasty way of combining these elements.

What about when you are asleep? Even though GH levels are lower than in younger years, nevertheless sleep is another powerful stimulus, like exercise, for GH release. GH has an anabolic effect. The best strategy to support muscle formation, over breakdown, is to take on board pre-sleep protein. Milk contains casein, which is an excellent source of a particular type of protein that aids muscle formation. It may be necessary to supplement this with a slow-release protein source, if you are seeking exercise adaptations for your muscles[16].

## Body composition

Your body is composed of many types of tissue. These can broadly be divided into metabolically active lean mass (muscles, bone and organs) and less metabolically active fat mass. Fat can be further subdivided into visceral fat (surrounding organs) and subcutaneous tissue fat (more superficial under the skin). While fat has an important role in protecting organs and acting as a dense energy store, nevertheless having too much or too little are both potentially unhealthy.

With declining hormone levels associated with middle age, there is a tendency for a loss of lean mass and an increase in fat mass, resulting in changes in body composition. There is also a decrease in insulin and leptin receptor sensitivity. This leads to a tendency to put on weight and a loss of satiety signalling, respectively. An expanding waistline increases the risk of cardiovascular disease and type 2 diabetes mellitus. A greater ratio of fat to lean mass can contribute to metabolic syndrome, which increases in incidence from middle age[17].

The good news is that exercise can help. A three-month intensive exercise programme for women in early menopause reduced centripetal obesity (subcutaneous and visceral fat)[18]. This finding reinforces the fact that exercise is extremely important in middle age: whether this is maintaining what you already doing, ensuring strength work is included, or increasing exercise levels if you are not doing something on a regular basis.

## Sleep more!

If this talk of exercise is making you feel tired, that is good thing! In a fascinating study of middle-aged men and women, it was found that sleep quality and quantity have an impact on both bone and muscle health[19]. How can sleep be a good thing for your musculoskeletal system? The answer, as ever, lies in your hormone networks. In addition to exercise being a powerful stimulus for GH release, so also is sleep. As we discussed above, GH, and specifically the active form IGF-1, is crucial for both bone and muscle health. Going to bed earlier, rather than later, was also beneficial. The benefits of sleep were found to be more in women who had not yet reached the menopause. Sleep helps increase leptin receptor sensitivity and sharpens up satiety signals. So, to ensure you are getting the most benefit from your nocturnal hormone networks, ensuring good sleep patterns is particularly important in middle age. Check out the top tips for "sleep hygiene" below.

Sleep patterns are important to prevent circadian misalignment and mitigate the potential subsequent risk of developing metabolic syndrome. In conjunction with circadian misalignment, sedentary lifestyle, overnutrition and declining hormone levels can contribute to metabolic syndrome[20]. This syndrome is a constellation of abdominal obesity, insulin resistance, dyslipidaemia and raised blood pressure. High levels of insulin are required to deal with excess energy intake relative to demand. Insulin resistance can then develop, reducing the ability to regulate blood sugar. This is a precursor to type 2 diabetes mellitus. Dyslipidaemia means more of the "bad" than the "good" cholesterol. The combination of all these factors increases the risk of heart disease and stroke.

During middle age it can be challenging to balance work, family and social commitments. As with the justice (male or female) from the Shakespeare quote, you may be advanced in your career and more time-restricted for exercising and sleeping. So, imbalances in behaviours can have a negative impact on hormone and therefore overall health. Making sleep a priority is important for your hormone health.

## Hormone stories: what happened next?

*Gerald was a 53-year-old man who had become something of a bon viveur in middle age and had noticed an expanding waistline. He got rather a shock standing on the weighing scales to find his body mass index (BMI) was hovering on the obese category. His blood pressure was somewhat raised. His blood test results were not comfortable viewing, with indicators of risk factors for metabolic syndrome. These included an adverse lipid profile, raised glycosylated haemoglobin and elevated liver enzyme, gamma-glutamyl transferase, which is associated with alcohol intake.*

*He resolved to take action, but where to start? We resolved that the best way to reduce his waistline and stave off metabolic syndrome would be through a combination of exercise and reducing energy intake, especially by cutting down on alcohol. Gerald embraced the challenge by joining a triathlon club and donating his "wine cellar" towards the forthcoming wedding of his daughter. Six months later Gerald was relishing taking part in sport again. He particularly enjoyed exercising with others and the variety of disciplines, which included regular strength training. He* reported sleeping better and generally feeling more "alive". Not only were his swim, bike and run times going down, so were his waistline, weight, blood pressure and the blood markers of metabolic syndrome risk.

**Tim** was a 51-year-old keen competitive, amateur cyclist, with a healthy BMI (body mass index). He intentionally lost body weight thinking this would improve his race performance but felt fatigued and suffered a stress fracture of his hip when he started running.

Was this a case of physiological decline of testosterone due to age or other factors? Blood tests showed that Tim had a lower level of testosterone than expected for his age and this was due to low energy availability (confirmed from clinical history and low levels of thyroid hormones and LH). Dual X-ray densitometry (DXA) scans showed that his BMD was significantly below that expected for his age. In other words, Tim had a relative energy deficiency in sport (RED-S). The priority for Tim was to restore energy availability through adjustments in nutrition and training. This improved internal production of testosterone to levels expected for his age. He started gradated skeletal loading exercise, alongside vitamin D supplementation to support bone health. Tim got back on his bike and felt much better.

**Katie** was 46 years of age and struggling with work and exercise training. As she was not having periods due to Mirena coil, there were no clues from the regularity of periods.

Were her symptoms of fatigue due to insufficient fuelling for her energy demands or reduced ovarian responsiveness? Blood tests came back indicating the latter, with raised levels of FSH and LH, and low oestradiol consistent with menopause. Thyroid function and all other markers that might be a cause of her symptoms were comfortably in the normal range. After discussing the results and having no contra-indications to HRT, Katie decided that she would like to try HRT and added transdermal oestradiol alongside the progestogen provided by the Mirena coil. Happily, this much improved her symptoms. Katie also took on board the recommendation to include more strength training and recovery time in her training schedule.

## Strategies to support your hormones in "middle age"

Here are the proactive steps you can take in terms of lifestyle choices you can make regarding exercise, nutrition and sleep to mitigate the outcomes of declining hormones

*Exercise*

- Including strength exercise in your weekly schedule becomes particularly important at this stage in your life to prevent sarcopenia (loss of muscle mass and function) and maintain a healthy body composition. This type of activity also indirectly supports bone health, alongside multidirectional loading exercise which has a direct positive effect on bone health.

*Nutrition*

- Timed protein intake is important for muscle health
  - After resistance exercise
  - Before bed

*Sleep and recovery*

- Revisit sleep hygiene strategies
  - Maintain consistent times for going to bed and getting up.
  - Take a milk drink before bed
- After 3 months of applying sleep hygiene strategies, if sleep remains a challenge, cognitive behavioural therapy (CBT) can be helpful. Consider "sleep scheduling" where you anchor the day by getting up at a consistent rising and try getting out of bed during the night if you can't sleep.

*Hormone replacement for women*

- It can be difficult to distinguish perimenopause symptoms from the stresses and strains of life.
- Do background research on hormone replacement therapy (HRT)[1].
- Transdermal forms of oestradiol combined with micronised progesterone are particularly good forms of HRT
- Doses of HRT can be personalised
- For women for whom HRT is contraindicated, or wish to pursue other options, there are non-pharmacological possibilities.

## *Hormone replacement for men*

- Start by reviewing your lifestyle choices
- It is important to exclude any underlying medical conditions
- Taking inappropriate testosterone, without full review of external factors and hormone networks, suppresses your own internal production and can have implications for fertility[21]

# Scene 6
## Old Age

> *"The lean and slipper'd pantaloon,*
> *With spectacles on nose and pouch on side,*
> *His youthful hose, well sav'd, a world too wide*
> *For his shrunk shank, and his big manly voice,*
> *Turning again toward childish treble, pipes*
> *And whistles in his sound."*
>
> *Shakespeare*

**Subtitle:** With increasing age come decreasing hormone levels. The declines in sex steroid hormones and growth hormone lead to a loss of muscle mass and function. Reduced muscle strength impairs the ability to stay active, compounding the situation. The twilight of hormone production also leads to weaker bones that are more prone to fracture. Increasing life expectancy and an ageing population highlight the importance of mitigating the negative effects of declining hormones on health and well-being. Effective strategies include adaptations of lifestyle factors, with attention to activity, nutrition and sleep.

### Hormone stories

*Colin* was a 71-year-old world-class age group swimmer. He was training in the pool every day, aiming to beat his rival at the next age group world championship. However, he reported feeling fatigued and some soreness in his shoulder. What do you think might be going on? What might help him in his quest to be a world champion?

*Jackie* was a 65-year-old woman, who was still working full time and said she did not have much time for exercise. She reached menopause at the age of 54 and had been taking HRT. Jackie reported that recently she had felt "unfit", finding it a struggle to carry heavy shopping. However, she lacked the confidence to join an exercise class in the gym.

## Hormone coda

The reason why Shakespeare describes the onset of old age as entering a second childhood is that hormone levels fall to those of a child. The timing of this change is set by the biochronometer with the longest timescale. Although chronological time moves forward, there is a reversal in hormone production.

Before puberty, boys and girls are on a level playing field when it comes to the key sex steroid hormones, having low testosterone and oestradiol, respectively. During adolescence there is a surge in these hormones which trigger divergent physical characteristics, appearance and performance that are sustained during adulthood. However, these differences regress later in life. Age-related hormone decline contributes to the tendency to revert to child-like appearance with "shrunk shank" (loss of muscle on leg) and "childish treble" voice.

Sex steroids also have a profound effect on internal physiological function, including substrate use (energy source). Children are less able to perform intense anaerobic exercise, because they have not yet developed the metabolism to use carbohydrate as a fuel source. This ability increases with adult levels of hormones but falls off again as hormone production declines later in life. Masters athletes often report losing their "top end" ability to sprint at high intensity.

Hormones also affect the ability to use fat as an energy source. Women, with a higher level of oestradiol, are better able to use fat as a fuel compared with men. This is helpful for long aerobic endurance exercise. However, after the menopause (average age 51), when oestradiol levels decline dramatically, men and women are once again on more of an even playing field when it comes to oestradiol[1].

### *Quality of life*

The World Health Organisation (WHO) defines quality of life (QOL) as "an individual's perception of their position in life in the context of the culture and value systems in which they live and in relation to their goals, expectations, standards and concerns". Health has an important bearing on the ability to live independently and perform the activities of daily life, work and sporting, cultural or social activities. The Center of Disease Control and Prevention (CDC) defines health-related quality of life (HRQOL) as "an individual's or a group's perceived physical and mental health over time".

An individual's HRQOL may become challenged with advancing age. Often this can be traced back to a decline in hormone function.

## *Hormone twilight*

If you were in any doubt about the importance of hormones for health, the physiological consequences of age-related hormone decline illustrate this crucial interplay between hormones, health and QOL. This is shown in Figure 16.1. A fall in hormone production causes loss of muscle mass. Reduced hormone levels have a negative effect on bone mass and alter body composition, favouring fat deposition over lean mass. These physical changes reduce muscle strength and exercise ability. More limited activity has adverse effects on hormones, bone, muscle and body composition[2]. In other words, a vicious circle can ensue, where lack of movement contributes to further loss of function and a lack of confidence to move. Age-related decline in hormone production and physical function can be compounded by pre-existing medical conditions, illness and suboptimal nutrition. Understanding how to mitigate these negative effects is very important, especially in view of increasing life expectancy.

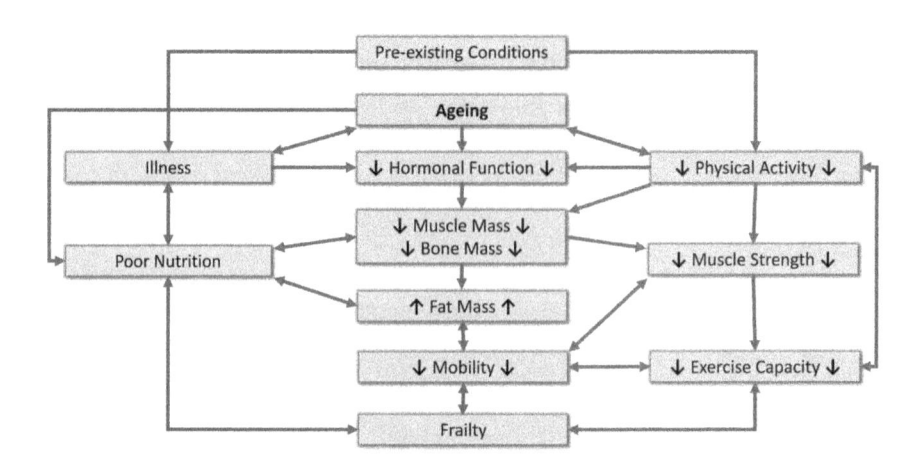

**Figure 16.1:** Model of ageing, hormones and physical function. Adapted from Copeland JL, Can J Appl Physiol 2004;29(1):76–89 2004

*Osteosarcopenia*

Osteosarcopenia means reduced health and function of the musculoskeletal system. This includes muscles, joints, bone and the neurological connections, which all contribute to make movement possible. Movement is fundamental to human survival and necessary to complete the activities of daily life, such as eating, washing and dressing. Loss of the ability to perform these tasks not only contributes to further physical decline shown in Figure 16.1 but also to emotional well-being. The net result is a reduction in quality of life. To understand how to optimise quality of life, it is important to consider the mechanisms behind age-related osteosarcopenia and examine the preventative strategies[3].

## *Muscle function*

Sarcopenia describes the loss of muscle mass, strength and function that occurs with ageing[4]. Reduced hormone levels impair the body's ability to respond to exercise stimulus and carry out ongoing repairs. Poor nutrition and reduced activity also play a part. Sarcopenia impairs physical function and can lead to disability. For example, the ability to get up from sitting to standing without using the arms of a chair is a straightforward test of muscle strength. Similarly, grip strength can be used as an assessment tool.

Resistance-based exercise has been found to have a beneficial effect on the catabolic, muscle-building hormone, insulin-like growth factor 1 (IGF-1) in both men and women[5]. In fact, weightlifting, carried out with the appropriate level of caution for elderly people, has been shown to increase IGF-1 in the skeletal muscle of frail men and women[6].

In a convincing demonstration of the beneficial effects of strength training for older people, a study put 16 men with an average age of 72 head-to-head with 14 men of average age 26 in a strength competition. As you might expect at the start of the study there were significant differences between the age groups in terms of muscle fibre size and capillary density. The younger men had bigger muscles supplied by more blood vessels bringing hormones and nutrients to the muscles. However, after the older men received 12 weeks of supervised resistance sessions, there was no longer any difference from the younger men. The older men saw an increase in the size of the type of muscle fibre for sprinting and improved blood supply (capillary bed density) for both the "fast-twitch" type II muscle fibres and the "slow-twitch" type I muscle fibre that is involved in endurance exercise. In other words, strength training in older men turned back the clock and improved the muscles involved in both fast movement and sustained endurance exercise to equal those of men less than half their age[7].

This type of strength work also has neurological benefits in terms of maintaining and in the case of this study, clearly improving the neuromuscular connections required for effective movement.

## *Bone health*

Bone health does not just depend on the mechanical loading of the skeleton to provide an osteogenic, bone-building stimulus. Hormones play an important role as discussed in "Act 1, Scene 7: Bare Bones". Oestradiol is particularly crucial for bone health. Bone is a dynamic tissue, with our skeleton being continuously "recycled" over our lifetime. Bone turnover is a balancing act between bone formation and bone resorption (breakdown). Oestradiol favours bone formation. As oestradiol levels decline with age in both men and women, the balance of bone turnover shifts to resorption. The net result is literally a loss of bone. Poor bone health increases the risk of a fragility fracture, which is a fracture sustained from a relatively low energy fall, for example from a standing height. Having weak bones is known as osteoporosis "brittle bone disease". Osteoporosis is also known as the "silent killer" causing a loss in quality of life and ultimately death[8].

Bone mineral density can be measured with a dual X-ray absorptiometry (DXA) scan and is used to assess bone health. Osteoporosis is defined according to the measurement from a DXA scan. The bone mineral density measurement is compared with its expected lifetime maximum (peak bone mass) attained around 20 years of age. This metric, known as the T-score, is expressed in standard deviations. Osteoporosis is defined as having a T-score of −2.5 or less, indicating a bone mineral density well below its peak. The Fracture Risk Assessment Tool (FRAX)* questionnaire can be used to predict the risk of fragility fracture in those over 40 years of age[9]. FRAX is based on recognised medical and lifestyle risk factors for poor bone health and T-score.

Oestradiol is the primary hormone affecting bone health. Although oestradiol decreases with advancing age in both men and women, its decline is most marked in women. This is because for women, the source of this most active form of oestrogen is the ovaries, which stop working at menopause (average age 51 years). This dramatic reduction in oestradiol in women is one of the main reasons why osteoporosis is more widespread in older women, compared with men. For example, in women, oestradiol can fall by around 100-fold after menopause. In contrast, male oestradiol remains reasonably steady throughout adult life, even after 50 years of age.

## Consequences of hormone twilight

### Osteoporosis

Older people tend to lose height. As bone health deteriorates, the vertebrae of the spine become compressed. In some cases, this impaction of vertebral bone results in a compression fracture. Wedge-shaped compression fractures of the spine are a well-recognised feature of osteoporosis. The so-called "dowager's hump" is a direct consequence of vertebral compression fractures. In addition to pain, vertebral compression fractures in the thoracic spine make it difficult to breath effectively.

Until relatively recently, weight training has been viewed cautiously for "brittle bones". However, an inspiring study demonstrated that menopausal women undertaking twice weekly heavy weightlifting exercise (five sets of five repetitions, >85% of one repetition maximum) did not sustain any fractures or injuries. They significantly improved their bone strength in the lumbar spine and maintained height, compared with a control group of women who did light strength work over the same eight-month period[10]. In addition to direct mechanical loading of the spine, improving back extensor muscle strength decreases the risk of vertebral compression fracture and so prevents loss of height[11].

### Quality of connective tissue

It is less well recognised that loss in height is also due to the effect of diminishing levels of oestradiol on collagen, a type of protein found in connective tissue. Connective tissue is a bit like internal adhesive tape, joining tissues together. This is one of the reasons you are more likely to get injured as you get older. Ligaments and tendons are made of collagen and give stability to all the joints in your body. If these stabilising structures are weaker, they are more likely to tear. In addition to being an injury in itself, a torn ligament reduces the stability of a joint. Add in some loss of balance, which occurs with advancing age, and a fall onto weakened bones can result in fracture.

Declining levels of oestradiol can lead to deterioration in the quality of collagen, which is a major constituent of the intervertebral discs. These discs are sandwiched between the vertebrae, providing cushioning within the spine.

Intervertebral discs can become squashed and protrude outwards, sometimes impinging on a nerve root coming off the spinal cord: a "slipped disc". With age, intervertebral discs lose their strength and integrity, making them more likely to be compressed. This contributes directly to loss of height and to the increased risk of vertebral compression fractures, as the discs lose their ability to absorb compression forces[12].

*Hip fracture*

When my sister returned from school one day, she found my grandmother on the floor in the kitchen, unable to get up. My grandmother explained that her cardigan had caught in a drawer and she had fallen. This demonstrates that sustaining a hip fracture involves a combination of factors: the likelihood of a fall and poor bone health.

The reason it is important to explore these risk factors is that a hip fracture is a significant injury requiring surgery and rehabilitation. Not only does this take its toll on an individual in terms of risk of surgery and hospitalisation, this type of fracture in the elderly also puts a big economic burden on healthcare. Having poor bone health is clearly a risk factor for fracture. However, having poor muscle function, sarcopenia, is also a contributor to hip fracture[13]. This is because having good muscle tone means that the pull of muscle on bone provides a stimulus to bone. Having good muscle tone also means you have the strength to maintain balance if you trip, in order to prevent a fall. This is closely related to proprioception: the awareness of your body in space. Feedback of spatial awareness includes feedback from muscles and joints. So simple balance-based exercises have an important part to play in fracture prevention, and balance is included as part of a fall risk assessment[14].

*Pharmaceutical options for bone health*

For women, provided there are no contraindications, HRT certainly is helpful in mitigating the bone loss due to menopause. HRT contains the bone-friendly hormone, oestradiol. However, HRT should not be started after 60 years of age just for prevention of osteoporotic fractures[15]. There are other medications that are used to support bone health for older men and women. These can be divided into those that prevent the breakdown of bone and those that encourage bone formation. The first category includes antiresorptive agents such as bisphosphonates and newer selective oestrogen receptor modulators (SERMS). In contrast, parathyroid hormone encourages bone formation[16]. The requirement and best form of medication are clinical decisions taken by a doctor in consultation with the individual. In all cases, lifestyle factors are the initial area to address.

*Body composition and metabolic health*

The age-related decline of anabolic ("tissue building") hormones, such as testosterone and growth hormone, leads to changes in body composition: a decrease in skeletal muscle and an increase in fat (adipose tissue). Skeletal muscle contains an abundance of mitochondria, the powerhouse of cells. This contrasts with the sparsity of mitochondria in adipose tissue. The result is a loss of metabolically active tissue that can present a potential challenge to blood glucose control. This in turn presents a risk to metabolic and cardiovascular health. Furthermore, visceral fat deposition, around the abdominal organs, is a contributing factor to metabolic syndrome, which is the constellation of poor blood glucose control, insulin resistance, high blood pressure, disrupted cholesterol profile and potentially "fatty" liver. Metabolic syndrome greatly increases the risk of cardiovascular disease[17].

Recent preliminary research reports that menopause presents a particular challenge to metabolic health[18]. Reduced levels of ovarian hormones, particularly oestradiol, is associated with a decreased response of cells to the hormones insulin and leptin. These hormones are important for effective and efficient metabolism by regulating blood glucose and satiety, respectively. This illustrates two important points about hormones. First, there is a synergistic effect between hormone networks. Oestradiol works in partnership with other hormones across many systems in the body. Second, even if hormone signals are being sent to cells, the responsiveness of these target cells determines the outcome. Menopause, with decline in oestradiol production, is due to the reduced response of the ovaries to pituitary hormone signals. Similarly, despite high levels of insulin and leptin, the cells can become resistant to paying attention to these signals. The outcome is that blood sugar levels will tend to run high and that satiety will not be registered by the hypothalamus. This means that the person may become a "volume eater", and blood glucose levels will not be well controlled. This will predispose to type 2 diabetes mellitus and depositing fat in the trunk area. On a positive note, taking HRT was shown to mitigate these metabolic issues. Also being aware of these challenges for metabolism with advancing age offers the opportunity to be proactive in timing and choice of food. Avoiding foods and drinks that cause "sugar spikes", which unfortunately does include alcohol, and avoiding quick fix weight reduction diets which ultimately lead to "weight cycling", compounding insulin resistance[19].

## *Ageing or disease?*

Part of the expected outcome of biological ageing is a change in the genetic machinery, such as telomere shortening (discussed further in the final scene), which contributes to decline in function in many systems in the body. Reduced function, whether of the endocrine, musculoskeletal, cardiovascular or neurological systems, or combinations of these predisposes to disease states.

For example, ageing causes reduced effectiveness of the immune system, resulting in a loss of "self-tolerance" at a cellular level. The immune system mistakes self-antigens (the tags on cells) for being "foreign". This could be partly due to faltering genetic machinery producing slightly defective proteins which truly do not have correct antigen tags. This prompts the immune system to lay siege to these mislabelled cells. The resultant increase in autoantibody production is considered to be a consequence of ageing, as opposed to an autoimmune disease.

Clearly, an age-compromised immune system is less resistant to disease. Increasing age sees involution (shrinking) of the thymus gland, which plays an important role in immune regulation. This could contribute to the increase in cancer with age[3].

## *Sex steroid hormone coda*

### *Menopause and beyond*

The word menopause derives from Greek word where "menos" means month and pausis "an ending". This is when the ovaries shut down and stop producing the sex steroids oestradiol and progesterone. With increasing life expectancy, a woman can spend a third or more of her life in the menopausal state. The dramatic drop in ovarian hormones can be very challenging, with around half of women experiencing physical and emotional issues adversely affecting their quality of life and a quarter reporting severe adverse impacts in terms of their personal and professional life[20].

With declining ovarian hormone levels come increased health risks across many systems including bone and cardiovascular health[21]. As described above, oestradiol is essential for bone health and plays an important role in cardiovascular health, maintaining a healthy lipid profile and the reactivity of the endothelial wall of arteries. From the age of menopause, with dramatically reduced oestradiol production, the risk of heart disease in women rises to match that of men. Cardiovascular disease is the main cause of death in menopausal women. Furthermore, as discussed above, osteoporosis has a big negative impact on health, especially in women. And yet, despite the longer life expectancy of women, health spending on women decreases relative to men from around the age of 50[22]. So, although women may live longer, it may be that their quality of life is lower.

HRT can improve the quality of life and the long-term health of women in terms of reduced overall mortality (death from all causes)[21]. As discussed in the previous scene, assessing the benefit of HRT in terms of quality of life and health, relative to risk, helps a woman arrive at an informed decision. Ideally starting HRT as soon as possible on reaching menopause is advisable to mitigate symptoms and provide cardiovascular and bone protection. There is no definitive time limit to how long to stay on HRT. Potentially this could be well into old age. This decision requires a joint decision between the woman and her prescribing doctor, adopting a personalised approach[23].

*Male hormone twilight*

In common with women, growth hormone declines with increasing age. However, when it comes to sex steroid hormones there is a big difference. Women experience a decrease in their predominant sex steroid oestradiol, down to as little of 1% of its prior level. In contrast, men after 50 years of age see a very modest decline in testosterone levels, with the expected range shifted downwards to about 85% of its youthful level. As discussed in Act 1, "Scene 5XY: Of Mice and Men", this is why testosterone "replacement" treatment is not advised unless there is clear medical evidence of failure to produce testosterone, justifying replacement. Artificially boosting testosterone above physiological levels can pose a risk rather than a benefit to health. For example, sustained high testosterone increases haemoglobin production and can render blood viscous and prone to clot formation, which increases the risk of stroke and heart attack. Furthermore, external sex steroid use increases liver activity, which is revealed on blood test with raised liver enzymes.

Rather, addressing the underlying cause of decreased testosterone production is a better approach. Increasing age can be associated with medical conditions (type 2 diabetes mellitus, obesity, medication) that can reduce testosterone production. Slipping into lifestyle choices, such as the lack of exercise (or in some cases excessive exercise) can also adversely impact testosterone levels[24]. Addressing the underlying cause of and modification of lifestyle behaviours can mitigate age-related decline in hormone production.

## Lifestyle factors for hormone health in older age

Making good lifestyle choices is always the first port of call for health. Taking regular exercise, maintaining body weight in a healthy range, not smoking and limiting intake of alcohol are important things you can do to sustain a good quality of life.

### *Exercise*

"Purposefully" doing exercise has become increasingly important with the increase in technology which reduces the physical demands of performing the activities of daily living. For example, the time saved by washing machines, dish washers and cars is often spent on activities like watching television, rather than deriving the health benefits of physical activity.

For menopausal women, exercise has been shown to support thermoregulation, alleviating the symptoms of hot flushes[25]. Exercise of moderate intensity in menopausal women improves metabolic health, by increasing insulin sensitivity and supporting a favourable body composition[26]. Taking at least two and a half hours of exercise per week also reduces the risk of breast cancer[21].

Strength exercise for both elderly men and women is a priority to mitigate the effects of declining anabolic hormones. This type of exercise, in synergy with nutrition, helps maintain favourable body composition and metabolic health. Furthermore, strength exercise is a preventative strategy for osteosarcopenia and crucial for optimising musculoskeletal function and quality of life.

Strength exercise is not limited to "pumping iron" in the gym. If this is not the place for you, there are many other options. Resistance exercise, using resistance bands, can be very effective across the full range of movement. This has the added advantage of not requiring expensive equipment, and it can be done at home. If you prefer a class setting, Pilates is a good choice. Swimming is an excellent form of exercise for hormone-driven aspects of cardiovascular and metabolic health. Although swimming does not mechanically load the skeleton to promote bone health, nevertheless, the pull of skeletal muscle on bone does provide some osteogenic (bone-building) benefit and is particularly helpful for those with joint issues that may limit other forms of strength training.

The elements of exercise specific for bone health and lowering the risk of falls and subsequent fracture are summed by in the appropriately named information from the Royal Osteoporosis Society "Strong, Straight, Steady"[27]. Strong and straight refer to benefits of strength exercise outlined above, which helps with bone strength and good posture. The steady element refers to good balance, which means that you are less likely to fall over. A fall, even a seemingly innocuous low energy fall from standing height, can result in fracture if bones are weak. Balance can be improved by including some proprioceptive type of exercise that requires awareness of where your body is in space. The simplest proprioception work is standing, with fingertips on a chair, and lifting alternate feet just of the floor.

## *Nutrition*

Eating a diet with a good range of food types and avoiding highly processed foods are important for maintaining healthy hormones. This becomes even more important when levels and responsiveness of hormones are declining with age.

Ensuring good protein intake supports muscle health, especially after an anabolic exercise stimulus[28]. Vitamin D supplementation is recommended for everyone living in northern latitudes and especially for older people who may be spending more time indoors[29].

## *Sleep*

Sleep quality and quantity can be affected by ageing. The master biological clock, the suprachiasmatic nucleus (SNC), controls the timed release of hormones and timing of physiological processes. The SNC itself starts to feel the effects of time with increasing age. This can result in a mistiming of hormone release that affects when older people feel sleepy and can fall asleep. Potentially reduced light-sensory input can also contribute to dysregulation. It is not that older people need less sleep, rather they may not be able to fall asleep so easily or they have disturbed sleep, rendering them less alert and productive in daylight hours. A vicious cycle of faulty biological timekeeping and mistimed hormone release can compound sleep problems with increasing years. The solution is to review the strategies of sleep hygiene. This includes establishing a bedtime routine and avoiding the use of electronic equipment late at night. A bedtime milk-based drink serves the dual role of providing the precursor tryptophan to make the sleep hormone melatonin and the protein casein to help with muscle repairs[30].

## Conclusions

Health related quality of life is challenged with advancing age, due to decline in hormone network function. It can be difficult to distinguish ageing from disease. These are often interdependent processes. Nevertheless, to maintain quality of life and prevent a vicious circle of declining function, there are positive steps that can be taken in the choice of exercise and nutrition to optimise health for age.

## Hormone stories: what happened next?

***Colin*** was the 71-year-old world swimmer who was feeling fatigued and had soreness in his shoulder. The first thing I recommended to Colin was to start doing some dry-land strength work. This is important to mitigate declining hormone levels, particularly IGF-1 and testosterone and support muscle strength and bone health. Although swimming is an excellent cardiovascular exercise, like cycling, this sport does not load the skeleton for bone health. We included some muscle activation exercises specific to swimming technique to ensure that he was engaging his latissimus dorsi muscles, which are part of a very substantial muscle group that offloads the smaller muscles around the shoulder joint. Some rotator cuff shoulder stability exercises were useful as a dry-land warm-up before swimming. Although Colin reported good nutritional strategies, he was happy to add some more foods with protein, especially milk before bed to favour muscle formation. Colin was not aware how important it is to take vitamin D supplementation, especially over winter months for bone, muscle and immune function.

***Jackie*** was a 60-year-old woman, working full time and lacking the confidence to take exercise classes. Although Jackie did not have a totally sedentary job, nevertheless taking at least two and a half hours per week of moderate intensity would certainly be beneficial for health and fitness. Furthermore, taking exercise decreases the risk of breast cancer in women in this age group. We agreed that Jackie could start off with brisk walks. Strength exercise training is important for bone health and body composition, so we discussed alternatives to attending a gym. Doing some Pilates with resistance bands was a good starting point. Jackie mentioned that she did like dancing. This is an excellent form of exercise for proprioception and bone health, because dancing involves changes of direction that promote both balance and bone strength. Jackie wished to continue taking HRT. We discussed the advice from the British Menopause Society that each woman should be treated as an individual, and there *is no set time for stopping HRT, provided no issues arise. Jackie was having regular breast screening and starting regular exercise supported the beneficial effects on HRT on long-term health.*

## Strategies to support your hormones in old age

### Exercise

- Strength-based exercise is important for body composition, as well as muscle and bone function
- Working on proprioception with balance-based skills is beneficial as a fall prevention strategy

### Nutrition

- Maintaining good eating habits
- Focus on protein intake to mitigate the effects of declining hormone levels
- Vitamin D supplementation increases in importance with ageing.
- Magnesium supplementation through the skin (e.g. spray) can help with muscle function and cramp prevention.

### Sleep

- Sleep is essential for health at all ages
- Review strategies to ensure good sleep

# Scene 7
## Dotage

> *"Second childishness and mere oblivion,*
> *Sans teeth, sans eyes, sans taste, sans everything."*
> Shakespeare

**Subtitle:** Dotage is a time in later old age associated with some loss of mental ability. This stage in life is often described as a second childhood. This is reflected in similarly low levels of hormones at both ends of the lifespan. On the other hand, ageing cells are totally different from the cells of a child. Aged cells are less responsive to hormones and more prone to "going wrong". This leads to a decline in physical and mental function. Nevertheless, ageing is a natural physiological process. Adaptation and maintaining social connections are important aspects of ageing "gracefully".

## Hormone stories

***Vivienne*** was a reasonably healthy 80-year-old who was not taking any regular medications. Although she was not able to "hop, skip and jump" anymore, being a retired language lecturer, she could still speak several languages and discuss literature. One morning she woke up to find that she could not communicate. Words came out, but in a way that did not make sense.

***Anthony*** was 82 years of age. He had had a very successful hip replacement. However, one morning he lost balance and fell in the bathroom. Fortunately, he did not fracture anything, but he continued to feel very unsteady, and his wife noticed that his speech was not as fluid as usual.

## Symmetry

Shakespeare was correct in describing dotage as a second childhood. Many of hormones fall to low levels as seen in prepubescent children. Fortunately, dental hygiene, visual and hearing aids have improved since Elizabethan times.

The fall in sex steroids in elderly people brings men and women back onto an even playing field. Low levels of oestradiol deprive women of the cardioprotective effect of this hormone. Cardiovascular disease is similar in older men and women and becomes the main cause of death in women[1]. Low levels of the anabolic ("muscle building") growth hormone contribute to sarcopenia (loss of muscle mass and function) and subsequent frailty. A decrease in metabolic rate and reduced physical activity can pose health challenges in old age.

## Longevity

Life expectancy has increased over time. Until 200 years ago, the average lifespan was around 30 years. Back in Roman times, there was only a 50% chance of reaching the age 5, with only about 10% of the population living into their 70s. In England, the Victorian age saw improvements in living conditions with clean drinking water and better nutrition, and in 1900 the average life expectancy was up to 50 years, with the main killer being infectious diseases, such as tuberculosis. The advent of immunisation and antibiotics after the Second World War fostered another increase in longevity[2].

In recent times, life expectancy has increased across the world from 66.8 years in 2000 to 73.4 years in 2019: an increase of more than 6 years[3]. However, do we really want to live longer in *"mere oblivion . . . sans everything"*? Longevity is less appealing if it comes at the expense of poor health and low quality of life. What we really want is healthy longevity, to be "hale and hearty" in old age. The World Health Organisation defines healthy life expectancy (HALE) as the average number of years in full health a person (usually at age 60) can expect to live based on current rates of ill-health and mortality. The arithmetic difference between life expectancy and healthy life expectancy gives an indication of how long a person is likely to live with health problems that impede everyday activity.

Although HALE has increased by 5.4 years, this has not kept pace with the 6.6 years increase in life expectancy.

Is there a limit to how far we can extend healthy life expectancy? To address this question, we need to consider the biological and disease processes involved with ageing and whether we need to look beyond only the physical aspects.

## What occurs with ageing?

We start to age from the moment of conception. There are many interrelated factors at play with biological ageing.

## Genetic machinery

With advancing age, the tail ends of the chromosomes that control the expression of DNA, the telomere regions, become shorter. They become damaged by oxidative stress. This means that in dotage the expression of DNA to make proteins is less effective and more prone to mistakes due to the combined effects of dwindling hormones and shortened telomeres. Interestingly, research conducted in space shows that low levels of magnesium can be associated with telomere shortening[4]. Happily, low magnesium is something that can easily be addressed on Earth, with magnesium being an ion that is readily absorbed through the skin, when applied as a spray or gel. Regrettably, magnesium is unlikely to be the elixir of youth, as there are other factors at play in the ageing process.

Even if the DNA material does not change, its expression can be altered by epigenetic effects. This is where changes occur to the molecules that wrap around DNA that affect the production of the intended protein. Methylation is an example of a molecular mechanism that has an epigenetic effect on DNA expression. Adding a methyl group near the promotor region ("start here") of a DNA molecule downregulates the ability of DNA to direct protein synthesis. This limits the ability of cells to rejuvenate, leaving ageing as the only option. This is the exact opposite of what happens at the start of life in the foetus where a wave of demethylation gives cells the ability and freedom to develop into a range of cell types, as discussed in Act 2, Scene 1.

On the other hand, indiscriminate demethylation occurring later in life can be linked to an increased risk of cancer. Cancer is where unhealthy cells become "immortal" and replicate at the expense of healthy cells. Age-related methylation drift is the term used to describe the indiscriminate methylation and demethylation of DNA, which can lead to faulty expression through this epigenetic mechanism. It has been suggested that age-related methylation drift could be delayed with calorie restriction[5]. The significance of the age-related changes in epigenetic methylation is that it is linked to the risk of diseases found in older age groups, such as cardiovascular and metabolic disease. Epigenetic biological age, rather than chronological age, has been proposed as an effective screening tool to identify those at risk of age-related disease and to target prevention strategies[6].

## Physiology of ageing

Although advances in medicine have greatly increased life expectancy, the incidence of diseases of old age has risen correspondingly. Understanding the physiology of ageing can help in extending healthy lifespans. As mentioned above, faulty genetic machinery leads to less accurate protein synthesis. This has a negative effect on many fundamental physiological processes, especially in the production of energy in the mitochondria, the powerhouses of the cells. Furthermore, the less efficient clearing of metabolic waste products leads to harmful accumulations, causing increased systemic inflammation. This can be aggravated by a build-up of senescent cells, whose normal function has been impaired by stress. Senescent cells play a useful short-term role in cleaning up damaged cells, but, if left unchecked, they start to damage healthy cells. Finally, cell communication can break down[2], as cells and tissues become less receptive and responsive to hormone messengers. The level of hormones themselves decline. The net effect of all these factors is a cumulative physiological malfunction in dotage.

## Disease processes in old age

With an ageing population, it is expected that by 2040 the number of people over 80 years will have tripled, thereby increasing the burden of chronic disease[7]. Disorders that are top of the list are cardiovascular, cardiometabolic and neurodegenerative diseases. Polypharmacy, the use of multiple medications, can result in interactions and potential unwanted side effects.

### *Cardiovascular and metabolic disease*

Cardiovascular disease (CVD) increases with age and is a leading cause of morbidity (disability) and mortality (death) in the elderly, followed by metabolic disease: type 2 diabetes mellitus[8]. The underlying aetiology of CVD is blockage of the arteries supplying oxygen and nutrients to important organs like the heart and brain. Lack of blood supply causes damage to cells (ischaemia) and ultimately cell death (infarction). This presents as a "heart attack" or stroke[9]. Atherosclerosis is the underlying process that causes CVD. The arteries become less flexible with age and potentially roughened on the inner surface where blood flows. Combined with high levels of circulating "unhealthy" cholesterol and inflammation, this leads to cholesterol deposits in the wall of arteries restricting blood flow[10].

For elderly postmenopausal women, low levels of oestrogen result in an increased risk of CVD to equal that of men. Oestrogen is a cardioprotective hormone that supports the reactivity of the artery walls and helps maintain a healthy lipid profile. Although there is no absolute age limit to taking Hormone Replacement Therapy (HRT), elderly women, potentially taking multiple medications, may find continuing HRT to be impractical[1].

Metabolic hormone issues, such as poor blood glucose control, magnify the risk of CVD. Insulin is the key hormone in blood glucose regulation. In type 2 diabetes mellitus (DM), although plenty of insulin is produced in response to high glucose levels in the blood, the cells become resistant to its action. This leads to sustained high levels of both glucose and insulin. This is more likely to occur in the elderly, as activity and energy demand decline, especially if nutrition exceeds activity levels and body composition has deteriorated. Low anabolic hormone levels (such as growth hormone and testosterone) result in a loss of lean body mass, compounded by reduced activity. Since lean body mass, specifically muscle, is the metabolically active type of tissue, reduced energy requirement should be matched by modified energy intake.

Staying as active as possible, even if limited to exercises sitting in a chair, and paying close attention to appropriate nutritional intake are both beneficial. Avoiding excessive calorie intake, with a particular emphasis on adequate protein, helps prevent insulin resistance and mitigates the loss of muscle mass and function (sarcopenia). In terms of hormone support, aside from HRT, vitamin D is a steroid hormone that all elderly people should supplement, as a healthy level cannot be obtained from diet alone. Away from the equator, the action of sunlight on the skin is limited, especially for elderly people spending much time indoors. Vitamin D is important for bone, muscle and immune function[11].

Magnesium intake has the potential to support health in old age, counterbalancing the effects of cumulative oxidative stress and inflammation[12]. Magnesium is well absorbed through the skin, so it can be taken very simply as a spray or as magnesium salts dissolved in a bath, at low expense. Evidence shows that magnesium mitigates many diseases, such as DM, cardiovascular disease and cardiac arrhythmia, osteoporosis and potentially neurodegenerative diseases[13].

## Neurodegenerative disease

Dementia is a syndrome reflecting progressive decline in brain function. This can include symptoms such as memory loss and cognitive decline including lack of mental sharpness, poor judgement and change in mood and emotional connection.

## Alzheimer's disease

Dementia includes brain vascular changes and Alzheimer's disease. Alzheimer's disease is characterised by the accumulation of type of protein in the brain called beta amyloid, which is linked to cognitive decline. Evidence shows that lack of sleep is associated with the deposition of beta amyloid, even before cognitive impairment is noted[14]. This is a significant finding as it provides a lifestyle prevention strategy. An additional hour of night-time sleep is associated with statistically significant reduction in the deposition of beta amyloid in the brain.

In a recent large study, lifestyle factors were found to have a significant effect on life expectancy and the number of years living with Alzheimers[15]. People who exercise, have cognitive engagement, eat healthily, don't smoke and drink modest amounts of alcohol not only live longer but live for more years without Alzheimer's disease. A 50% reduction in years lived without Alzheimer's dementia over 65 years of age was observed.

## Parkinson's disease

Parkinson's disease is a process that affects the control of movement, together with effects on cognition and emotion[16]. Initially movement issues can start on one side, so it can be tricky to distinguish from a stroke. In fact, problems with cerebral blood flow can cause "vascular Parkinson's" disease[17]. There can be other causes of Parkinsonism, such as medication. However, Parkinson's disease is specifically where degeneration of dopaminergic neurons located in substantia nigra (a particular area of the brain) causes the characteristic symptoms. Dopamine is a neurotransmitter, a very short-range hormone acting as a signalling molecule between nerve cells, particularly in the brain. Low levels of cerebral dopamine cause Parkinson's disease.

In practice, Parkinson's is a clinical diagnosis based on movement patterns. Typically, the person displays slow movement (bradykinesia) and walks with a shuffling gait, with poor balance and stiffness. Often, initiation of movement is the most challenging. Once underway, it becomes hard to stop. At rest, there can be a slight tremor, most noticeable in the hands, often described as a "pill rolling tremor".

However, Parkinson's disease is not just a condition affecting movement. The autonomic nervous system can be adversely impacted, causing swallowing issues and problems with constipation and bladder control. Erratic blood pressure control can result in postural hypotension, where a drop in blood pressure on standing compounds issues with balance. Changes in emotion and mental sharpness often occur as Parkinson's progresses. Associated problems with sleep can lead to a vicious circle, with fatigue contributing to suboptimal function.

Treatment is typically with medication to increase dopamine. The introduction of L-Dopa in the 1950s transformed the lives of many suffering from Parkinson's and earned Arvid Carlsson a Nobel Prize in 2000. L-Dopa is combined with carbidopa to mitigate side effects, such as a drop in blood pressure and nausea. Carbidopa is a decarboxylase inhibitor that prevents the peripheral breakdown of L-Dopa, allowing more to cross the blood-brain barrier to reach the target area.

## Potential age-reversing medical interventions

There are several candidate interventions for preventing the decline in function associated with ageing. Some are realistic while others are ephemeral fountains of youth. Starting with the more fanciful, "parabiosis" draws inspiration from experiments where a plasma transfusion from a young mouse rejuvenated an old mouse[18]. The mechanism is thought to be blood-borne factors reactivating gene expression, including the hormone insulin-like growth factor (IGF-1)[19]. Another avenue is the equivalent of a "factory reset" for cells, giving them the possibility to become pluripotent again, like the cells in a foetus, allowing them to develop into any type of cell that is in demand. However, this approach could come with the potential peril of the sorcerer's apprentice; the uncontrolled generation of an army of individual cells all doing the same thing or potentially different things.

The rejuvenation of cells could be a strategy for organ regeneration. For example, pluripotent cells might be able to transform into heart muscle cells to replace damaged heart tissue. This would certainly be preferable to a heart transplant, where the recipient must take powerful immunosuppressive drugs, if an available organ can be found. The downside is that to be most effective in restoring cardiac cell potential, these cells need to be primed by preparing with medication. Individuals at risk of suffering a cardiovascular event would have to be identified in order to do this cell priming, before the heart muscle is damaged.

However, the rate-limiting step in all these potential age-reversing interventions is the brain. It is not just a case of rejuvenating an organ. The brain holds the unique memories and personality of an individual. Successful ageing is not limited to preventing physical and physiological decline.

## What is successful ageing?

Successful ageing is characterised by adaptation. Ageing is not a disease; it is a natural physiological process. Ageing is as natural as growth and development at the start of life. Even if physical ability declines with senescence, research has found that the most content older people are those who put a higher value on well-being and social function than physical ability. In other words, the happiest old people accept a decline in physical function and adapt to this change[20].

Japan has a large elderly population with some of the healthiest, happiest old people. How do Japanese people age successfully? As defined at the beginning of this book, health is not just an absence of disease. Health is a positive sense in each of its physical, mental and social aspects. Accepting the physical limitations of old age and prioritising social health has been a successful strategy for old people in Japan[21].

Coming back a full circle, rather than focusing efforts on preventing ageing once it has already started, it is far more effective to start making anti-ageing interventions while you are still young, particularly modifiable lifestyle factors[22]. In the young there is more potential for anti-ageing strategies to have effect, rather than waiting for the arrival of Shakespeare's second childhood.

## Hormone stories: what happened next?

*Vivienne was a reasonably healthy 80-year-old retired language lecturer who woke up to find that she could not communicate. Words came out, but in a way that did not make sense.*

*On admission to the hospital, Vivienne received a CT of the head that showed a stroke on the left side of the brain. A lack of blood supply had caused neurons to die in that area of the brain where speech is controlled. Damage to the speech motor region, Broca's area, results in slurred speech, called dysarthria. This is often connected with control of swallowing called dysphagia. Damage to the adjacent speech* sensory region, Wernicke's area, causes problems with language expression: not being able to find the right words and meaning. As these speech areas are adjacent to each other, a stroke in this area of the brain often affects all aspects of speech.

Vivienne was left very frustrated and frightened. She had gone to bed as a fluent linguist and woken up unable to communicate. Cardiovascular disease occurs frequently in old people. In women the lack of oestrogen following menopause increases this risk. Happily, for Vivienne with patience, perseverance and speech therapy she regained her power of communication and boosted her confidence by doing challenging Latin translation from her grandson's textbooks! Future stroke prevention was addressed by controlling blood pressure with antihypertensive medication and starting lipid-lowering medication.

**Anthony** was the 82-year-old with a hip replacement who lost his balance in the bathroom. He continued to feel very unsteady and lost fluency of speech.

Anthony attended hospital and had a CT scan that revealed a small cerebellar stroke. The cerebellum is an area of the brain that controls movement. This is not a common area for a stroke to occur and produces characteristic symptoms including dizziness and loss of balance, jerky movement and issues with disjointed speech.

Anthony had been coming to see me for Pilates following his hip replacement. So, following his stroke we focused on balance and proprioception (awareness of where the body is in space). Initially this was sitting in a chair and then progressed to standing work. He gradually returned to his normal routine of going for a regular morning walk with his wife. After working with a speech therapist, he was able to recite some very tricky tongue twisters!

## Strategies to support your hormones in old age

### Sleep

- Sleep remains an important factor in aligning biochronometers in old age.
- Although advanced age can present challenges to good sleep patterns, pursuing good quality and quantity of night-time sleep reduces the risk of cardiometabolic and neurodegenerative disease.

### Nutrition

- Maintaining an intake of a variety of food groups is positive for health in advancing age.
- Attention to food preparation may be required, especially for those with varying degrees of dysphagia (difficulty swallowing).

- Intake of protein is a priority to mitigate sarcopenia.
- Year-round vitamin D supplementation is recommended. This is available in tablet, liquid and spray form.

## *Exercise*

- Physical activity remains as important as ever in supporting hormone health. This may be limited to moving limbs sitting in a chair. Nevertheless, this is valuable and preferable to total inactivity.

# Coda

> *"If we could give every individual the right amount of nourishment and exercise, not too little and not too much, we would have found the safest way to health."*
>
> *Hippocrates*

**Subtitle:** In essence Hippocrates was correct that our lifestyle behaviours determine our health. Now, over two thousand years later, we know why. Hormones are the vital link between all our modes of interaction with the external environment and our internal physical and mental health. Hormones set in motion our path towards personal optimal health so we can each attain our full potential.

Over two thousand years ago, Hippocrates was correct that the balance of our behaviours determines our health. However, he was not aware of what mediates this interaction between our lifestyle choices and genetic expression. That would have to wait another two thousand years until the description of hormones that "set in motion" our path to health. Hormones are the intermediaries and governors of the interplay between nature and nurture.

Although DNA contains the blueprint to life, these instructions remain inert and unread until they are brought to life by hormones. Hormonal messages enter the cell nucleus and determine gene expression, thereby controlling the selection and timing of protein production. Enzymes, the biological catalysts that regulate all the physiological processes of life, are built out of these of proteins.

Hormone networks are dynamic, adapting to changes in our lifestyles throughout life. To personalise health, each of us needs to understand how our own personal hormones operate. In the future, the advice offered in this book will be enhanced by artificial intelligence techniques that augment and individualise hormone intelligence.

Understanding the intricacies of the hormone players that determine our physical and mental health allows us to pursue the safest way to personal health and performance.

# References

## References Act 1, Scene 1 What is Health?

1. What is health? The ability to adapt. *The Lancet.* 2009; 373 (9666): 781. https://doi.org/10.1016/S0140-6736(09)60456-6. https://www.thelancet.com/journals/lancet/article/PIIS0140-6736(09)60456-6/fulltext
2. Machteld H, André K, Lawrence G et al. How should we define health? *BMJ.* 2011; 343: d4163. https://www.bmj.com/bmj/section-pdf/187291?path=/bmj/343/7817/Analysis.full.pdf
3. Ruth KS, Day FR, Hussain J et al. Genetic insights into biological mechanisms governing human ovarian ageing. *Nature.* 2021. https://doi.org/10.1038/s41586-021-03779-7
4. Bell J, Spector T. A twin approach to unravelling epigenetics. *Trends in Genetics.* 2011; 27 (3): 116–125. ISSN 0168-9525. https://doi.org/10.1016/j.tig.2010.12.005
5. Khoury M. Nobody is average but what to do about it? The challenge of individualized disease prevention based on genomics. Posted on July 2, 2014, Director, Office of Public Health Genomics, Centers for Disease Control and Prevention. https://blogs.cdc.gov/genomics/2014/07/02/nobody-is-average/?utm_content=buffer1ab48&utm_medium=social&utm_source=twitter.com&utm_campaign=buffer
6. Langenberg C, Sharp SJ, Franks PW, Scott RA, Deloukas P et al. Gene-lifestyle interaction and type 2 diabetes: the EPIC InterAct Case-CohortStudy. *PLoS Med.* 2014; 11 (5): e1001647. https://doi.org/10.1371/journal.pmed.1001647Academic

## References Act 2, Scene 2 Hormones 4 Health

1. Wass J, Owen K., eds. *Oxford Handbook Endocrinology and Diabetes.* Third Edition, 2014. Chapter 13 Diabetes. Oxford University Press.
2. Keay N, Bracken RM. Managing type 1 diabetes in the active population. *Br J Sports Med.* 2020; 54: 809–810.
3. Vasileiou, M., Thyroid disease assessment and management: summary of NICE guidance. *BMJ.* 2020; 368. https://doi.org/10.1136/bmj.m41 (Published 29 January 2020) Cite this as: BMJ 2020; 368: m41.
4. Keay N. Thyroid function in athletes and dancers. *Br J Sports Med.* 2020. https://blogs.bmj.com/bjsm/2020/03/12/thyroid-function-in-athletes-and-dancers/
5. Longobardi S, Keay N, Ehrnborg C et al. Growth Hormone (GH) effects on bone and collagen turnover in healthy adults and its potential as a marker of GH abuse in sports: a double blind, placebo-controlled study. *J Clin Endocrinol Metab.* 2000; 85 (4): 1505–1512. https://doi.org/10.1210/jcem.85.4.6551

# References Act 1, Scene 3 Harnessing Hormones

1. Warburton DE, Nicol CW, Bredin SS. Health benefits of physical activity: the evidence. *CMAJ.* 2006 Mar 14; 174 (6): 801–809. https://doi.org/10.1503/cmaj.051351. PMID: 16534088; PMCID: PMC1402378.
2. Safdar A, Tarnopolsky MA. Exosomes as mediators of the systemic adaptations to endurance exercise. *Cold Spring Harb Perspect Med.* 2018 Mar 1; 8 (3): a029827. https://doi.org/10.1101/cshperspect.a029827. PMID: 28490541; PMCID: PMC5830902.
3. Magliulo L, Bondi D, Pini N et al. The wonder exerkines—novel insights: a critical state-of-the-art review. *Mol Cell Biochem.* 2021. https://doi.org/10.1007/s11010-021-04264-5
4. Moore SC, Patel AV, Matthews CE et al. Leisure time physical activity of moderate to vigorous intensity and mortality: a large, pooled cohort analysis. *PLoS Med.* 2012; 9: e1001335. https://doi.org/10.1371/journal.pmed.1001335
5. Sturgiss E, Jay M, Campbell-Scherer D et al. Challenging assumptions in obesity research. BMJ 2017; 359. https://doi.org/10.1136/bmj.j5303
6. Xiong, Qin MD1, Hu, Xiang MD1, Xu, Yiting MD1, Zhang, Xueli MD1, Pan, Xiaoping BS1, Xiao, Yunfeng BS2, Ma, Xiaojing MD, PhD1, Bao, Yuqian MD1, Jia, Weiping MD, PhD1. Association of visceral fat area with the presence of depressive symptoms in Chinese postmenopausal women with normal glucose tolerance. *Menopause.* 2017; 24 (11): 1289–1294. https://doi.org/10.1097/GME.0000000000000917
7. Arhire L, Mihalache L, Covasa M. Irisin: a hope in understanding and managing obesity and metabolic syndrome. *Front. Endocrinol.* 2019. https://doi.org/10.3389/fendo.2019.00524
8. Massachusetts Hospital. The hormone irisin is found to confer benefits of exercise on cognitive function. https://www.massgeneral.org/news/press-release/The-hormone-irisin-is-found-to-confer-benefits-of-exercise-on-cognitive-function
9. Keay N. Body composition for health and sports performance. *Br J Sports Med.* blog 2017.
10. McCarthy, O, Pitt, JP, Keay, N et al. Passing on the exercise baton: what can endocrine patients learn from elite athletes? *Clin Endocrinol (Oxf).* 2022; 96: 781–792. https://doi.org/10.1111/cen.14683
11. Rynders C, Blanc S, DeJong N et al. Sedentary behaviour is a key determinant of metabolic inflexibility. *J Physiol.* 2018; 596: 1319–1330. https://doi.org/10.1113/JP273282
12. Dishman RK, McDowell CP, Herring MP. Customary physical activity and odds of depression: a systematic review and meta-analysis of 111 prospective cohort studies. *British Journal of Sports Medicine.* 2021; 55: 926–934.
13. All-Party Parliamentary Group on Arts, Health and Wellbeing Creative Health: The Arts for Health and Wellbeing. https://www.culturehealthandwellbeing.org.uk/appg-inquiry/
14. Beer N, Dimmock, J, Jackson B et al. Providing choice in exercise influences food intake at the subsequent meal. *Med Sci Sports Exerc.* 2017; 49 (10): 2110–2118. https://doi.org/10.1249/MSS.0000000000001330
15. McNally S, Nunan D, Dixon A, Maruthappu M, Butler K, Gray M et al. Focus on physical activity can help avoid unnecessary social care. *BMJ.* 2017; 359: j4609. https://doi.org/10.1136/bmj.j4609
16. Keay N. The role of pilates supporting sports performance. *Pilates Foundation Essay* 2016. https://nickykeayfitness.files.wordpress.com/2016/10/pilates-foundation-essay.pdf
17. Hesselink M, Schrauwen-Hinderling V, Schrauwen P. Skeletal muscle mitochondria as a target to prevent or treat type 2 diabetes mellitus. *Nat Rev Endocrinol.* 2016; 12: 633–645. https://doi.org/10.1038/nrendo.2016.104

# References

18. Nunes-Silva A, Freitas-Lima LC. The association between physical exercise and Reactive Oxygen Species (ROS) production. *J Sports Med Doping Stud*. 2015; 5: 152. https://doi.org/10.4172/2161-0673.1000152
19. Eat Well NHS guidelines accessed 2021. https://www.nhs.uk/live-well/eat-well/
20. Eat Well guide UK Government 2018. https://www.gov.uk/government/publications/the-eatwell-guide/the-eatwell-guide-how-to-use-in-promotional-material
21. Eckel RH, Grundy SM, Zimmet PZ. The metabolic syndrome. *Lancet*. 2005 Apr 16–22; 365 (9468): 1415–1428. https://doi.org/10.1016/S0140-6736(05)66378-7. PMID: 15836891.
22. British Association of Sport and Exercise Medicine. Health 4 Performance. Relative energy deficiency in sport (RED-S). http://health4performance.co.uk/
23. Slater J, McLay-Cooke R, Brown R, Black K. Female recreational exercisers at risk for low energy availability. *Int J Sport Nutr Exerc Metab*. 2016; 26 (5): 421–427. https://doi.org/10.1123/ijsnem.2015-0245
24. Aragon AA, Schoenfeld BJ, Wildman R et al. International society of sports nutrition position stand: diets and body composition. *J Int Soc Sports Nutr*. 2017; 14: 16. https://doi.org/10.1186/s12970-017-0174-y
25. Townsend,R, Elliott-Sale K, Currell K et al. The effect of postexercise carbohydrate and protein ingestion on bone metabolism. *Translational Journal of the ACSM*. 2017; 2 (20): 129–137. https://doi.org/10.1249/TJX.0000000000000045
26. Keay N. Sleep for health and sports performance. *Br J Sports Med*. 2017. https://blogs.bmj.com/bjsm/2017/02/07/sleep-health-sports-performance/
27. Watson N, Badr M, Belenky G et al. Recommended amount of sleep for a healthy adult: a joint consensus statement of the American Academy of Sleep Medicine and Sleep Research Society. *J Clin Sleep Med*. 2015; 11 (6): 591–592.
28. Paruthi S, Brooks LJ, D'Ambrosio C et al. Recommended amount of sleep for pediatric populations: a consensus statement of the American academy of sleep medicine. *J Clin Sleep Med*. 2016; 12 (6): 785–786. Published 2016 Jun 15. https://doi.org/10.5664/jcsm.5866
29. Keay N. Lifestyle Choices for optimising health: exercise, nutrition, sleep. *Br J Sports Med*, blog 2017. https://blogs.bmj.com/bjsm/2017/11/20/lifestyle-choices-optimising-health-exercise-nutrition-sleep/
30. Malhotra A, Redberg RF, Meier P. Saturated fat does not clog the arteries: coronary heart disease is a chronic inflammatory condition, the risk of which can be effectively reduced from healthy lifestyle interventions. *Br J Sports Med*. 2017; 51: 1111–1112.
31. Yu Wei, Cheng Ji-Dong. Uric acid and cardiovascular disease: an update from molecular mechanism to clinical perspective. *Frontiers in Pharmacology*. 2020; 11: 1607.
32. Burke L, Ross M, Garvican-Lewis L et al. Low carbohydrate, high fat diet impairs exercise economy and negates the performance benefit from intensified training in elite race walkers. *J Physiol*. 2017 May 1; 595 (9): 2785–2807. https://doi.org/10.1113/JP273230. Epub 2017 Feb 14. PMID: 28012184; PMCID: PMC5407976.
33. Zinn C, Wood M, Williden M et al. Ketogenic diet benefits body composition and well-being but not performance in a pilot case study of New Zealand endurance athletes. *J Int Soc Sports Nutr*. 2017 Jul 12; 14: 22. https://doi.org/10.1186/s12970-017-0180-0. PMID: 28706467; PMCID: PMC5506682.
34. Croteau E, Castellano CA, Fortier M et al. A cross-sectional comparison of brain glucose and ketone metabolism in cognitively healthy older adults, mild cognitive impairment and early Alzheimer's disease. *Exp Gerontol*. 2018 Jul 1; 107: 18–26. https://doi.org/10.1016/j.exger.2017.07.004. Epub 2017 Jul 12. PMID: 28709938.

35. Sabag A, Chnag D, Johnson N. Growth hormone as a potential mediator of aerobic exercise-induced reductions in visceral adipose tissue. *Front Physiol.* 2021. https://doi.org/10.3389/fphys.2021.623570
36. Keay N. Temporal considerations in Endocrine/Metabolic interactions Part 2. *Br J Sports Med.* 2017. https://blogs.bmj.com/bjsm/2017/10/03/temporal-considerations-endocrinemetabolic-interactions-part-2/
37. Harris M, Kuo C-H. Scientific challenges on theory of fat burning by exercise. *Front Physiol.* 2021. https://doi.org/10.3389/fphys.2021.685166
38. Keay N. One road to Rome: exercise. *Br J Sports Med.* 2017. https://blogs.bmj.com/bjsm/2017/08/24/one-road-rome-exercise/
39. D'Antona. Editorial: possible mechanisms to explain abdominal fat loss effect of exercise training other than fatty acid oxidation front. *Physiol.* 2021. https://doi.org/10.3389/fphys.2021.789463

# References Act 1 Scene 4 It's all in the Timing

1. The Nobel Prize in Physiology or Medicine 2017 Circadian biological clocks. https://www.nobelprize.org/prizes/medicine/2017/press-release/
2. Keay N. Temporal considerations in Endocrine/Metabolic interactions Part 1. *Br J Sports Med.* 2017. https://blogs.bmj.com/bjsm/2017/09/29/temporal-considerations-endocrinemetabolic-interactions-part-1/
3. Gamble K, Berry R, Frank S et al. Circadian clock control of endocrine factors. *Nat Rev Endocrinol.* 2014; 10: 466–475. https://doi.org/10.1038/nrendo.2014.78
4. Ikegami K, Refetoff S, Van Cauter E et al. Interconnection between circadian clocks and thyroid function. *Nat Rev Endocrinol.* 2019; 15: 590–600. https://doi.org/10.1038/s41574-019-0237-z
5. Keay N, Overseas A, Francis G. Indicators and correlates of low energy availability in male and female dancers. *BMJ Open Sport & Exercise Medicine.* 2020; 6: e000906. https://doi.org/10.1136/bmjsem-2020-000906
6. Caetano G, Bozinovic I, Dupont C et al. Impact of sleep on female and male reproductive functions: a systematic review. *Fertility and Sterility.* 2021; 115 (3). https://doi.org/10.1016/j.fertnstert.2020.08.1429
7. Mericq V, Martinez-Aguayo A, Uauy R et al. Long-term metabolic risk among children born premature or small for gestational age. *Nat Rev Endocrinol.* 2017; 13: 50–62. https://doi.org/10.1038/nrendo.2016.127
8. McCarthy O, Pitt J, Keay N et al. Passing on the exercise baton: what can endocrine patients learn from elite athletes? *Clinical Endocrinology.* 2022. https://doi.org/10.1111/cen.14683
9. Clarke D, Skiba P. Rationale and resources for teaching the mathematical modeling of athletic training and performance. *Adv Physiol Educ.* 2013; 37: 134–152. https://doi.org/10.1152/advan.00078.2011
10. Impey SG, Hearris MA, Hammond KM et al. Fuel for the work required: a theoretical framework for carbohydrate periodization and the glycogen threshold hypothesis. *Sports Med.* 2018; 48 (5): 1031–1048. https://doi.org/10.1007/s40279-018-0867-7. PMID: 29453741; PMCID: PMC5889771.
11. Burke L. Ketogenic low-CHO, high-fat diet: the future of elite endurance sport? *J. Physiol.* 2020. https://doi.org/10.1113/JP278928

## References

12. Nikbakhtian S, Reed A, Obika B et al. Accelerometer-derived sleep onset timing and cardiovascular disease incidence: a UK Biobank cohort study. *European Heart Journal - Digital Health*. 2021; ztab088. https://doi.org/10.1093/ehjdh/ztab088
13. Westerterp-Plantenga, M. Sleep, circadian rhythm and body weight: parallel developments. *Proc Nutr Soc*. 2016; 75 (4): 431–439. https://doi.org/10.1017/S0029665116000227
14. Keay N. Temporal considerations in endocrine/metabolic interactions Part 2. *Br J Sports Med*. 2017. https://blogs.bmj.com/bjsm/2017/10/03/temporal-considerations-endocrinemetabolic-interactions-part-2/
15. Ruddick-Collins L, Morgan P, Johnstine A. Mealtime: a circadian disruptor and determinant of energy balance? *Journal of Endocrinology*. 2020. https://doi.org/10.1111/jne.12886
16. Smith H, Betts J. Nutrient timing and metabolic regulation. *Journal of Physiology*. 2022 https://doi.org/10.1113/JP280756
17. Zouhal H, Saeidi A, Salhi A et al. Exercise training and fasting: current insights. *Open Access J Sports Med*. 2020; 11: 1–28. Published 2020 Jan 21. https://doi.org/10.2147/OAJSM.S224919
18. Townsend R, Elliott-Sale K, Currell K et al. The effect of postexercise carbohydrate and protein ingestion on bone metabolism. *Translational Journal of the ACSM*. 2017; 2 (20): 129–137. https://doi.org/10.1249/TJX.0000000000000045
19. Keay N. Internal biological clocks and sport performance. *Br J Sports Med*. 2017. https://blogs.bmj.com/bjsm/2017/10/17/internal-biological-clocks-sport-performance/
20. Frimpong E, Mograss M, Zvionow T, Dang-Vu TT. The effects of evening high-intensity exercise on sleep in healthy adults: a systematic review and meta-analysis. *Sleep Med Rev*. 2021; 60: 101535. https://doi.org/10.1016/j.smrv.2021.101535. Epub ahead of print. PMID: 34416428.
21. Arciero P, Ives S, Mohr A et al. Exercise reduces abdominal fat and blood pressure in women; Evening exercise increases muscular performance in women and lowers blood pressure in men. *Front Physiol*. 2022. https://doi.org/10.3389/fphys.2022.893783
22. Rynders C, Blanc S, DeJong N et al. Sedentary behaviour is a key determinant of metabolic inflexibility. *J Physiol*. 2018; 596: 1319–1330. https://doi.org/10.1113/JP273282
23. Keay N. Addiction to Exercise – what distinguishes a healthy level of commitment from exercise addiction? *Br J Sports Med*. 2017. https://blogs.bmj.com/bjsm/2017/08/03/addiction-exercise-distinguishes-healthy-level-commitment-exercise-addiction/
24. Thomas J, Kern P, Bush H et al. Circadian rhythm phase shifts caused by time exercise vary with phenotype. *JCI Insight*. 2020; 5 (3): e134270. https://doi.org/10.1172/jci.insight.134270
25. Jakubowicz D, Barnea M, Wainstein J, Froy O. Effects of caloric intake timing on insulin resistance and hyperandrogenism in lean women with polycystic ovary syndrome. *Clin Sci (Lond)*. 2013 Nov; 125 (9): 423–32. https://doi.org/10.1042/CS20130071. PMID: 23688334.
26. Leproult R, Van Cauter E. Effect of 1 week of sleep restriction on testosterone levels in young healthy men. *JAMA*. 2011; 305 (21): 2173–2174. https://doi.org/10.1001/jama.2011.710
27. Swanson C, Shea S, Kohrt W et al. Sleep restriction with circadian disruption negatively alter bone turnover markers in women. *The Journal of Clinical Endocrinology & Metabolism*. 2020; 105 (7): 2456–2463. https://doi.org/10.1210/clinem/dgaa232
28. Swanson C. Sleep disruptions and bone health: what do we know so far? *Curr Opin Endocrinol Diabetes Obes*. 2021; 28 (4): 348–353. https://doi.org/10.1097/MED.0000000000000639

29. Dorsey A, de Lecea L, Jennings KJ. Neurobiological and hormonal mechanisms regulating women's sleep. *Front Neurosci.* 2021 Jan 14; 14: 625397. https://doi.org/10.3389/fnins.2020.625397. PMID: 33519372; PMCID: PMC7840832. https://www.ncbi.nlm.nih.gov/pmc/articles/PMC7840832/
30. Bedrosian T, Nelson R. Timing of light exposure affects mood and brain circuits. *Transl Psychiatry.* 2017; 7: e1017. https://doi.org/10.1038/tp.2016.262

# References Act 1, Scene 5XY Of Mice and Men

1. Hirschberg A. Female hyperandrogenism and elite sport. *Endocrine Connections.* 2020, 9 (4): R81–R92.
2. De Ronde W, Pols H, Van Leeuwen J et al. The importance of oestrogens in males. *Clinical Endocrinology.* 2003; 58: 529–542.
3. Petak S, Nankin H, Spark R et al. American association of clinical endocrinologists. medical guidelines for clinical practice for the evaluation and treatment of hypogonadism in adult male patients—2002 update. *Endocrine Practice.* 2002; 8 (6): 439–456. ISSN 1530-891X, https://doi.org/10.4158/EP.8.6.439
4. Oxford Handbook of Endocrinology and Diabetes. Reproductive Endocrinology Chapter 4 Third Edition, Edited by Prof J. Wass.
5. Leproult R, Van Cauter E. Effect of 1 week of sleep restriction on testosterone levels in young healthy men. *JAMA.* 2011; 305 (21): 2173–2174. https://doi.org/10.1001/jama.2011.710
6. Metabolic Syndrome NHS. https://www.nhs.uk/conditions/metabolic-syndrome/ and https://patient.info/doctor/metabolic-syndrome
7. Rosario P, Davide M, Enrico R et al. Metabolic disorders and male hypogonadotropic hypogonadism. *Frontiers in Endocrinology.* 2019; 10: 345. https://www.frontiersin.org/article/10.3389/fendo.2019.00345, https://doi.org/10.3389/fendo.2019.00345 ISSN1664-2392
8. Keay N. Optimal Health including male athletes. *Br J Sports Med.* 2017. https://blogs.bmj.com/bjsm/2017/04/04/optimal-health-including-male-athletes-part-2-relative-energy-deficiency-sports/
9. Keay N. Update on relative energy deficiency in sports (RED-S). *Br J Sports Med.* 2018. https://blogs.bmj.com/bjsm/2018/05/30/2018-update-relative-energy-deficiency-in-sport-red-s/
10. Management of the Menopause. *British Menopause Society.* Sixth Edition
11. Bhasin S, Cunningham G, Hayes F et al. Testosterone therapy in men with androgen deficiency syndromes: an endocrine society clinical practice guideline. *The Journal of Clinical Endocrinology & Metabolism.* 2010; 95 (6): 2536–2559. https://doi.org/10.1210/jc.2009-2354
12. Vermeulen A. Androgen replacement therapy in the aging male—a critical evaluation. *The Journal of Clinical Endocrinology & Metabolism.* 2001; 86 (6): 2380–2390. https://doi.org/10.1210/jcem.86.6.7630
13. De Ronde W, Smit D. Anabolic androgenic steroid abuse in young males. *Endocrine Connections.* 2020; 9 (4): R102–R111.
14. Rasmussen J, Selmer C, Østergren P et al. Former abusers of anabolic androgenic steroids exhibit decreased testosterone levels and hypogonadal symptoms years after cessation: a case-control study. *PLoS ONE.* 2016; 11: e0161208. https://doi.org/10.1371/journal.pone.0161208

# References Act 1, Scene 5XX Of Mice, Men and Women

1. Soldin O, Chung S, Mattison D. Sex differences in drug disposition. *J Biomed Biotechnol.* 2011, Article ID 187103. https://doi.org/10.1155/2011/187103
2. Khamis R, Ammari T, Mikhail G. Gender differences in coronary heart disease. Education in Heart. Acute coronary syndromes. *BMJ Heart.* http://doi.org/10.1136/heartjnl-2014-306463
3. Sheel AW. Sex differences in the physiology of exercise: an integrative perspective. *Exp Physiol.* 2016; 101: 211–212.
4. Harrison CL, Hirschberg AL, Moholdt T. Editorial: exercise and sport: their influences on women's health across the lifespan. *Front Physiol.* 2021; 11: 615468. Published 2021 Jan 20. https://doi.org/10.3389/fphys.2020.615468
5. Costello JT, Bieuzen F, Bleakley CM. Where are all the female participants in Sports and Exercise Medicine research? *Eur J Sport Sci.* 2014; 14: 847–851.
6. Bruinvels G, Burden RJ, McGregor AJ et al. Sport, exercise and the menstrual cycle: where is the research? *Br J Sports Med.* 2017; 51: 487–488.
7. Wass J, Owen K. *Oxford handbook of endocrinology and diabetes.* Chapter 4 Third Edition. Oxford University Press.
8. de Ronde W, Pols Huibert AP, van Leeuwen Johannes PTM, de Jong Frank H. The importance of oestrogens in males. *Clin Endocrinol.* 2003; 58: 529–542.
9. Heikura IA, Uusitalo AL, Stellingwerff T, Bergland D, Mero AA, Burke LM. Low energy availability is difficult to assess but outcomes have large impact on bone injury rates in elite distance athletes. *Int J Sport Nutr Exerc Metab.* 2018; 28 (4): 403–411.
10. Royal Osteoporosis Society Causes of osteoporosis and broken bones. https://theros.org.uk/information-and-support/osteoporosis/causes/. Accessed 2021 Mar 21.
11. Li D, Hitchcock CL, Barr SI, Yu T, Prior JC. Negative spinal bone mineral density changes and subclinical ovulatory disturbances—prospective data in healthy premenopausal women with regular menstrual cycles. *Epidemiol Rev.* 2014; 36: 137–147.
12. Martin D, Timmins K, Cowie C et al. Injury incidence across the menstrual cycle in international footballers. In *Frontiers in Sports and Active Living 2021.* ISSN 2624-9367.
13. Novella S, Mompeon A, Hermenegildo. Mechanisms underlying the influence of oestrogen on cardiovascular physiology in women. *J Physiol.* 2019; 597 (19): 2873–4886.
14. Rickenlund, A, Eriksson, MJ, Schenck-Gustafsson, K., Lindén Hirschberg, A. Amenorrhea in female athletes is associated with endothelial dysfunction and unfavorable lipid profile. *J Clin Endocrinol Metab.* 2005; 90 (3): 1354–1359. https://doi.org/10.1210/jc.2004-1286
15. Prior J. Progesterone within ovulatory menstrual cycles needed for cardiovascular protection: an evidence-based hypothesis. *Journal of Restorative Medicine.* 2014; 3 (1). https://doi.org/10.14200/jrm.2014.3.0106
16. Baker L, Meldrum K, Wang M et al. The role of estrogen in cardiovascular disease. *J. Surg. Res., Research Review* 2003; 115 (2): 325–344. https://doi.org/10.1016/S0022-4804(03)00215-4
17. Rehbein E, Hornung J, Sundström Poromaa I, Derntl B. Shaping of the female human brain by sex hormones: a review. *Neuroendocrinology.* 2021; 111 (3): 183–206. https://doi.org/10.1159/000507083. Epub 2020 Mar 11. PMID: 32155633.
18. Barth C, Villringer A, Sacher J. Sex hormones affect neurotransmitters and shape the adult female brain during hormonal transition periods. *Front Neurosci.* 2015; 9: 37. https://doi.org/10.3389/fnins.2015.00037

19. Tornberg ÅB, Melin A, Koivula FM, Johansson A, Skouby S, Faber J, Sjödin A. Reduced neuromuscular performance in amenorrheic elite endurance athletes. *Med Sci Sports Exerc.* 2017; 49 (12): 2478–2485. https://doi.org/10.1249/MSS.0000000000001383. PMID: 28723842.
20. Dorsey A, de Lecea L, Jennings KJ. Neurobiological and hormonal mechanisms regulating women's sleep. *Front Neurosci.* 2021 Jan 14; 14: 625397. https://doi.org/10.3389/fnins.2020.625397. PMID: 33519372; PMCID: PMC7840832. https://www.ncbi.nlm.nih.gov/pmc/articles/PMC7840832/
21. Ioannis E. Messinis, Ovarian feedback, mechanism of action and possible clinical implications. *Human Reproduction Update.* 2006; 12 (5): 557–571. https://doi.org/10.1093/humupd/dml020
22. Prior JC. Ovulatory disturbances: they do matter. *Can J Diagn.* 1997; 14: 64–82.
23. Oosthuyse T, Bosch AN. The effect of the menstrual cycle on exercise metabolism: implications for exercise performance in eumenorrhoeic women. *Sports Med.* 2010 Mar 1; 40 (3): 207–227. https://doi.org/10.2165/11317090-000000000-00000. PMID: 20199120.
24. Isacco L, Duché P, Boisseau N. Influence of hormonal status on substrate utilization at rest and during exercise in the female population. *Sports Med.* 2012 Apr 1; 42 (4): 327–342. https://doi.org/10.2165/11598900-000000000-00000. PMID: 22380007.
25. Wohlgemuth K, Arieta L, Brewer G et al. Sex differences and considerations for female specific nutritional strategies: a narrative review. *J Int Soc Sports Nutr.* 2021; 18: 27. https://doi.org/10.1186/s12970-021-00422-8
26. Janse de Jonge XA. Effects of the menstrual cycle on exercise performance. *Sports Med.* 2003; 33 (11): 833–851. https://doi.org/10.2165/00007256-200333110-00004. PMID: 12959622.
27. Hulton A, Malone J, Campbell I et al. The effect of the menstrual cycle and hyperglycaemia on hormonal and metabolic responses during exercise. *Eur J Appl Physiol.* 2021. https://doi.org/10.1007/s00421-021-04754-w
28. National Institute of Clinical Excellence guidelines Premenstrual Syndrome. Revised May 2019. Accessed Mar 2021.
29. Rocha AL, Oliveira FR, Azevedo RC et al. Recent advances in the understanding and management of polycystic ovary syndrome. *F1000Res.* 2019; 8: F1000 Faculty Rev-565. Published 2019 Apr 26. https://doi.org/10.12688/f1000research.15318.1
30. Liu AY, Petit MA, Prior JC. Exercise and the hypothalamus: ovulatory adaptations. In Hackney A., Constantini N. (eds), *Endocrinology of Physical Activity and Sport. Contemporary Endocrinology.* Humana, Cham, 2020. https://doi.org/10.1007/978-3-030-33376-8_8
31. Bruinvels G, Goldsmith E, Blagrove R et al. Prevalence and frequency of menstrual cycle symptoms are associated with availability to train and compete: a study of 6812 exercising women recruited using the Strava exercise app. *Br J Sports Med.* 2020. https://doi.org/10.1136/bjsports-2020-102792
32. Findlay RJ, Macrae EHR, Whyte IY et al. How the menstrual cycle and menstruation affect sporting performance: experiences and perceptions of elite female rugby players. *Br J Sports Med.* 2020; 54: 1108–1113.
33. McNulty KL, Elliott-Sale KJ, Dolan E et al. The effects of menstrual cycle phase on exercise performance in eumenorrheic women: a systematic review and meta-analysis. *Sports Med.* 2020; 50: 1813–1827.
34. Grieger JA, Norman RJ. Menstrual cycle length and patterns in a global cohort of women using a mobile phone app: retrospective cohort study. *J Med Internet Res.* 2020 Jun 24; 22 (6): e17109. https://doi.org/10.2196/17109. PMID: 32442161; PMCID: PMC7381001.

35. Fehring R, Scheinder M, Raviele K. Variability in the phases of the menstrual cycle. *Clinical Research*. 2005; 35 (3): 376–384. https://doi.org/10.1111/j.1552-6909.2006.00051.x
36. Janse DE, Jonge X, Thompson B, Han A. Methodological recommendations for menstrual cycle research in sports and exercise. *Med Sci Sports Exerc*. 2019; 51 (12): 2610–2617. https://doi.org/10.1249/MSS.0000000000002073. PMID: 31246715.
37. Elliott-Sale K, Minahan C, de Jonge X et al. Methodological considerations for studies in sport and exercise science with women as participants: a working guide for standards of practice for research on women. *Sports Med*. 2021. https://doi.org/10.1007/s40279-021-01435-8
38. Keay N, Lanfear M, Francis G. Clinical application of interactive monitoring of indicators of health in professional dancers. *J Forensic Biomech*. 2021; 12 (5). No:1000380. https://doi.org/10.1101/2021.09.25.21263895
39. Management of the Menopause. Sixth Edition. British Menopause Society.
40. Ruth K, Day F, Hussain J et al. Genetic insights into biological mechanisms governing human ovarian ageing. *Nature*. 2021. https://doi.org/10.1038/s41586-021-03779-7
41. Zondervan KT. Genomic analysis identifies variants that can predict the timing of menopause. *Nature*. 2021;596(7872):345-346. doi: 10.1038/d41586-021-01710-8. PMID: 34349269.
42. Keay N. Hormone intelligence for female dancers, athletes and exercisers. *Br J Sports Med*. 2021. https://blogs.bmj.com/bjsm/2021/06/28/hormone-intelligence-for-female-dancers-athletes-and-exercisers/
43. Keay N. Fingerprinting hormones St John's College Cambridge 2021. https://johnian.joh.cam.ac.uk/news/fingerprinting-hormones/

# References Act 1 Scene 6 Hormone Supermodels

1. van der Schaar M, "Machine learning for individualised medicine", Chapter 10 of the 2018 Annual Report of the Chief Medical Officer. Health 2040 – Better Health Within Reach. Accessed 2021. https://assets.publishing.service.gov.uk/government/uploads/system/uploads/attachment_data/file/767549/Annual_report_of_the_Chief_Medical_Officer_2018_-_health_2040_-_better_health_within_reach.pdf#page=161
2. Revolutionising Healthcare Engagement Sessions for Clinicians. Presented by the van der Schaar Lab: machine learning and AI for medicine, Cambridge University. Accessed 2021. https://www.vanderschaar-lab.com/engagement-sessions/revolutionizing-healthcare/
3. Van de Schoot R, Depaoli S, King R et al. Bayesian statistics and modelling. *Nat Rev Methods Primers*. 2021; 1: 1. https://doi.org/10.1038/s43586-020-00001-2
4. Independent report by Artificial Intelligence Council UK Government January 2021. Accessed June 2021. https://www.gov.uk/government/groups/ai-council
5. Liu AY, Petit MA, Prior JC. Exercise and the hypothalamus: ovulatory adaptations. In Hackney A, Constantini N (eds), *Endocrinology of Physical Activity and Sport*. Contemporary Endocrinology. Humana, Cham, 2020. https://doi.org/10.1007/978-3-030-33376-8_8
6. Keay N, Lanfear M, Francis G. Clinical application of monitoring indicators of female dancer health, including application of artificial intelligence in female hormone networks. *Internal Journal of Sports Medicine and Rehabilitation*. 2022; 5: 24. https://doi.org/10.28933/ijsmr-2022-04-2205
7. Keay N, Craghill E, Francis G. Female football specific energy availability questionnaire and menstrual cycle hormone monitoring. *Sports Injr Med*. 2022; 6: 177. https://doi.org/10.29011/2576-9596.100177

8. Keay N. Hormone intelligence for female dancers, athletes and exercisers. *British Journal of Sport and Exercise Medicine*. June 2021. https://blogs.bmj.com/bjsm/2021/06/28/hormone-intelligence-for-female-dancers-athletes-and-exercisers/
9. Keay N, Francis G, Fingerprinting hormones. *St John's College, Cambridge University*. June 2021. https://johnian.joh.cam.ac.uk/news/fingerprinting-hormones/

# References Act 1, Scene 7 Bare Bones

1. Tucker K, Morita K, Qiao N et al. Colas, but not other carbonated beverages, are associated with low bone mineral density in older women: the Framingham Osteoporosis Study. *Am J Clin Nutr*. 2006 Oct; 84 (4): 936–42. https://doi.org/10.1093/ajcn/84.4.936. PMID: 17023723.
2. Ahn H, Park Y. Sugar-sweetened beverage consumption and bone health: a systematic review and meta-analysis. *Nutr J*. 2010; 20: 41. https://doi.org/10.1186/s12937-021-00698-1
3. Keay N, Francis G, Hind K. Bone health risk assessment in a clinical setting: an evaluation of a new screening tool for active populations. *MedRxiv*. 2019. https://doi.org/10.1101/2020.08.07.20170142
4. Santos L, Elliott-Sale KJ, Sale C. Exercise and bone health across the lifespan. *Biogerontology*. 2017; 18: 931–946. https://doi.org/10.1007/s10522-017-9732-6
5. Locatelli V, Bianchi V. Effect of GH/IGF-1 on bone metabolism and osteoporosis. *International Journal of Endocrinology*. 2014. https://doi.org/10.1155/2014/235060
6. Hernandez C, Beaupré G, Carter D. A theoretical analysis of the relative influences of peak BMD, age-related bone loss and menopause on the development of osteoporosis. *Osteoporos Int*. 2003; 14: 843–847. https://doi.org/10.1007/s00198-003-1454-8
7. Keay N. The modifiable factors affecting bone mineral accumulation in girls: the paradoxical effect of exercise on bone. *Nutr Bull*. 2000; 25: 219–222. https://doi.org/10.1046/j.1467-3010.2000.00051.x.
8. Keay N. Dancing through adolescence. *Editorial, British Journal of Sports Medicine*. September 1998; 32 (3): 196–197.
9. Keay N. Fogelman I, Blake G. Bone mineral density in professional female dancers. *Br J Sports Med*. 1997; 31: 1437. https://doi.org/10.1136/bjsm.31.2.143pmid:http://www.ncbi.nlm.nih.gov/pubmed/9192130
10. De Souza MJ, West S, Jamal S et al. The presence of both an energy deficiency and estrogen deficiency exacerbate alterations of bone metabolism in exercising women. *Bone*. 2008; 43 (1): 140–148. ISSN 8756-3282, https://doi.org/10.1016/j.bone.2008.03.013
11. Li D, Hitchcock C, Barr S et al. Negative spinal bone mineral density changes and subclinical ovulatory disturbances—prospective data in healthy premenopausal women with regular menstrual cycles. *Epidemiol Rev*. 2014; 36: 137–147.
12. Tenforde A, Parziale A, Popp K et al. Low bone mineral density in male athletes is associated with bone stress injuries at anatomic sites with greater trabecular composition. *Am J Sports Med*. 2017; 46 (3): 036354651773058. https://doi.org/10.1177/0363546517730584
13. Swanson, Christine M. Sleep disruptions and bone health: what do we know so far? *Curr Opin Endocrinol Diabetes Obes*. August 2021; 28 (4): 348–353. https://doi.org/10.1097/MED.0000000000000639
14. Management of the Menopause. *Chapter 11 Osteoporosis prevention and treatment*. British Menopause Society. Sixth Edition.

15. Hutson MJ, O'Donnell E, Brooke-Wavell K et al. Effects of low energy availability on bone health in endurance athletes and high-impact exercise as a potential countermeasure: a narrative review. *Sports Med.* 2021 Mar; 51 (3): 391–403. https://doi.org/10.1007/s40279-020-01396-4. PMID: 33346900; PMCID: PMC7900047.
16. Warden SJ, Edwards WB, Willy RW. Preventing bone stress injuries in runners with optimal workload. *Curr Osteoporos Rep.* 2021. https://doi.org/10.1007/s11914-021-00666-y
17. Keay N. Cyclists: make no bones about it. *Br J Sports Med.* 2018. https://blogs.bmj.com/bjsm/2018/02/27/cyclists-make-no-bones/
18. Wolman R, Clark P, McNally E, Harries M, Reeve J. Menstrual state and exercise as determinants of spinal trabecular bone density in female athletes. *BMJ.* 1990; 301: 516. https://doi.org/10.1136/bmj.301.6751.516
19. Keay N, Francis G, Hind K. Low energy availability assessed by a sport-specific questionnaire and clinical interview indicative of bone health, endocrine profile and cycling performance in competitive male cyclists. *BMJ Open Sport & Exercise Medicine.* 2018; 4: e000424. https://doi.org/10.1136/bmjsem-2018-000424
20. Keay N, Francis G, Entwistle I et al. Clinical evaluation of education relating to nutrition and skeletal loading in competitive male road cyclists at risk of relative energy deficiency in sports (RED-S): 6-month randomised controlled trial. *BMJ Open Sport & Exercise Medicine.* 2019; 5: e000523. https://doi.org/10.1136/ bmjsem-2019-000523
21. Francis G. Don't ride your bike like an astronaut Science4performance. https://science4performance.com/2019/04/05/dont-ride-your-bike-like-an-astronaut/
22. British Association of Sports and Exercise Medicine website Health4Performance.co.uk. http://health4performance.co.uk/healthcare-professionals/
23. Papageorgiou M, Dolan E, Elliott-Sale KJ et al. Reduced energy availability: implications for bone health in physically active populations. *Eur J Nutr.* 2018; 57, 847–859. https://doi.org/10.1007/s00394-017-1498-8
24. Keay N. Returning to sport/dance: restoring energy availability in RED-S. *Br J Sports Med.* 2019. https://blogs.bmj.com/bjsm/2019/03/26/returning-to-sport-dance-restoring-energy-availability-in-red-s/
25. Keay N. Synergistic interactions of steroid hormones. *Br J Sports Med.* 2018. https://blogs.bmj.com/bjsm/2018/09/11/synergistic-interactions-of-steroid-hormones/
26. Owens D, Allison R, Close G. Vitamin D and the athlete: current perspectives and new challenges. *Sports Med.* 2018; 48: 3–16. https://doi.org/10.1007/s40279-017-0841-9
27. Sonneville K, Gordon C, Kocher M et al. Vitamin D, Calcium, and dairy intakes and stress fractures among female adolescents. *Arch Pediatr Adolesc Med.* 2012; 166 (7): 595–600. https://doi.org/10.1001/archpediatrics.2012.5
28. Lappe J, Cullen D, Haynatzki G et al. Calcium and Vitamin D supplementation decreases incidence of stress fractures in female navy recruits. *J Bone Miner Res.* 2009; 23 (5): 741–749. https://doi.org/10.1359/jbmr.080102
29. Keay N. Surprisingly low levels of Vitamin D in cyclists. *Br J Sports Med.* 2018. https://blogs.bmj.com/bjsm/2018/11/28/surprisingly-low-levels-of-vitamin-d-in-cyclists/
30. Heikura I, Uusitalo A, Stellingwerff T et al. Low energy availability is difficult to assess but outcomes have large impact on bone injury rates in elite distance athletes. *Int J Sport Nutr Exerc Metab.* 2018; 28 (4): 403–411. https://journals.humankinetics.com/view/journals/ijsnem/28/4/article-p403.xml
31. Wolman R, Wyon M, Koutedakis Y et al. Vitamin D status in professional ballet dancers: winter vs. summer. *J Sci Med Sport.* 2013; 16 (5): 388–391. https://doi.org/10.1016/j.jsams.2012.12.010

32. Wyon M, Koutedakis Y, Wolman R et al. The influence of winter vitamin D supplementation on muscle function and injury occurrence in elite ballet dancers: a controlled study. *J Sci Med Sport*. 2014; 17 (1): 8–12. ISSN 1440-2440, https://doi.org/10.1016/j.jsams.2013.03.007
33. Martineau AR, Jolliffe DA, Hooper RL et al. Vitamin D supplementation to prevent acute respiratory tract infections: systematic review and meta-analysis of individual participant data. *BMJ*. 2017; 356: i6583. https://doi.org/10.1136/bmj.i6583
34. He CS, Handzlik M, Fraser WD et al. Influence of vitamin D status on respiratory infection incidence and immune function during 4 months of winter training in endurance sport athletes. *Exerc Immunol Rev*. 2013; 19: 86–101. PMID: 23977722.
35. Beck B, Daly R, Singh M, Taaffe D. Exercise and Sports Science Australia (ESSA) position statement on exercise prescription for the prevention and management of osteoporosis. *J Sci Med Sport*. 2017 May; 20 (5): 438–445. https://doi.org/10.1016/j.jsams.2016.10.001. Epub 2016 Oct 31. PMID: 27840033.
36. Royal osteoporosis society: strong, steady and straight an expert consensus statement on physical activity and exercise for osteoporosis. https://theros.org.uk/media/0o5h1l53/ros-strong-steady-straight-quick-guide-february-2019.pdf

# References Act 1, Scene 8 Mind the gut

1. Keay N, Overseas A, Francis G. Indicators and correlates of low energy availability in male and female dancers. *BMJ Open Sport & Exercise Medicine*. 2020; 6: e000906. https://doi.org/10.1136/bmjsem-2020-000906
2. De Souza MJ, Hontscharuk R, Olmsted M et al. Drive for thinness score is a proxy indicator of energy deficiency in exercising women. *Appetite*. 2007; 48 (3): 359–367. https://doi.org/10.1016/j.appet.2006.10.009. Epub 2006 Dec 20. PMID: 17184880.
3. Jurov I, Keay N, Hadžić V et al. Relationship between energy availability, energy conservation and cognitive restraint with performance measures in male endurance athletes. *J Int Soc Sports Nutr*. 2021; 18 (24). https://doi.org/10.1186/s12970-021-00419-3
4. Keay N. Addiction to Exercise – what distinguishes a healthy level of commitment from exercise addiction? *Br J Sports Med*. 2017. https://blogs.bmj.com/bjsm/2017/08/03/addiction-exercise-distinguishes-healthy-level-commitment-exercise-addiction/
5. Mountjoy M, Sundgot-Borgen JK, Burke LM et al. IOC consensus statement on relative energy deficiency in sport (RED-S): 2018 update. *Br J Sports Med*. 2018; 52: 687–697.
6. Laughlin G, Yen S. Hypoleptinemia in women athletes: absence of a diurnal rhythm with amenorrhea. *J Clin Endocrinol Metab*. 1997; 82 (1): 318–321. https://doi.org/10.1210/jcem.82.1.3840
7. Popovic V, Duntas LH. Leptin, TRH and ghrelin: influence on energy homeostasis at rest and during exercise. *Horm Metab Res*. 2005; 37 (9): 533–537. https://doi.org/10.1055/s-2005-870418. PMID: 16175489.
8. Van de Wielle R, Michels N. Longitudinal associations of leptin and adiponectin with heart rate variability in children. *Front Physiol*. 2017. https://doi.org/10.3389/fphys.2017.00498
9. Bresalier R, Chapkin R. Human microbiome in health and disease: the good, the bad, and the bugly. *Dig Dis Sci*. 2020; 65: 671–673. https://doi.org/10.1007/s10620-020-06059-y
10. Valdes AM, Walter J, Segal E, Spector TD. Role of the gut microbiota in nutrition and health. *BMJ*. 2018; 361: k2179. https://doi.org/10.1136/bmj.k2179

## References

11. Keay N. Inflammation: why and how much? *British Association of Sport and Exercise Medicine*. 2017. https://basem.co.uk/inflammation-why-and-how-much/
12. Thaiss C, Levy M, Korem T et al. Microbiota diurnal rhythmicity programs host transcriptome oscillations. *Cell*. 2016; 167 (6): 1495–1510
13. Hartstra A, Nieuwdorp M, Herrema H. Interplay between gut microbiota, its metabolites and human metabolism: dissecting cause from consequence. *Trends in Food Science & Technology*. 2016; 57: 233–243. ISSN 0924-2244, https://doi.org/10.1016/j.tifs.2016.08.009
14. Liu R, Hong J, Xu X et al. Gut microbiome and serum metabolome alterations in obesity and after weight-loss intervention. *Nat Med*. 2017; 23: 859–868. https://doi.org/10.1038/nm.4358
15. Al-Asmakh M, Anuar F, Zadjali F et al. Gut microbial communities modulating brain development and function. *Gut Microbes*. 2012; 3 (4): 366–373. https://doi.org/10.4161/gmic.21287
16. Goodpaster B, Sparks L. Metabolic flexibility in health and disease. *Cell Metabolism*. 2017; 25 (5): 1027–1036. doi:https://doi.org/10.1016/j.cmet.2017.04.015
17. Clark A, Mach N. The crosstalk between the gut microbiota and mitochondria during exercise. *Front Physiol*. 2017 May 19; 8: 319. https://doi.org/10.3389/fphys.2017.00319. PMID: 28579962; PMCID: PMC5437217.
18. Petersen LM, Bautista EJ, Nguyen H et al. Community characteristics of the gut microbiomes of competitive cyclists. *Microbiome*. 2017; 5: 98. https://doi.org/10.1186/s40168-017-0320-4
19. Keay N. Balance of recovery and adaptation for sport performance 2016. https://nickykeayfitness.com/2016/12/11/balance-of-recovery-and-adaptation-for-sport-performance/
20. Keay N. What has your gut microbiome ever done for you? *Nickykeayfitness* 2017. https://nickykeayfitness.com/2017/09/01/what-has-your-gut-microbiota-ever-done-for-you/
21. Purchiaroni F, Tortora A, Gabrielli M et al. The role of intestinal microbiota and the immune system. *Eur Rev Med Pharmacol Sci*. 2013; 17 (3): 323–333. PMID: 23426535.
22. Qinghui M, Jay K, Christopher R et al. Leaky gut as a danger signal for autoimmune diseases. *Front. Immunol*. 2017; 8: 598. https://www.frontiersin.org/article/10.3389/fimmu.2017.00598, https://doi.org/10.3389/fimmu.2017.00598
23. Quiroga R, Nistal E, Estébanez B et al. Exercise training modulates the gut microbiota profile and impairs inflammatory signaling pathways in obese children. *Exp Mol Med*. 2020; 52: 1048–1061. https://doi.org/10.1038/s12276-020-0459-0
24. Royal Society of Medicine. Endocrine division webinar on microbiome and endocrine dysfunction. 26–28 April 2022
25. Mihrshahi S, Ding D, Gale J et al. Vegetarian diet and all-cause mortality: evidence from a large population-based Australian cohort - the 45 and up study. *Prev Med*. 2017; 97: 1–7. https://doi.org/10.1016/j.ypmed.2016.12.044
26. Lim S, Kim E, Kim A et al. Nutritional factors affecting mental health. *Clinical Nutrition Research*. 2016; 5 (3): 143–152. https://doi.org/10.7762/cnr.2016.5.3.143
27. Keay N. Synergistic interactions of steroid hormones. *Br J Sports Med*. 2018. https://blogs.bmj.com/bjsm/2018/09/11/synergistic-interactions-of-steroid-hormones/
28. Suez J, Korem T, Zeevi D et al. Artificial sweeteners induce glucose intolerance by altering the gut microbiota. *Nature*. 2014; 514 (7521): 181–186. https://doi.org/10.1038/nature13793
29. Nutrition Society. Fuelling gut microbes Webinar April 2022.

30. Rodriguez-Daza M, Pulido-Mateos E, Lupien-Meilleur J et al. Polyphenol-mediated gut microbiota modulation: toward prebiotics and further. *Front Nutr.* 2021. https://doi.org/10.3389/fnut.2021.689456
31. Zmora N, Suez J, Elinav E. You are what you eat: diet, health and the gut microbiota. *Nat Rev Gastroenterol Hepatol.* 2019; 16: 35–56. https://doi.org/10.1038/s41575-018-0061-2

# References Act 1 Scene 9 A Balancing Act

1. Westerterp-Plantenga, M. Sleep, circadian rhythm and body weight: parallel developments. *Proc Nutr Soc.* 2016; 75 (4): 431–439. https://doi.org/10.1017/S0029665116000227
2. Pega F, Náfrádi B, Momen N et al. Global, regional, and national burdens of ischemic heart disease and stroke attributable to exposure to long working hours for 194 countries, 2000–2016: a systematic analysis from the WHO/ILO Joint Estimates of the Work-related Burden of Disease and Injury. *Environ Int.* 2021; 106595. ISSN 0160-4120, https://doi.org/10.1016/j.envint.2021.106595
3. Cornier M-C, Dabelea D, Hernandez T et al. The metabolic syndrome. *Endocrine Reviews.* 2008; 29 (7): 777–822. https://doi.org/10.1210/er.2008-0024
4. Hooper D, Snyder A, Hackney A. The endocrine system in overtraining. In Hackney A., Constantini N. (eds), *Endocrinology of Physical Activity and Sport 2020. Contemporary Endocrinology*. Humana, Cham. https://doi.org/10.1007/978-3-030-33376-8_27
5. Meeusen R, Duclos M, Foster C et al. Prevention, diagnosis and treatment of the overtraining syndrome: joint consensus statement of the European College of Sport Science (ECSS) and the American College of Sports Medicine (ACSM). *Eur J Sport Sci.* 2013; 13 (1): 1–24. https://doi.org/10.1080/17461391.2012.730061
6. Adlercreutz H, Harkonen M, Kuoppasalmi K et al. Effect of training on plasma anabolic and catabolic steroid hormones and their response during physical exercise. *Int. J. Sports Med.* 1986; 7 (SUPPL. 1): 27–28. https://doi.org/10.1055/s-2008-1025798
7. Banfi G, Dolci A. Free testosterone/cortisol ratio in soccer: usefulness of a categorization of values. *J Sports Med Phys Fitness.* 2006 Dec; 46 (4): 611–616. PMID: 17119528
8. Liu A, Petit M, Prior J et al. Global, regional, and national burdens of ischemic heart disease and stroke attributable to exposure to long working hours for 194 countries, 2000–2016: a systematic analysis from the WHO/ILO Joint Estimates of the Work-related Burden of Disease and Injury. *Environ Int.* 2021: 106595. ISSN 0160-4120, https://doi.org/10.1016/j.envint.2021.106595
9. Budgett R, Hiscock N, Arida RM, Castell LM. The effects of the 5-HT2C agonist m-chlorophenylpiperazine on elite athletes with unexplained underperformance syndrome (overtraining). *Br J Sports Med.* 2010 Mar; 44 (4): 280–283. https://doi.org/10.1136/bjsm.2008.046425
10. Smith LL. Tissue trauma: the underlying cause of overtraining syndrome? *J Strength Cond Res.* 2004; 1: 185–193. https://doi.org/10.1519/1533-4287(2004)018<0185:tttuco>2.0.co;2. PMID: 14971991.
11. Longobardi S., Keay N., Ehrnborg C et al. Growth Hormone (GH) effects on bone and collagen turnover in healthy adults and its potential as a marker of GH abuse in sports: a double blind, placebo-controlled study. *J Clin Endocrinol Metab.* 2020 85 (4): 1505–1512. https://doi.org/10.1210/jcem.85.4.6551
12. Meeusen R, Duclos M, Gleeson M et al. Prevention, diagnosis and treatment of the Overtraining Syndrome. *Eur J Sport Sci.* 2006; 6 (1): 1–14. https://doi.org/10.1080/17461390600617717

13. Armstrong LE, VanHeest JL. The unknown mechanism of the overtraining syndrome: clues from depression and psychoneuroimmunology. *Sports Med.* 2002; 32 (3): 185–209. https://doi.org/10.2165/00007256-200232030-00003. PMID: 11839081.
14. Gabbett TJ, Nassis GP, Oetter E et al. The athlete monitoring cycle: a practical guide to interpreting and applying training monitoring data. *Br J Sports Med.* 2017; 51: 1451–1452.
15. Lane AR, Duke JW, Hackney AC. Influence of dietary carbohydrate intake on the free testosterone: cortisol ratio responses to short-term intensive exercise training. *Eur J Appl Physiol.* 2010; 108 (6): 1125–1131. https://doi.org/10.1007/s00421-009-1220-5. Epub 2009 Dec 20. PMID: 20091182.
16. Schaal K, VanLoan MD, Hausswirth C, Casazza GA. Decreased energy availability during training overload is associated with non-functional overreaching and suppressed ovarian function in female runners. *Appl Physiol Nutr Metab.* 2021 Mar 2. https://doi.org/10.1139/apnm-2020-0880. Epub ahead of print. PMID: 33651630.
17. Keay N. Addiction to exercise – what distinguishes a healthy level of commitment from exercise addiction? *Br J Sports Med.* 2017. https://blogs.bmj.com/bjsm/2017/08/03/addiction-exercise-distinguishes-healthy-level-commitment-exercise-addiction/

# References Act 1 Scene 10 In the Red

1. Drinkwater BL, Nilson K, Chesnut CH et al. Bone mineral content of amenorrheic and eumenorrheic athletes. *N Engl J Med.* 1984; 311: 277–281. https://doi.org/10.1056/NEJM198408023110501
2. Otis CL, Drinkwater B, Johnson M, Loucks A, Wilmore J. American College of Sports Medicine position stand. The Female Athlete Triad. *Med. Sci. Sports Exerc.* 1997; 29 (5): i–ix. https://doi.org/10.1097/00005768-199705000-00037
3. De Souza MJ, Nattiv A, Joy E et al. 2014 Female Athlete Triad Coalition Consensus Statement on Treatment and Return to Play of the Female Athlete Triad: 1st international conference held in San Francisco, California, May 2012 and 2nd International Conference held in Indianapolis, Indiana, May 2013. *Br J Sports Med.* 2014; 48: 289.
4. De Souza MJ, Toombs R, Scheid J, O'Donnell E, WestS, Williams N. High prevalence of subtle and severe menstrual disturbances in exercising women: confirmation using daily hormone measures. *Hum Reprod.* 2010; 25: 491–503.
5. Mountjoy M, Sundgot-Borgen J, Burke L et al. The IOC consensus statement: beyond the Female Athlete Triad—Relative Energy Deficiency in Sport (RED-S). *Br J Sports Med.* 2014; 48: 491–497.
6. Mountjoy M, Sundgot-Borgen J, Burke, L et al. International Olympic Committee (IOC) Consensus Statement on Relative Energy Deficiency in Sport (RED-S): 2018 update. *Int J Sport Nutr Exerc Metab.* 28 (4): 316–331. Retrieved May 25, 2021, from http://journals.humankinetics.com/view/journals/ijsnem/28/4/article-p316.xml
7. Keay N, Francis G. Infographic. Energy availability: concept, control and consequences in relative energy deficiency in sport (RED-S). *Br J Sports Med.* 2019; 53: 1310–1311.
8. Loucks A, Thuma J. Luteinizing hormone pulsatility is disrupted at a threshold of energy availability in regularly menstruating women. *J Clin Endocrinol Metab.* 2003; 88 (1): 297–311. https://doi.org/10.1210/jc.2002-020369
9. Lanfranco F, Minetto MA. The male reproductive system, exercise, and training: endocrine adaptations. In Hackney A, Constantini N (eds), *Endocrinology of Physical Activity and Sport. Contemporary Endocrinology.* Humana, Cham, 2020. https://doi.org/10.1007/978-3-030-33376-8_7

## References

10. Laughlin GA, Yen SSC. Hypoleptinemia in women athletes: absence of a diurnal rhythm with amenorrhea. *J Clin Endocrinol Metab*. 1997; 82 (1): 318–321. https://doi.org/10.1210/jcem.82.1.3840
11. Loucks AB, Heath EM. Induction of low-T3 syndrome in exercising women occurs at a threshold of energy availability. *Am J Physiol Regul Integr Comp Physiol*. 1994; 266 (3): 35–3. https://doi.org/10.1152/ajpregu.1994.266.3.r817
12. Staal S, Sjödin A, Fahrenholtz I, Bonnesen K, Melin A. Low RMRratio as a surrogate marker for energy deficiency, the choice of predictive equation vital for correctly identifying male and female ballet dancers at risk. *Int J Sport Nutr Exerc Metab*. 2018; 28 (4): 412–418. Retrieved May 24, 2021, from http://journals.humankinetics.com/view/journals/ijsnem/28/4/article-p412.xml
13. Frisch RE, Gotz-Welbergen AV, McArthur JW et al. Delayed menarche and amenorrhea of college athletes in relation to age of onset of training. *JAMA*. 1981; 246 (14): 1559–1563. https://doi.org/10.1001/jama.1981.03320140047029
14. Thong F, McLean C, Graham T. Plasma leptin in female athletes: relationship with body fat, reproductive, nutritional, and endocrine factors. *J Appl Physiolo*. 2000; 88: 2037–2044. https://doi.org/10.1152/jappl.2000.88.6.2037
15. Jurov I, Keay N, Hadžić V et al. Relationship between energy availability, energy conservation and cognitive restraint with performance measures in male endurance athletes. *J Int Soc Sports Nutr*. 2021; 18: 24. https://doi.org/10.1186/s12970-021-00419-3
16. Williams N, Leidy H, Hill B et al. Magnitude of daily energy deficit predicts frequency but not severity of menstrual disturbances associated with exercise and caloric restriction. *Am J Physiol*. 2015; 308 (1): E29–39. https://doi.org/10.1152/ajpendo.00386.2013
17. Exercise and the hypothalamus: ovulatory adaptations. Lui A. In Hackney A, Constantini N (eds), *Endocrinology of Physical Activity and Sport. Contemporary Endocrinology*. Humana, Cham, 2020. https://doi.org/10.1007/978-3-030-33376-8_8
18. Cooper K, Ackerman K. Endocrine implications of relative energy deficiency in sport. In Hackney A, Constantini N (eds), *Endocrinology of Physical Activity and Sport. Contemporary Endocrinology*. Humana, Cham, 2020. https://doi.org/10.1007/978-3-030-33376-8_17
19. Areta JL, Taylor HL, Koehler K. Low energy availability: history, definition and evidence of its endocrine, metabolic and physiological effects in prospective studies in females and males. *Eur J Appl Physiol*. 2021 Springer Science and Business Media Deutschland GmbH. https://doi.org/10.1007/s00421-020-04516-0
20. Townsend R, Elliot-Sale K, Currell K et al. The effect of postexercise carbohydrate and protein ingestion on bone metabolism. *Med Sci Sports Exerc*. 2017; 49 (6): 1209–1218. https://doi.org/10.1249/MSS.0000000000001211
21. Ihle R, Loucks A. Dose-response relationships between energy availability and bone turnover in young exercising women. *J. Bone Miner. Res*. 2004; 19 (8): 1231–1240.
22. Heikura I, Uusitalo A, Stellingwerff T et al. Low energy availability is difficult to assess but outcomes have large impact on bone injury rates in elite distance athletes. *Int J Sport Nutr Exerc Metab*. 2018; 28 (4): 403–411. Retrieved May 28, 2021, from http://journals.humankinetics.com/view/journals/ijsnem/28/4/article-p403.xml
23. Keay N. The modifiable factors affecting bone mineral accumulation in girls: the paradoxical effect of exercise on bone. *Nutr Bull*. 2000; 25 (3): 219–222.
24. Ackerman K, Nazem T, Chapko D et al. Bone microarchitecture is impaired in adolescent amenorrhoeic athletes compared with eumenorrheic athletes and nonathletic controls. *J Clin Endocrinol Metab*. 2011; 96 (10): 3123–3133. https://doi.org/10.1210/jc.2011-1614

25. Ackerman K, Cano S, De Nardo M et al. Fractures in relation to menstrual status and bone parameters in young athletes. *Med Sci Sports Exerc*. 2015; 47 (8): 1577–1586. https://doi.org/10.1249/MSS.0000000000000574
26. O'Donnell E, Goodman J, Harvey P. Cardiovascular consequences of ovarian disruption: a focus on functional hypothalamic amenorrhea in physically active women. *J Clin Endocrinol Metab*. 2011; 96 (12): 3638–3648. https://doi.org/10.1210/jc.2011-1223
27. Torstveit M, Fahrenholtz I, Stenqvist T et al. Within-day energy deficiency and metabolic perturbation in male endurance athletes. *Int J Sport Nutr Exerc Metab*. 2018 Jul 1; 28 (4): 419–427. https://doi.org/10.1123/ijsnem.2017-0337. Epub 2018 Jun 26. PMID: 29405793.
28. Fahrenholtz I, Sjödin A, Benardot D et al. Within-day energy deficiency and reproductive function in female endurance athletes. *Scand J Med Sci Sports*. 2018; 28 (3): 1139–1146. https://doi.org/10.1111/sms.13030. Epub 2018 Feb 5. PMID: 29205517.
29. Keay N, Francis G, Hind K. Low energy availability assessed by a sport-specific questionnaire and clinical interview indicative of bone health, endocrine profile and cycling performance in competitive male cyclists. *BMJ Open Sport & Exercise Medicine*. 2018; 4: e000424. https://doi.org/10.1136/bmjsem-2018-000424
30. Russo I, Gatta P, Garnhan et al. Assessing overall exercise recovery processes using carbohydrate and carbohydrate-protein containing recovery beverages. *Front Physiol*. 2021. https://doi.org/10.3389/fphys.2021.628863
31. Deutz R, Benardot D, Martin D et al. Relationship between energy deficits and body composition in elite female gymnasts and runners. *Med Sci Sports Exerc*. 2000; 32 (3): 659–668. https://doi.org/10.1097/00005768-200003000-00017
32. Keay N, Overseas A, Francis G. Indicators and correlates of low energy availability in male and female dancers. *BMJ Open Sport & Exercise Medicine*. 2020; 6: e000906. https://doi.org/10.1136/bmjsem-2020-000906
33. Gibbs J, Williams N, Mallinson R et al. Effect of high dietary restraint on energy availability and menstrual status. *Med Sci Sports Exerc*. 2013; 45 (9): 1790–1797 https://doi.org/10.1249/MSS.0b013e3182910e11
34. De Souza MJ, Hontscharuk R, Olmsted M, Kerr G, Williams NI. Drive for thinness score is a proxy indicator of energy deficiency in exercising women. *Appetite*. 2007; 48 (3): 359–367. https://doi.org/10.1016/j.appet.2006.10.009. Epub 2006 Dec 20. PMID: 17184880.
35. Vescovi J, Scheid J, Hontscharuk R et al. Cognitive dietary restraint: impact on bone, menstrual and metabolic status in young women. *Physiol Behav*. 2008; 95 (1–2): 48–55. https://doi.org/10.1016/j.physbeh.2008.04.003. Epub 2008 Apr 11. PMID: 18508099.
36. Bedford J, Prior J, Barr S. A prospective exploration of cognitive dietary restraint, subclinical ovulatory disturbances, cortisol, and change in bone density over two years in healthy young women. *J Clin Endocrinol Metab*. 2010; 95 (7): 3291–3299. https://doi.org/10.1210/jc.2009-2497
37. Torstveit M, Fahrenholtz I, Lichtenstein M et al. Exercise dependence, eating disorder symptoms and biomarkers of Relative Energy Deficiency in Sports (RED-S) among male endurance athletes. *BMJ Open Sport & Exercise Medicine*. 2019; 5: e000439. https://doi.org/10.1136/bmjsem-2018-000439
38. Jurov I, Keay N, Hadžić V et al. Relationship between energy availability, energy conservation and cognitive restraint with performance measures in male endurance athletes. *J Int Soc Sports Nutr*. 2021; 18: 24. https://doi.org/10.1186/s12970-021-00419-3

# References

39. Vanheest J, Rodgers C, Mahoney C et al. Ovarian suppression impairs sport performance in junior elite female swimmers. *Med Sci Sports Exerc.* 2014; 46 (1): 156–166. https://doi.org/10.1249/MSS.0b013e3182a32b72. PMID: 23846160.
40. Tornberg Å, Melin A, Koivula F, Johansson A et al. Reduced neuromuscular performance in amenorrhoeic elite endurance athletes. *Med Sci Sports Exerc.* 2017; 49 (12): 2478–2485. PubMed ID: 28723842
41. Keay N, Francis G, Entwistle I et al. Clinical evaluation of education relating to nutrition and skeletal loading in competitive male road cyclists at risk of relative energy deficiency in sports (RED-S): 6-month randomised controlled trial. *BMJ Open Sport & Exercise Medicine.* 2019; 5: e000523. https://doi.org/10.1136/bmjsem-2019-000523
42. Keay N, Fogelman I, Blake G. Bone mineral density in professional female dancers. *Br J Sports Med.* 1997; 31: 143–147.
43. Burke L, Lundy B, Fahrenholtz, I, Melin A. Pitfalls of Conducting and Interpreting Estimates of Energy Availability in Free-Living Athletes. *Int J Sport Nutr Exerc Metab.* 2018; 28 (4): 350–363. Retrieved May 31, 2021, from http://journals.humankinetics.com/view/journals/ijsnem/28/4/article-p350.xml
44. Keay N. What are the challenges for female dancers? Female Athlete Conference 2021. Strategies for Health and Performance.
45. Melin A, Tornberg ÅB, Skouby S et al. The LEAF questionnaire: a screening tool for the identification of female athletes at risk for the female athlete triad. *Br J Sports Med.* 2014; 48: 540–545.
46. Wells K, Jeacocke N, Appaneal R et al. The Australian Institute of Sport (AIS) and National Eating Disorders Collaboration (NEDC) position statement on disordered eating in high performance sport. *Br J Sports Med.* 2020; 54: 1247–1258.
47. Stellingwerff T, Heikura IA, Meeusen R et al. Overtraining Syndrome (OTS) and Relative Energy Deficiency in Sport (RED-S): shared pathways, symptoms and complexities. *Sports Med.* 2021. https://doi.org/10.1007/s40279-021-01491-0
48. Plateau CR, Arcelus J, Meyer C. Detecting eating psychopathology in female athletes by asking about exercise: use of the compulsive exercise test. *Eur Eat Disord Rev.* 2017; 25: 618–624. https://doi.org/10.1002/erv.2561pmid:http://www.ncbi.nlm.nih.gov/pubmed/29057602
49. Stenqvist T, Torstveit M, Faber J, Melin A. Impact of a 4-Week Intensified Endurance Training Intervention on Markers of Relative Energy Deficiency in Sport (RED-S) and Performance Among Well-Trained Male Cyclists. *Front Endocrinol (Lausanne)* 2020; 11: 512365. https://doi.org/10.3389/fendo.2020.512365
50. Schaal K, VanLoan M, Hausswirth C, Casazza G. Decreased energy availability during training overload is associated with non-functional overreaching and suppressed ovarian function in female runners. *Appl Physiol Nutr Metab.* https://doi.org/10.1139/apnm-2020-0880
51. Mountjoy M, Sundgot-Borgen J, Burke L et al. The IOC relative energy deficiency in sport clinical assessment tool (RED-S CAT). *Br J Sports Med.* 2015; 49: 1354.
52. Berga S, Marcus M, Loucks T, Hlastala S, Ringham R, Krohn M. Recovery of ovarian activity in women with functional hypothalamic amenorrhea who were treated with cognitive behaviour therapy. *Fertil Steril.* 2003; 80: 976–981.
53. De Souza MJ, Mallinson R, Strock N et al. Randomised controlled trial of the effects of increased energy intake on menstrual recovery in exercising women with menstrual disturbances: the 'REFUEL' study. Human Reproduction 2021; deab149, https://doi.org/10.1093/humrep/deab149

54. Impey S et al. Fuel for the work required: a practical approach to amalgamating train-low paradigms for endurance athletes. *Physiological Reports*. 2019; e12803.
55. Keay N, Lanfear M. Insights into novel monitoring of dancer health and performance at Scottish Ballet. International Association of Dance Medicine and Science Conference 2021.
56. Keay N, Lanfear M, Francis G. Clinical application of interactive monitoring of indicators of health in professional dancers. *J Forensic Biomech*. 2021, 12 (5). No:1000380. https://doi.org/10.1101/2021.09.25.21263895
57. Keay N, Lanfear M, Francis G. Clinical application of monitoring indicators of female dancer health, including application of artificial intelligence in female hormone networks. *Internal Journal of Sports Medicine and Rehabilitation*, 2022; 5:24. DOI: 10.28933/ijsmr-2022-04-2205
58. Keay N. Thyroid function in athletes and dancers. *Br J Sports Med*. 2020. https://blogs.bmj.com/bjsm/2020/03/12/thyroid-function-in-athletes-and-dancers/
59. Gordon C, Ackerman K, Berga S et al. Functional hypothalamic amenorrhea: an endocrine society clinical practice guideline. *J Clin Endocrinol Metab*. 2017; 102 (5): 1413–1439. https://doi.org/10.1210/jc.2017-00131
60. Ackerman KE, Singhal V, Baskaran C et al. Oestrogen replacement improves bone mineral density in oligo-amenorrhoeic athletes: a randomised clinical trial. *Br J Sports Med*. 2019; 53: 229–236.
61. National Institute of Clinical Excellence (NICE) Clinical Knowledge Summaries (CKS). Accessed February 2022. cks.nice.org.uk/topics/amenorrhoea/management/secondary-amenorrhoea/#manging-oesteoporosis-risk
62. Kuikman M, Mountjoy M, Stellingwerff T et al. A review of nonpharmacological strategies in the treatment of relative energy deficiency in sport. *Int J Sport Nutr Exerc Metab*. 2021; 31 (3): 268–275. https://doi.org/10.1123/IJSNEM.2020-0211

# References Act 2 Scene 1 Infancy

1. Hoet J, Hanson M. Intrauterine nutrition: its importance during critical periods for cardiovascular and endocrine development. *J Physiol*. 1999; 514: 617–627.
2. Mericq V, Martinez-Aguayo A, Uauy R et al. Long-term metabolic risk among children born premature or small for gestational age. *Nat Rev Endocrinol*. 2017; 13: 50–62. https://doi.org/10.1038/nrendo.2016.127
3. Fleming T, Velazquez M, Eckert J et al. Nutrition of females during the peri-conceptional period and effects on foetal programming and health of offspring. *Animal Reproduction Science*. 2012; 130 (3–4): 193–197. https://doi.org/10.1016/j.anireprosci.2012.01.015
4. Godfrey K, Lillycrop K, Burdge G et al. Epigenetic mechanisms and the mismatch concept of the developmental origins of health and disease. *Pediatr Res*. 2007; 61: 5–10. https://doi.org/10.1203/pdr.0b013e318045bedb
5. West-Eberhard MJ. *Developmental Plasticity and Evolution*. Oxford University Press, New York, 2003.
6. Barker D, Osmond C. Infant mortality, childhood nutrition, and Ischaemic heart disease in England and Wales. *The Lancet*. 1986; 327 (8489): 1077–1081. https://doi.org/10.1016/S0140-6736(86)91340-1
7. Barker D J P. Fetal origins of coronary heart disease. *BMJ*. 1995; 311: 171. https://doi.org/10.1136/bmj.311.6998.171
8. Painter R, de Rooij S, Bossuyt P et al. Early onset of coronary artery disease after prenatal exposure to the Dutch famine. *The American Journal of Clinical Nutrition* 2006; 84 (2): 322–327. https://doi.org/10.1093/ajcn/84.2.322

9. Stanner S, Bulmer K, Andres C et al. Does malnutrition in utero determine diabetes and coronary heart disease in adulthood? Results from the Leningrad siege study, a cross sectional study. *BMJ*. 1997; 315: 1342–1349.
10. Barker D, Gluckman P, Harding J et al. Fetal nutrition and cardiovascular disease in adult life. *The Lancet*. 1993; 341 (8850): 938–941. https://doi.org/10.1016/0140-6736(93)91224-A
11. Hales CN, Barker DJP, The thrifty phenotype hypothesis: type 2 diabetes. *British Medical Bulletin* 2001; 60 (1): 5–20. https://doi.org/10.1093/bmb/60.1.5
12. Eriksson JG. The fetal origins hypothesis–10 years on. *BMJ*. 2005; 330 (7500): 1096–1097. https://doi.org/10.1136/bmj.330.7500.1096
13. Diabetes Mellitus. *Oxford Handbook of Endocrinology and Diabetes*. Third Edition. 2016 Edited by Professor John Wass.
14. Endocrinology in Pregnancy. *Oxford Handbook of Endocrinology and Diabetes*. Third Edition. 2016 Edited by Professor John Wass.
15. Persson I et al. Influence of perinatal factors on the onset of puberty in boys and girls: Implications for interpretation of link with risk of long term diseases. *Am. J. Epidemiol.* 1999; 150: 747–755.
16. Sloboda DM, Hart R, Doherty DA, Pennell CE, Hickey M. Age at menarche: influences of prenatal and postnatal growth. *J. Clin. Endocrinol. Metab.* 2007; 92: 46–50.
17. Rich-Edwards J, Kleinman K, Michels K et al. Longitudinal study of birth weight and adult body mass index in predicting risk of coronary heart disease and stroke in women. *BMJ*. 2005; 330: 1115https://doi.org/10.1136/bmj.38434.629630.E0
18. Gluckman PD, Hanson MA. *Mismatch; how our world no longer fits our bodies*. Oxford University Press, Oxford, 2006.
19. Gluckman PD, Hanson MA. The developmental origins of the metabolic syndrome. *Trends Endocrinol Metab*. 2004; 15: 183–187.

## References Act 2 Scene 2 Childhood

1. Weber DR, Leonard MB, Zemel BS. Body composition analysis in the pediatric population. *Pediatr Endocrinol Rev*. 2012; 10 (1): 130–139.
2. Paediatric Endocrinology. *Oxford Handbook of Diabetes and Endocrinology*. Third Edition. 2016 Edited Professor J. Wass.
3. Bergeron MF, Mountjoy M, Armstrong N et al. International Olympic Committee consensus statement on youth athletic development. *British Journal of Sports Medicine*. 2015; 49: 843–851.
4. Keay N. Mini-series part 2: young people: neuromuscular skills for sport performance. *British Journal of Sports Medicine*. 2017. https://blogs.bmj.com/bjsm/2017/07/24/young-people-neuromuscular-skills-sport-performance/
5. Keay N. Exercise and fitness in young people – what factors contribute to long term health? *British Journal of Sports Medicine*. 2017. https://blogs.bmj.com/bjsm/2017/07/14/exercise-fitness-young-people-factors-contribute-long-term-health/
6. James S, McLanahan S, Schneper L et al. Sleep duration and telomere length in children. *Journal of Pediatrics*. 2017; 187: P247–252.E1.
7. Paruthi S, Brooks LJ, D'Ambrosio C et al. Recommended amount of sleep for pediatric populations: a consensus statement of the American academy of sleep medicine. *J Clin Sleep Med*. 2016; 12 (6): 785–786. Published 2016 Jun 15. https://doi.org/10.5664/jcsm.5866

8. Westerterp-Plantenga M. Sleep, circadian rhythm and body weight: parallel developments. *Proceedings of the Nutrition Society.* 2016; 75 (4): 431–439. https://doi.org/10.1017/S0029665116000227
9. Nightingale CM, Rudnicka AR, Donin AS et al. Screen time is associated with adiposity and insulin resistance in children. *Archives of Disease in Childhood.* 2017; 102: 612–616. https://adc.bmj.com/content/102/7/612
10. Haapala E, Väistö J, Lintu N et al. Physical activity and sedentary time in relation to academic achievement in children. *Journal of Science and Medicine in Sport.* 2017; 20 (6): 583–589. https://doi.org/10.1016/j.jsams.2016.11.003
11. Haapala E, Lintu N, Eloranta A-M et al. Mediating effects of motor performance, cardiorespiratory fitness, physical activity, and sedentary behaviour on the associations of adiposity and other cardiometabolic risk factors with academic achievement in children. *Journal of Sports Sciences.* 2018; 36 (20): 2296–2303. https://doi.org/10.1080/02640414.2018.1449562
12. Isacco L, Duché P, Boisseau N. Influence of hormonal status on substrate utilization at rest and during exercise in the female population. *Sports Med.* 2012; 42 (4): 327–342. https://doi.org/10.2165/11598900-000000000-00000. PMID: 22380007.
13. Childhood obesity: A growing pandemic. *The Lancet Diabetes & Endocrinology.* 2022; 10 (1). ISSN 2213-8587. https://doi.org/10.1016/S2213-8587(21)00314-4
14. Hall K, Ayuketah A, Brychta R et al. Ultra-processed diets cause excess calorie intake and weight gain: an inpatient randomized controlled trial of ad libitum food intake. *Cell Metabolism.* 2019; 30 (1): 67–77.e3. ISSN 1550-4131. https://doi.org/10.1016/j.cmet.2019.05.008
15. Keay N. Synergistic Interactions of steroid hormones. *British Journal of Sports Medicine* 2018. https://blogs.bmj.com/bjsm/2018/09/11/synergistic-interactions-of-steroid-hormones/

# References Act 2, Scene 3 Teenager

1. *Oxford Handbook of Endocrinology and Diabetes.* Third edition. 2016 Edited by Professor J. Wass. Chapter 7, Paediatric Endocrinology. Oxford University Press.
2. Naulé L, Maione L, Kaiser U. Puberty, a sensitive window of hypothalamic development and plasticity. *Endocrinology.* 2021; 162 (1): bqaa209. https://doi.org/10.1210/endocr/bqaa209. PMID: 33175140; PMCID: PMC7733306.
3. Fechner P. The biology of puberty: new developments in sex differences. In C. Hayward (Ed.), *Gender Differences at Puberty 2003 Cambridge Studies on Child and Adolescent Health,* pp. 17–28. Cambridge: Cambridge University Press. https://doi.org/10.1017/CBO9780511489716.003
4. Frisch RE, Gotz-Welbergen AV, McArthur JW et al. Delayed menarche and amenorrhea of college athletes in relation to age of onset of training. *JAMA.* 1981; 246 (14): 1559–1563. https://doi.org/10.1001/jama.1981.03320140047029
5. Jenkins P, Taylor L, Keay N. Decreased serum leptin levels in female dancers are affected by menstrual status. Annual Meeting of the Endocrine Society. June 1998.
6. Ackerman K, Slusarz K, Guereca G et al. Higher ghrelin and lower leptin secretion are associated with lower LH secretion in young amenorrhoeic athletes compared with eumenorrheic athletes and controls. *American Journal of Physiology Endocrinology and Metabolism.* 2012; 302 (7): E800–E806.

## References

7. Keay N. What's so good about menstrual cycles? *British Journal of Sports and Exercise Medicine.* 2019. https://blogs.bmj.com/bjsm/2019/02/08/whats-so-good-about-menstrual-cycles/
8. Peper J, Brouwer R, Schnack H et al. Sex steroids and brain structure in pubertal boys and girls. *Psychoneuroendocrinology.* 2009; 34 (3): 332–342. https://doi.org/10.1016/j.psyneuen.2008.09.012
9. Piekarski DJ, Johnson CM, Boivin JR et al. Does puberty mark a transition in sensitive periods for plasticity in the associative neocortex? *Brain Res.* 2017; 1654 (Pt B): 123–144. https://doi.org/10.1016/j.brainres.2016.08.042
10. Minsky M. Why people think computers can't. *AI Magazine.* 1982; 3 (4): 3. https://doi.org/10.1609/aimag.v3i4.376
11. Laube C, van den Bos W, Fandakova Y. The relationship between pubertal hormones and brain plasticity: implications for cognitive training in adolescence. *Dev Cogn Neurosci.* 2020; Apr; 42: 100753. https://doi.org/10.1016/j.dcn.2020.100753
12. Keay N. Sleep for health and sports performance. *British Journal of Sports and Exercise Medicine.* 2017. https://blogs.bmj.com/bjsm/2017/02/07/sleep-health-sports-performance/
13. Westerterp-Plantenga M. Sleep, circadian rhythm and body weight: parallel developments. *Proceedings of the Nutrition Society.* 2016; 75 (4): 431–439. https://doi.org/10.1017/S0029665116000227
14. Hilton L, Loucks A. Low energy availability, not exercise stress, suppresses the diurnal rhythm of leptin in healthy young women. *American Journal of Physiology-Endocrinology and Metabolism.* 2000; 278 (1): E43–E49. https://doi.org/10.1152/ajpendo.2000.278.1.E43
15. Keay N. The modifiable factors affecting bone mineral accumulation in girls: the paradoxical effect of exercise on bone. *Nutr Bull.* 2000; 25: 219–222. https://doi.org/10.1046/j.1467-3010.2000.00051.x
16. Ackerman K, Cano Sokoloff N, DE Nardo Maffazioli G et al. Fractures in relation to menstrual status and bone parameters in young athletes. *Med Sci Sports Exerc.* 2015; 47 (8): 1577–1586. https://doi.org/10.1249/MSS.0000000000000574
17. Ackerman K, Nazem T, Chapko D et al. Bone microarchitecture is impaired in adolescent amenorrhoeic athletes compared with eumenorrheic athletes and nonathletic controls. *The Journal of Clinical Endocrinology & Metabolism.* 2011; 96 (10): 3123–3133. https://doi.org/10.1210/jc.2011-1614
18. Hernandez C, Beaupré G, Carter D. A theoretical analysis of the relative influences of peak BMD, age-related bone loss and menopause on the development of osteoporosis. *Osteoporosis Int.* 2003; 14: 843–847. https://doi.org/10.1007/s00198-003-1454-8
19. Keay N, Fogelman I. Blake G bone mineral density in professional female dancers. *British Journal of Sports Medicine.* 1997; 31: 143–147.
20. Keay N. Exercise and fitness in young people – what factors contribute to long term health? *British Journal of Sports and Exercise Medicine.* 2017. https://blogs.bmj.com/bjsm/2017/07/14/exercise-fitness-young-people-factors-contribute-long-term-health/
21. Keay N. Optimising Health, Fitness and Sports Performance for young people. *British Journal of Sports and Exercise Medicine.* 2017. https://blogs.bmj.com/bjsm/2017/06/30/optimising-health-fitness-sports-performance-young-people/
22. Keay N. Young people: neuromuscular skills for Sport Performance. *British Journal of Sports and Exercise Medicine.* 2017. https://blogs.bmj.com/bjsm/2017/07/24/young-people-neuromuscular-skills-sport-performance/
23. Professor Daniel Wolpert, Royal Society Ferrier Lecture 2021. How the brain controls the body.

24. Training as a high-performing female athlete – Team. Sport Ready Academy. Online course https://www.sportreadyacademy.com/p/training-as-a-high-performing-female-athlete1/?preview=logged_out
25. Training as a high-performing female athlete – Individual athlete. Sport Ready Academy. Online course https://www.sportreadyacademy.com/p/training-as-a-high-performing-female-athlete
26. Training as a high-performing female dancer – Team. Sport Ready Academy. Online course https://www.sportreadyacademy.com/p/training-as-a-high-performing-female-dancer-team?affcode=510837_zabxigc8
27. Training as a high-performing female dancer – Individual dancer. Sport Ready Academy. Online course https://www.sportreadyacademy.com/p/training-as-a-high-performing-female-dancer

# References Act 2 Scene 4 Young Person

1. Cornier M-C, Dabelea D, Hernandez T et al. The Metabolic syndrome. *Endocrine Reviews*. 2008; 29 (7): 777–822. https://doi.org/10.1210/er.2008-0024
2. McNulty K, Elliott-Sale K, Dolan E et al. The effects of menstrual cycle phase on exercise performance in Eumenorrheic women: a systematic review and meta-analysis. *Sports Med*. 2020; 50: 1813–1827.
3. Dasa M, Kristoffersen M, Ersvær E et al. The female menstrual cycles effect on strength and power parameters in high-level female team athletes. *Front. Physiol*. 2021; 12: 600668. https://doi.org/10.3389/fphys.2021.600668
4. Julian R, Skorski S, Hecksteden A et al. Menstrual cycle phase and elite female soccer match-play: influence on various physical performance outputs. *Science and Medicine in Football*. 2020. https://doi.org/10.1080/24733938.2020.1802057
5. Rael B, Alfaro-Magallanes VCM, Romero-Parra N et al. IronFEMME study group. Menstrual cycle phases influence on cardiorespiratory response to exercise in endurance-trained females. *Int. J. Environ. Res. Public Health*. 2021; 18: 860. https://doi.org/10.3390/ijerph18030860
6. Julian R, Sargent D. Periodisation: tailoring training based on the menstrual cycle may work in theory but can they be used in practice? *Science and Medicine in Football*. 2020; 4: 253–254. https://doi.org/10.1080/24733938.2020.1828615
7. Wohlgemuth K, Arieta L, Brewer G et al. Sex differences and considerations for female specific nutritional strategies: a narrative review. *J Int Soc Sports Nutr*. 2021; 18: 27. https://doi.org/10.1186/s12970-021-00422-8
8. Green L, O'Brien P, Panay N, Craig M. On behalf of the Royal College of obstetricians and gynaecologists. Management of premenstrual syndrome. *BJOG*. 2017; 124: e73–e105.
9. Endometriosis: diagnosis and management NICE guideline CKS. Updated 2020 https://cks.nice.org.uk/topics/endometriosis/
10. Harrison C, Hirschberg A, Moholdt T. Editorial: exercise and sport: their influences on women's health across the lifespan. *Front Physiol*. 2021; 11: 615468. https://doi.org/10.3389/fphys.2020.615468
11. Rotterdam ESHRE/ASRM-Sponsored PCOS Consensus Workshop Group: revised 2003 consensus on diagnostic criteria and long-term health risks related to polycystic ovary syndrome. Fertil Steril. 2004; 81 (1): 19–25.

12. Kristensen SL, Ramlau-Hansen CH, Ernst E, Olsen SF, Bonde JP, Vested A, Toft G. A very large proportion of young Danish women have polycystic ovaries: Is a revision of the Rotterdam criteria needed? *Human Reproduction*. 2010; 25 (12): 3117–3122. https://doi.org/10.1093/humrep/deq273
13. Rocha AL, Oliveira FR, Azevedo RC et al. Recent advances in the understanding and management of polycystic ovary syndrome. *F1000Res*. 2019; 8: F1000. https://doi.org/10.12688/f1000research.15318.1
14. Franks S. Diagnosis of Polycystic Ovarian Syndrome: in defense of the Rotterdam criteria. *The Journal of Clinical Endocrinology & Metabolism*. 2006; 91 (3): 786–789. https://doi.org/10.1210/jc.2005-2501
15. Patten R, Boyle A, Moholdt T et al. Exercise interventions in polycystic ovary syndrome: a systematic review and meta-analysis. *Frontiers in Physiology*. 2020; 11: 606. https://www.frontiersin.org/article/10.3389/fphys.2020.00606; https://doi.org/10.3389/fphys.2020.00606
16. International evidence-based guideline for the assessment and management of polycystic ovary syndrome 2018. Copyright Monash University, Melbourne Australia 2018. Accessed June 2021.
17. Your Contraception Guide National Health Service. Accessed February 27 2021.
18. Behre H, Zitzmann M, Anderson R et al. Efficacy and safety of an injectable combination hormonal contraceptive for men. *The Journal of Clinical Endocrinology & Metabolism*. 2016; 101 (12): 14779–14788. https://doi.org/10.1210/jc.2016-2141
19. US Food and Drug Administration "black box warning". https://www.accessdata.fda.gov/drugsatfda_docs/label/2004/20246s025lbl.pdf
20. Meier C, Brauchli Y, Jick S et al. Use of depot medroxyprogesterone acetate and fracture risk. *The Journal of Clinical Endocrinology & Metabolism*. 2010; 95 (11): 4909–4916. https://doi.org/10.1210/jc.2010-0032
21. Contraceptives, hormonal National Institute of Clinical Excellence guidelines accessed March 6, 2021. https://cks.nice.org.uk/topics/contraception-assessment/management/assessment-for-contraception/
22. Beksinska M, Smit J. Hormonal contraception and bone mineral density. *Expert Review of Obstetrics & Gynecology*. 2011; 6 (3): 305–319. https://doi.org/10.1586/eog.11.19
23. Gordon C, Ackerman K, Berga S et al. Functional hypothalamic amenorrhea: an endocrine society clinical practice guideline. *Journal of Clinical Endocrinology and Metabolism*. 2017 102 (5): 1413–1439. https://doi.org/10.1210/jc.2017-00131
24. National Institute of Clinical Excellence (NICE) Clinical Knowledge Summaries (CKS) Accessed February 2022 cks.nice.org.uk/topics/amenorrhoea/management/secondary-amenorrhoea/#manging-oesteoporosis-risk
25. Cheng J, Santiago A, Kristen A. Menstrual irregularity, hormonal contraceptive use, and bone stress injuries in collegiate female athletes in the United States. *American Academy of Physical Medicine and Rehabilitation*. 2020. https://doi.org/10.1002/pmrj.12539
26. Myllyaho M, Ihalainen J, Hackney A et al. Hormonal contraceptive use does not affect strength, endurance, or body composition adaptations to combined strength and endurance training in women. *J Strength Cond Res*. 2021; 35 (2): 449–457. https://doi.org/10.1519/JSC.0000000000002713. PMID: 29927884. https://pubmed.ncbi.nlm.nih.gov/29927884/
27. Larsen B, Cox A. Coley inflammation and oral contraceptive use in female athletes before the Rio Olympic games front. *Physiol*. 2020. https://doi.org/10.3389/fphys.2020.00497

28. One Dance UK. Pregnancy and the dancer information sheet 19. https://www.onedanceuk.org/wp-content/uploads/2017/11/DUK-Info-Sheet-19-Pregnancy-information-for-dancers.pdf
29. Keay N. The role of Pilates in Sports Performance. *Pilates Foundation Essay.* https://nickykeayfitness.files.wordpress.com/2016/10/pilates-foundation-essay.pdf
30. Keeping well in pregnancy NHS guide. https://www.nhs.uk/pregnancy/keeping-well/

# References Act 2 Scene 5 Middle Age

1. Copeland JL. Exercise in Older Adults: The Effect of Age on Exercise Endocrinology. *Endocrinology of Physical Activity and Sport.* Third Edition. 2020 Edited by Hackney A, Constantini N. Humana Press.
2. National Institute of Clinical Excellence. *Menopause: Diagnosis and Management Update 2019.* Accessed March 2021.
3. Royal College of Obstetricians and Gynaecologists. *Treatment for symptoms of the menopause.* RCOG, 2018.
4. Janice Rymer, Kate Brian, Lesley Regan. HRT and breast cancer risk. Editorial. *BMJ* 2019; 367: l5928 doi: 10.1136/bmj.l5928 (Published 11 October 2019).
5. Gordon C, Ackerman K, Berga S et al. Functional hypothalamic amenorrhea: An endocrine society clinical practice guideline. *Journal of Clinical Endocrinology and Metabolism.* 2017; 102 (5): 1413–1439.
6. NICE guidelines https://cks.nice.org.uk/topics/amenorrhoea/management/secondary-amenorrhoea/#managing-osteoporosis-risk
7. Shapiro S, Farmer RDT, Mueck AO, et al. Does hormone replacement therapy cause breast cancer? An application of causal principles to three studies. *BMJ Sexual & Reproductive Health.* 2011; 37: 165–172.
8. Understanding the risk of breast cancer. Women's Health Concern, British Menopause Society. https://thebms.org.uk/wp-content/uploads/2016/04/WHC-UnderstandingRisksofBreastCancer-MARCH2017.pdf
9. British Menopause Society & Women's Health Concern 2020 recommendations on hormone replacement therapy in menopausal women. https://thebms.org.uk/publications/consensus-statements/bms-whcs-2020-recommendations-on-hormone-replacement-therapy-in-menopausal-women/ Accessed April 2021.
10. European Society of Human Reproduction and Embryology. Guideline on the management of premature ovarian insufficiency. 2015. https://www.eshre.eu/Guidelines-and-Legal/Guidelines/Management-of-premature-ovarian-insufficiency.aspx Accessed May 2021
11. Testosterone replacement in menopause British Menopause Society Guidelines Accessed May 2022 https://thebms.org.uk/publications/tools-for-clinicians/testosterone-replacement-in-menopause/
12. Bhasin S, Brito JP, Cunningham GR et al. Testosterone therapy in men with hypogonadism: An endocrine society clinical practice guideline. *J Clin Endocrinol Metab.* 2018; 103 (5): 1715–1744. doi: 10.1210/jc.2018-00229. PMID: 29562364.
13. Keay N, Francis G, Entwistle I, et al Clinical evaluation of education relating to nutrition and skeletal loading in competitive male road cyclists at risk of relative energy deficiency in sports (RED-S): 6-month randomised controlled trial. *BMJ Open Sport & Exercise Medicine.* 2019; 5: e000523. doi: 10.1136/bmjsem-2019-000523

14. Hameed M, Harridge S, Goldspink G. Sarcopenia and Hypertrophy: A Role for Insulin-Like Growth Factor-1 in Aged Muscle? *Exercise and Sport Sciences Reviews*. 2002; 30 (1): 15–19.
15. Traylor DA, Gorissen SHM, Phillips SM. Perspective: Protein requirements and optimal intakes in aging: Are we ready to recommend more than the recommended daily allowance? *Adv Nutr*. 2018; 9 (3): 171–182. doi:10.1093/advances/nmy003
16. Trommelen J, van Loon LJ. Pre-sleep protein ingestion to improve the skeletal muscle adaptive response to exercise training. *Nutrients*. 2016; 8 (12): 763. doi:10.3390/nu8120763
17. Cornier M-C, Dabelea D, Hernandez T et al. The metabolic syndrome. *Endocrine Reviews*. 1 December 2008; 29 (7): 777–822. https://doi.org/10.1210/er.2008-0024
18. Mandrup C, Roland C, Egelund Jon et al. Effects of high-intensity exercise training on adipose tissue mass, glucose uptake and protein content in pre- and post-menopausal women. *Frontiers in Sports and Active Living*. 2020; (2): 60. https://www.frontiersin.org/article/10.3389/fspor.2020.00060 DOI 10.3389/fspor.2020.00060
19. Lucassen EA, de Mutsert R, le Cessie S, Appelman-Dijkstra NM, Rosendaal FR, van Heemst D, et al. Poor sleep quality and later sleep timing are risk factors for osteopenia and sarcopenia in middle-aged men and women: The NEO study. *PLoS ONE*. 2017; 12 (5): e0176685. https://doi.org/10.1371/journal.pone.0176685
20. Marc-Andre Cornier, Dana Dabelea, Teri L. Hernandez, Rachel C. Lindstrom, Amy J. Steig, Nicole R. Stob, Rachael E. Van Pelt, Hong Wang, Robert H. Eckel, The metabolic syndrome. *Endocrine Reviews*. 2008; 29 (7): 777–822. https://doi.org/10.1210/er.2008-0024
21. Corona G, Goulis DG, Huhtaniemi I, Zitzmann M, Toppari J, Forti G, Vanderschueren D, Wu FC. European Academy of Andrology (EAA) guidelines on investigation, treatment and monitoring of functional hypogonadism in males: endorsing organization: European Society of Endocrinology. *Andrology*. 2020; (5): 970–987. https://doi.org/10.1111/andr.12770. Epub 2020 Mar 20. PMID: 32026626.

# References Act 2 Scene 6 Old age

1. Isacco L, Duché P, Boisseau N. Influence of hormonal status on substrate utilization at rest and during exercise in the female population. *Sports Med*. 2012; 42 (4): 327–342. https://doi.org/10.2165/11598900-000000000-00000. PMID: 22380007.
2. Scott JM, Downs M, Buxton R et al. Disuse-induced muscle loss and rehabilitation: the National Aeronautics and Space Administration Bed Rest Study. *Crit Care Explor*. 2020; 2 (12): e0269. Published 2020 Nov 24. https://doi.org/10.1097/CCE.0000000000000269
3. Royal Society of Medicine conference on Biology of Ageing 21/4/22. https://www.rsm.ac.uk/
4. Volpi E, Nazemi R, Fujita S. Muscle tissue changes with aging. *Curr Opin Clin Nutr Metab Care*. 2004; 7 (4): 405–410. https://doi.org/10.1097/01.mco.0000134362.76653.b2
5. Goldspink G, Harridge S. Growth factors and muscle ageing. *Experimental Gerontology*. 2004; 39 (10): 1433–1438. ISSN 0531-5565. https://doi.org/10.1016/j.exger.2004.08.010
6. Fiatarone-Singh M, Ding, Manfredi W, Solares T et al. Insulin-like growth factor 1 in skeletal muscle after weightlifting exercises in frail elders. *Am. J. Physiol*. 1999; 277 (Endocrinol. Metab. 40): E135–E143.

# References

7. Verdijk L, Snijders T, Holloway TM et al. Resistance training increases skeletal muscle capillarization in healthy older men. *Med Sci Sports Exerc.* 2016; 48 (11): 2157–2164. https://doi.org/10.1249/MSS.0000000000001019. PMID: 27327032.
8. Royal Osteoporosis Society. https://theros.org.uk/information-and-support/ Accessed April 2022.
9. Kanis JA, Johnell O, Oden A et al. FRAX™ and the assessment of fracture probability in men and women from the UK. *Osteoporosis Int.* 2008; 19: 385–397. https://doi.org/10.1007/s00198-007-0543-5
10. Watson S, Weeks B, Weis L et al. High-intensity resistance and impact training improves bone mineral density and physical function in postmenopausal women with osteopenia and osteoporosis: the LIFTMOR randomized controlled trial. *JBMR.* 2018; 33 (2): 211–220. https://doi.org/10.1002/jbmr.3284
11. Sinaki M, Itoi E, Wahner H et al. Stronger back muscles reduce the incidence of vertebral fractures: A prospective 10-year follow-up of postmenopausal women. *Bone.* 2002; 30 (6): 836–841. https://doi.org/10.1016/S8756-3282(02)00739-1
12. Calleja-Agius J, Brincat M. Menopause-related changes in the musculoskeletal system, cartilages and joints. In Genazzani AR, Brincat M (eds.), *Frontiers in Gynecological Endocrinology.* 2014. ISGE Series. Springer, Cham. https://doi.org/10.1007/978-3-319-03494-2_19
13. Kramer I, Snijders T, Smeets J et al. Extensive type II muscle fiber atrophy in elderly female hip fracture patients. *The Journals of Gerontology.* 2017; Series A, 72 (10): 1369–1375. https://doi.org/10.1093/gerona/glw253
14. Close JCT, Lord SR. Fall assessment in older people. *BMJ.* 2011; 343: d5153. https://doi.org/10.1136/bmj.d5153
15. Management of the Menopause. *Chapter 11 Osteoporosis prevention and management Sixth Edition.* British Menopause Society 2017.
16. Compston J, Cooper A, Cooper C et al. The National Osteoporosis Guideline Group (NOGG). UK clinical guideline for the prevention and treatment of osteoporosis. *Arch Osteoporos.* 2017; 12: 43. https://doi.org/10.1007/s11657-017-0324-5
17. Marc-Andre Cornier, Dana Dabelea, Teri L. Hernandez et al. The metabolic syndrome. *Endocrine Reviews.* 2008; 29 (7): 777–822. https://doi.org/10.1210/er.2008-0024
18. Bermingham K, Linenberg I, Hall W et al. Menopause is associated with postprandial metabolism, metabolic health and lifestyle: the ZOE PREDICT study. *Preprint Lancet.* Available at SSRN: https://ssrn.com/abstract 4051462; http://dx.doi.org/10.2139/ssrn.4051462
19. British Menopause Society meeting. Hot topics in menopause care. May 2022. https://thebms.org.uk/
20. Rymer J, Brian K, Regan L. HRT and breast cancer risk. *Editorial BMJ.* 2019; 367: l5928. https://doi.org/10.1136/bmj.l5928
21. *Management of Menopause.* Sixth Edition. British Menopause Society, 2017.
22. *Public hospital spending in England: evidence from National Health Service administrative records.* Institute of Fiscal Studies 2015.
23. National Institute of Clinical Excellence. *Menopause: Diagnosis and Management.* Update 2019. Accessed March 2021. https://www.nice.org.uk/guidance/ng23/chapter/Recommendations
24. Vermeulen A. Androgen replacement therapy in the aging male—A critical evaluation. *The Journal of Clinical Endocrinology & Metabolism.* 2001; 86 (6): 2380–2390. https://doi.org/10.1210/jcem.86.6.7630

25. Bailey T, Cable T, Aziz N et al. Exercise training reduces the acute physiological severity of post-menopausal hot flushes. *Journal of Physiology*. 2016; 594 (3): 657–667. https://doi.org/10.1113/JP271456
26. Mandrup C, Roland C, Egelund J et al. Effects of high-intensity exercise training on adipose tissue mass, glucose uptake and protein content in pre- and post-menopausal women. *Frontiers in Sports and Active Living*. 2020 (2): 60. https://www.frontiersin.org/article/10.3389/fspor.2020.00060; https://doi.org/10.3389/fspor.2020.00060
27. Royal Osteoporosis Society. Strong, Straight, Steady. https://theros.org.uk/media/0o5h1l53/ros-strong-steady-straight-quick-guide-february-2019.pdf. Accessed March 21, 2021.
28. Traylor DA, Gorissen SHM, Phillips SM. Perspective: protein requirements and optimal intakes in aging: are we ready to recommend more than the recommended daily allowance? *Adv Nutr*. 2018; 9 (3): 171–182. https://doi.org/10.1093/advances/nmy003
29. Royal Osteoporosis Society. Vitamin D and Bone Health. https://strwebprdmedia.blob.core.windows.net/media/ef2ideu2/ros-vitamin-d-and-bone-health-in-adults-february-2020.pdf. Accessed June 2021.
30. Sleep Foundation. Ageing and Sleep. https://www.sleepfoundation.org/aging-and-sleep. Accessed April 2022.

# References Act 2 Scene 7 Dotage

1. *Management of Menopause*. Sixth Edition. British Menopause Society.
2. The Fountain of Youth. Economist podcast, March 15, 2022. https://overcast.fm/+JXrSh_yEo
3. Life Expectancy and Healthy Life Expectancy. *The Global Heath Observatory*. World Health Organisation. Accessed April 2022.
4. Rowe WJ. Correcting magnesium deficiencies may prolong life. *Clin Interv Aging*. 2012; 7: 51–54. https://doi.org/10.2147/CIA.S28768. Epub 2012 Feb 16. PMID: 22379366; PMCID: PMC3287408.
5. Maegawa S, Lu Y, Maegawa T et al. Caloric restriction delays age-related methylation drift. *Nat Commun*. 2017; 8: 539. https://doi.org/10.1038/s41467-017-00607-3
6. Bocklandt S, Lin W, Sehl M et al. Epigenetic predictor of age. *PLoS ONE*. 2011; 6: e14821.
7. Social Affairs. Population Division. *World Population Ageing 2007*. United Nations Publications, 2007.
8. Vos T, Flaxman AD, Naghavi M et al. Years lived with disability (YLDs) for 1160 sequelae of 289 diseases and injuries 1990–2010: A systematic analysis for the Global Burden of Disease Study 2010. *The Lancet*. 2012; 380 (9859): 2163–2196.
9. Cardiovascular Disease (CVD). NHS. https://www.nhs.uk/conditions/cardiovascular-disease/. Accessed April 2022.
10. Malhotra A, Redberg RF, Meier P. Saturated fat does not clog the arteries: Coronary heart disease is a chronic inflammatory condition, the risk of which can be effectively reduced from healthy lifestyle interventions. *British Journal of Sports Medicine*. 2017; 51: 1111–1112.
11. Keay N. Synergistic Interactions of Steroid Hormones. *British Journal of Sports Medicine*. 2018. https://blogs.bmj.com/bjsm/2018/09/11/synergistic-interactions-of-steroid-hormones/
12. Barbagallo M, Dominguez LJ. Magnesium and aging. *Curr Pharm Des*. 2010; 16 (7): 832–839. https://doi.org/10.2174/138161210790883679. PMID: 20388094.

*References*

13. Gröber U, Schmidt J, Kisters K. Magnesium in prevention and therapy. *Nutrients*. 2015; 7: 8199–8226. https://doi.org/10.3390/nu7095388
14. Insel PS, Mohlenhoff BS, Neylan TC et al. Association of sleep and β-Amyloid pathology among older cognitively unimpaired adults. *JAMA Netw Open*. 2021; 4 (7): e2117573. https://doi.org/10.1001/jamanetworkopen.2021.17573
15. Dhana K, Franco OH, Ritz EM, Ford CN, Desai P, Krueger KR et al. Healthy lifestyle and life expectancy with and without Alzheimer's dementia: Population based cohort study. *BMJ*. 2022; 377: e068390. https://doi.org/10.1136/bmj-2021-068390
16. Jankovic J. Parkinson's disease: Clinical features and diagnosis. *Journal of Neurology, Neurosurgery & Psychiatry*. 2008; 79: 368–376.
17. Tolosa E, Wenning G, Poewe W. The diagnosis of Parkinson's disease. *The Lancet Neurology*. 2006; 5 (1): 75–86. ISSN 1474-4422. https://doi.org/10.1016/S1474-4422(05)70285-4
18. Pálovics R, Keller A, Schaum N et al. Molecular hallmarks of heterochronic parabiosis at single-cell resolution. *Nature*. 2022; 603: 309–314. https://doi.org/10.1038/s41586-022-04461-2
19. Conese M, Carbone A, Beccia E, Angiolillo A. The fountain of youth: a tale of parabiosis, stem cells, and rejuvenation. *Open Med (Wars)*. 2017; 12: 376–383. https://doi.org/10.1515/med-2017-0053
20. von Faber M, Bootsma-van der Wiel A, van Exel E et al. Successful aging in the oldest old: who can be characterized as successfully aged? *Arch Intern Med*. 2001; 161 (22): 2694–2700. https://doi.org/10.1001/archinte.161.22.2694. PMID: 11732934.
21. Japan is searching for the secrets to healthy old age. https://www.economist.com/asia/2022/02/05/japan-is-searching-for-the-secrets-to-healthy-old-age February 2022.
22. Belsky D, Caspi A, Houts R et al. Quantification of biological aging in young adults. *Proceedings of the National Academy of Sciences*. 2015; 112 (30): E4104–E4110. https://doi.org/10.1073/pnas.1506264112

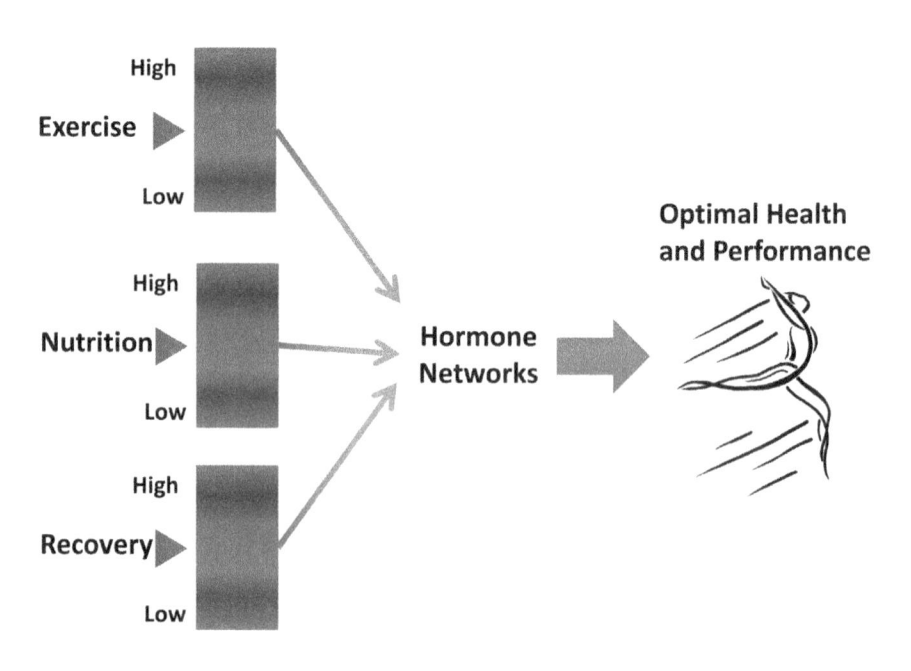

Balancing lifestyle factors for hormone health to optimise health and performance

# Glossary

**Genotype:** the complete collection of genes in the DNA of an individual.
**Phenotype:** the external appearance of an individual resulting from the interaction of genotype and environment.
**Karyotype:** the complete collect of chromosomes in an individual.
**Woman/women/female** refers to the biological sex of a person carrying the XX karyotype.
**Man/men/male** refers to the biological sex of a person carrying the XY karyotype.
**Gametes:** sperm and eggs, which are haploid cells containing a single set of chromosomes.
**Gonads:** the testes in men and ovaries in women, where the gametes are made.

## Hormone systems

**Hormone**: a chemical substance released into the bloodstream from a ductless hormone-producing gland. Hormones bind to cells to exert physiological responses.
**Endocrine system**: all the hormone-producing glands, along with the hormones they produce.
**Neuroendocrine system**: partnership between the nervous system and endocrine system to produce a physiological response such as in the "let down reflex" in breast feeding.

## Modes of action of biological chemicals

**Autocrine:** the action of a biological chemical on the cell that produced it.
**Paracrine:** the action of a biological chemical on neighbouring cells, adjacent to where it is produced.
**Endocrine:** the action of a hormone on cells distant from where it was produced.
**Anabolic:** promoting tissue formation, for example increasing muscle and bone.
**Catabolic:** promoting tissue breakdown, for example decreasing muscle and bone.

## Hormone control mechanisms

**Homeostasis:** the biological process of maintaining the internal milieu at a consistent state for physiological processes to occur. For example, maintenance of blood glucose concentrations within a range.
**Feedback loop:** a biological mechanism that maintains homeostasis.
**Biochronometer:** a biological timekeeper.
**Supra chiasmic nucleus (SCN):** the master biochronometer, located in the hypothalamus.

## Hormones axes

**Hypothalamic-pituitary axis (HP axis)** The hypothalamus and pituitary are located in the brain. The hypothalamus acts as the neuroendocrine gatekeeper integrating internal and external cues. As this information is processed, the appropriate hormone signals are sent to the pituitary gland. The pituitary gland, the conductor of the endocrine orchestra, sends appropriate hormone signals to endocrine glands throughout the body. Both the hypothalamus and pituitary glands receive feedback from peripheral hormones of the endocrine system.

## Reproductive axis

**Gonadotrophin-releasing hormone (GnRH):** a hormone released from the hypothalamus to act on the pituitary gland.
**Follicle-stimulating hormone (FSH):** a hormone released from the pituitary gland, in response to GnRH, acting on the ovaries in women to support the maturation of eggs and the testes in men to support sperm production.
**Luteinising hormone (LH):** a hormone released from the pituitary gland, in response to GnRH, acting on the ovaries in women and the testes in men. A sharp surge in LH triggers ovulation in women.
**Oestrogen:** a category of sex steroid hormones principally associated with the female reproductive system. The US spelling is estrogen.
**Oestradiol:** and most active form oestrogen produced by the ovaries and placenta in women. In men oestradiol is derived from the aromatisation of testosterone. The US spelling is estradiol.

**Progesterone:** a sex steroid hormone produced by the ovaries and placenta in women to maintain the endometrial lining of the uterus. In men progesterone is produced in the testes.

**Testosterone:** a sex steroid hormone produced by the testes in men and by the ovaries in women. It has an anabolic effect on tissues.

## Thyroid axis

**Thyrotrophin-releasing hormone (TRH):** a hormone released by the hypothalamus, acting on the pituitary gland.

**Thyroid-stimulating hormone (TSH):** a hormone released by the pituitary, in response to TRH from the hypothalamus, acting on the thyroid gland.

**Thyroxine (T4):** a hormone produced by the thyroid gland, in response to TSH, which contributes to determining metabolic rate.

**Triiodothyronine (T3):** a hormone produced by the thyroid gland, in response to TSH. There is also some peripheral tissue conversion of T4 to T3.

## Growth hormone axis

**Growth hormone-releasing hormone (GHRH):** a hormone released by the hypothalamus, acting on the pituitary gland.

**Growth hormone (GH):** a hormone released by the pituitary in response to GHRH from the hypothalamus.

**Insulin-like growth factor 1 (IGF-1):** a hormone derived from conversion of GH peripherally, once GH has been released by the pituitary gland and has an anabolic effect.

## Adrenal axis

**Hypothalamic-pituitary-adrenal axis (HPA)**

**Corticotrophin-releasing hormone (CRH):** a hormone released by the hypothalamus, acting on the pituitary gland.

**Adrenocorticotrophic hormone (ACTH):** a hormone released by the pituitary, acting on the adrenal cortex of the adrenal gland.

**Cortisol:** a steroid hormone released from the adrenal cortex in response to ACTH.

## Menstrual states (and their adjectival forms)

**Eumenorrhoea (eumenorrhoeic):** the expected menstrual state of a healthy woman of reproductive age, where the gap between menstrual periods is 22 to 35 days

**Amenorhoea (amenorrhoeic):** a lack of menstrual periods.

    **Primary amenorrhoea:** the absence of establishment of menstrual periods. There are some differences in the definitions. To take account of these differences, the National Institute for Health (NICE), Care Excellence Clinical Knowledge Summaries (CKS) 2022 advise the following. "To assess girls who have not established menstruation by the age of 13 years and have no secondary sexual characteristics and girls who have not established menstruation by the age of 15 years and have normal secondary sexual characteristics."

    **Secondary amenorrhoea:** the absence the of menstrual periods in a previously regular menstruating woman. There are some differences in definitions. The National Institute for Health (NICE), Care Excellence Clinical Knowledge Summaries (CKS) 2022 advise assessing for an underlying cause of secondary amenorrhoea "if there is cessation of menstruation for 3–6 months in women with previously normal and regular menses, or for 6–12 months in women with previous oligomenorrhoea."

**Perimenopause:** the time over which the ovaries loose responsiveness, culminating in menopause.

**Oligomenorrhoea:** where the gap between periods is more than 35 days and/or where a woman has fewer than 9 periods per calendar year.

**Polymenorrhoea:** where the gap between menstrual periods is less than 21 days.

**Menopause:** the point in time when menstrual periods stop due to lack of response from the ovaries. Typically this occurs around the age of 51, with some years of variation around this age. Menopause is confirmed retrospectively, 12 months after the last menstrual period.

## Female specific

**Functional hypothalamic amenorrhoea (FHA):** the lack of periods due to an imbalance in behaviours causing downregulation of the HP axis, in the absence of any physiological or medical cause of amenorrhoea.

**Subclinical anovulatory cycle:** a menstrual cycle where ovulation does not occur, despite regular menstrual periods.

**Primary ovarian insufficiency (POI):** reduced ovarian responsiveness and function, occurring before the age of 40.

**Hormone replacement therapy (HRT):** medication with the aim of restoring female hormones oestradiol and progesterone to physiological levels comparable to women with regular ovulatory cycles. This is typically for women in perimenopause and menopause, although can be used for bone protection in those with FHA.

**Combined oral contraceptive pill (COCP):** a combination of synthetic forms of oestradiol and progesterone that supresses ovulation. Withdrawal bleeds can occur. The National Institute for Health and Care Excellence (NICE), Care Excellence Clinical Knowledge Summaries (CKS) 2022 advise against COCP in women with FHA.

## Sleep hygiene strategies

- Aim for eight hours of sleep per night. Go to bed and get up at consistent times – set an alarm for bedtime, well before midnight!
- Establish a bedtime routine to ensure good sleep hygiene
- Explore what helps you wind down: reading, listening to music, taking a bath
- A milk drink at bedtime contains tryptophan to make the sleep hormone melatonin and the protein casein to aid muscle repair and formation
- Avoid electronic devices close to bedtime, as the frequency of light disrupts the production of melatonin
- Avoid alcohol or stimulants such as caffeine, nicotine or late exercise
- Sleep in a well-ventilated room

## Further steps for persistent sleep problems

- Cognitive Behavioural therapy (CBT)
- "Sleep scheduling" anchors the day with consistent morning rising time and getting out of bed until sleepy at night

## Exercise training

**Exerkines:** substances including peptides, nucleic acids, and metabolites that are release by metabolically active tissues of muscle, bone and gut during exercise.

**Periodisation:** structuring and scheduling of exercise training, in combination with appropriate nutrition and recovery strategies, to derive the maximal beneficial effects.

**Supercompensation:** positive adaptation from exercise training derived after sufficient recovery from a training stimulus.

**Functional overreaching (FOR):** where training stimulus is matched by sufficient recovery to produce supercompensation. This results in improved exercise performance over time.

**Non-functional overreaching (NFOR):** where the training stimulus is not synchronised with sufficient recovery, resulting in stagnation of performance.

**Overtraining syndrome (OTS):** the consequence of cumulative NFOR over time.

## Metabolism

**Substrate:** the type of molecule used for cellular respiration. For example, glucose, fatty acids or amino acids (found in foods containing carbohydrate, fat and protein).

**Metabolic rate:** the rate at which cellular respiration occurs. If measured in totally rested, fasted state this is basal metabolic rate (BMR). If measured later in the day after some light movements of daily living, not fasted this is resting metabolic rate (RMR).

**Body mass index (BMI):** an assessment of body mass versus weight calculated by dividing weight in kg by the square of height measured in metres. Note this does not account for body composition.

**Metabolic syndrome:** a constellation of factors including insulin resistance, hypertension and obesity which increases the risk of developing cardiometabolic disease, such as diabetes mellitus type 2, "heart attack" and stroke.

**Insulin resistance:** the reduced response of cells to insulin, associated with development of type 2 diabetes mellitus as the underlying aetiology.

**Metabolic flexibility:** the ability to generate energy flexibly using a variety of substrate types.

**Adipose tissue:** fat tissue.

**Adikopines:** a family of hormones produced by adipose tissue, such as leptin.

# Bone

**Dual X-ray absorptiometry (DXA):** a type of scan, using very low level ionising radiation, to assess bone health: primarily bone mineral density. Typically, the lumbar spine and hip are scanned. DXA can also be used to assess body composition.

**Bone mineral density (BMD):** the quantified assessment of bone health from a DXA scan.

- **T-Score:** the number of standard deviations away from the BMD for a young healthy person.
- **Z-Score:** is the number of standard deviations away from the BMD for a person of the same age.

**Osteogenic:** stimulus that promotes bone formation, such as mechanical loading of bone through movement.

**Bone formation:** the process of building up bone.

**Bone resorption:** the process of breaking down bone tissue.

**Bone turnover:** the balance of bone formation and bone resorption.

# Gut

**Microbiota:** a community of micro-organisms.

**Microbiome:** the sum of the genetic material of all the microbes in a particular environment.

**Prebiotic:** a food that provides nutrition for the gut microbiota.

**Probiotic:** fermented food favourable to gut microbiota.

# Unbalanced behaviours

**Functional hormone disorder:** Reversible effects of external lifestyle behaviours on hormone networks, in contrast to hormone disruption caused by medical conditions.

**Low energy availability:** where energy availability is insufficient to meet the demands of fundamental physiology processes.

**Relative energy deficiency in sport (RED-S):** the clinical syndrome of downregulated physiological function, as a result of low energy availability. This can have adverse effects on both health and performance

**Restrictive eating:** an eating behaviour that restricts the intake of overall calories or certain food types.

**Disordered eating:** disrupted eating behaviour, which does not meet the diagnostic criteria of an eating disorder.

**Eating disorder:** a clinical condition determined by a specialist, according to certain diagnostic criteria.

## Selected endocrine conditions

**Diabetes Mellitus (DM):** the most common endocrine condition, where there is difficulty in controlling blood glucose levels. This could be due to reduced production of insulin (type 1 DM) or reduced response of cells to insulin (type 2 DM).

**Polycystic ovary syndrome (PCOS):** the most common endocrinopathy in women of reproductive age. PCOS is diagnosed according to the Rotterdam criteria, consisting of two out of the three symptoms and signs of: irregular periods, clinical, biochemical evidence of raised androgens, multiple follicles meeting criteria on pelvic ultrasound, in the absence of any other condition causing multiple follicles. There is a metabolic component (insulin resistance) of PCOS.

## Some organisations

**World Health Organisation (WHO):** an organisation that collates data on trends in population health across the world.

**National Institute for Health and Care Excellence (NICE):** an executive public body of the Department of Health and Social Care in England, providing evidence-based recommendations developed by independent committees, including professionals and lay members.

**Clinical Knowledge Summaries (CKS):** regularly updated clinical guidelines provided by NICE, offering a summary of the current evidence base and advice on best practice.

**World anti-doping agency (WADA):** an international organisation that co-ordinates and monitors drug-free sport. WADA provides a yearly updated list of substances banned in sport, which may confer a performance enhancement and risk the health of the athlete.

**Therapeutic use exemption (TUE):** documentation provided by a medical doctor to allow an athlete to use a medication on the banned list, for proven medical reasons.